Pathophysiology

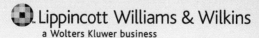

Lippincott Williams & Wilkins
a Wolters Kluwer business

Philadelphia · Baltimore · New York · London
Buenos Aires · Hong Kong · Sydney · Tokyo

STAFF

EXECUTIVE PUBLISHER
Judith A. Schilling McCann, RN, MSN

EDITORIAL DIRECTOR
William J. Kelly

CLINICAL DIRECTOR
Joan M. Robinson, RN, MSN

SENIOR ART DIRECTOR
Arlene Putterman

EDITORIAL PROJECT MANAGER
Catherine E. Harold

CLINICAL PROJECT MANAGER
Eileen Cassin Gallen, RN, BS

COPY EDITORS
Heather Ditch, Amy Furman,
Dona Perkins

DESIGNERS
Debra Moloshok (book design),
Matie Anne Patterson (project
manager)

DIGITAL COMPOSITION SERVICES
Diane Paluba (manager),
Joyce Rossi Biletz, Donna S. Morris

MANUFACTURING
Patrica K. Dorshaw (director),
Beth J. Welsh

EDITORIAL ASSISTANTS
Megan L. Aldinger, Karen J. Kirk,
Linda K. Ruhf

DESIGN ASSISTANT
Georg Purvis 4th

INDEXER
Dianne Prewitt

The clinical treatments described and recommended in this publication are based on research and consultation with nursing, medical, and legal authorities. To the best of our knowledge, these procedures reflect currently accepted practice. Nevertheless, they can't be considered absolute and universal recommendations. For individual applications, all recommendations must be considered in light of the patient's clinical condition and, before administration of new or infrequently used drugs, in light of the latest package-insert information. The authors and publisher disclaim any responsibility for any adverse effects resulting from the suggested procedures, from any undetected errors, or from the reader's misunderstanding of the text.

LPNPatho010306

Library of Congress Cataloging-in-Publication Data

LPN expert guides. Pathophysiology.
   p. ; cm.
   Includes bibliographical references and index.
   1. Pathology—Handbooks, manuals, etc.
2. Practical nursing—Handbooks, manuals, etc. I. Lippincott Williams & Wilkins. II. Title: Pathophysiology
   [DNLM: 1. Pathophysiology—Handbooks. 2. Nursing, Practical—methods—Handbooks. WY 49 L9245 2006]
RB30.L66 2006
616'.07—dc22   2005034580
ISBN 1-58255-895-7 (alk. paper)

Contents

Contributors and consultants

Katrina D. Allen, RN, MSN, CCRN
Nursing Instructor
Faulkner State Community College
Bay Minette, Ala.

Janice W. Chapman, RN, MSN
Health Careers Site Coordinator & Instructor
Reid State College
Atmore, Ala.

Tricia Duff, LPN, I.V. certified
Coumadin Nurse
Concord (N.H.) Hospital

Richard R. Gibbs, LVN
Staff Nurse, Rehab Unit
Mesquite (Tex.) Community Hospital

Charla K. Hollin, RN, BSN
Nursing Program Director
Rich Mountain Community College
Mena, Ark.

Donna Kearns, LPN, BEd, MEd, EdD
Chair, Special Services Department
University of Central Oklahoma
Edmond, Okla.

Noel C. Piano, RN, MS
Instructor
Lafayette School of Practical Nursing
Williamsburg, Va.

Dina Nicole Salvatore, LPN
Charge Nurse
Windemere Nursing & Rehabilitation Center
Oak Bluffs, Mass.

Kendra S. Seiler, RN, MSN
Nursing Instructor
Rio Hondo Community College
Whittier, Calif.

Georgia A. Simmons, RN, BSN
Practical Nursing Instructor
Ivy Tech State College
Madison, Ind.

Julie Traynor, MSN, RN
Director, Dakota Practical Nursing Program
Lake Region State College
Devils Lake, N.D.

1

PATHOPHYSIOLOGY BASICS

Understanding cells

The cell is the body's basic building block, the smallest living component of an organism. Millions of cells form highly specialized units that function together as:
- tissues, such as muscle, blood, and bone
- organs, such as the brain, heart, and liver
- integrated body systems, such as the central nervous system (CNS), cardiovascular system, and digestive system.

CELL COMPONENTS
Each cell contains structures known as *organelles,* each with specific functions. (See *A look at cell components,* page 2.) Organelles are held in an aqueous substance called *cytoplasm,* which is bounded by the cell membrane.

The *nucleus* is the largest organelle. It controls cell activity and stores deoxyribonucleic acid (DNA), which carries genetic material and is responsible for cellular reproduction, also known as *division.* Other organelles include:
- *ribosomes* and the *endoplasmic reticulum,* which synthesize proteins and metabolize fat inside the cell
- the *Golgi apparatus,* which contains enzymes that function in cellular metabolism
- *lysosomes,* which contain digestive enzymes that permit cytoplasmic digestion
- *mitochondria,* which make adenosine triphosphate, the energy that fuels cellular activity.

A look at cell components

This illustration shows cell components and structures. Each part helps maintain the cell's life and homeostasis.

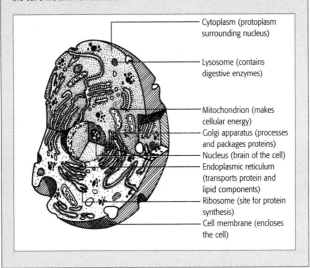

Cytoplasm (protoplasm surrounding nucleus)

Lysosome (contains digestive enzymes)

Mitochondrion (makes cellular energy)

Golgi apparatus (processes and packages proteins)

Nucleus (brain of the cell)

Endoplasmic reticulum (transports protein and lipid components)

Ribosome (site for protein synthesis)

Cell membrane (encloses the cell)

CELL DIVISION AND REPRODUCTION

Cell reproduction occurs in two stages. In the first stage, called *mitosis,* the nucleus and genetic material divide. In the second stage, called *cytokinesis,* the cytoplasm divides, starting during late anaphase or telophase. At the end of cytokinesis, the cell produces two daughter cells. (See *Phases of cell reproduction.*)

Before it divides, a cell must double its mass and content. This occurs during the growth phase, called *interphase.* Chromatin — the small, slender rods that give the nucleus its granular appearance — begins to form. Replication and duplication of DNA occur during the four phases of mitosis:

1. prophase
2. metaphase
3. anaphase
4. telophase.

Phases of cell reproduction

These illustrations show the phases of cell reproduction.

PROPHASE

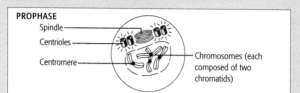

Spindle
Centrioles
Centromere
Chromosomes (each composed of two chromatids)

METAPHASE

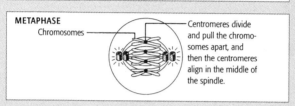

Chromosomes
Centromeres divide and pull the chromosomes apart, and then the centromeres align in the middle of the spindle.

ANAPHASE

Centromeres separate and pull chromosomes toward opposite sides of the cell.

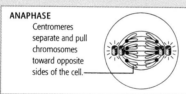

TELOPHASE

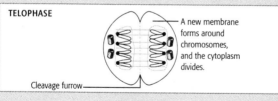

A new membrane forms around chromosomes, and the cytoplasm divides.

Cleavage furrow

CYTOKINESIS

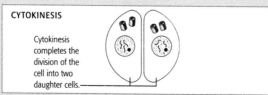

Cytokinesis completes the division of the cell into two daughter cells.

Prophase

In this first phase of cell division, chromosomes coil and shorten, and the nuclear membrane dissolves. Each chromosome is made up of a pair of strands called *chromatids,* which are connected by a spindle of fibers called a *centromere.*

Metaphase

In metaphase, centromeres divide, pulling the chromosomes apart. The centromeres then align in the middle of the spindle.

Anaphase

Centromeres now begin to separate and pull the newly replicated chromosomes toward opposite sides of the cell. By the end of anaphase, 46 chromosomes are present on each side of the cell.

Telophase

During telophase, a new membrane forms around each set of 46 chromosomes. The spindle fibers disappear, cytokinesis occurs, and the cytoplasm divides, producing two identical new daughter cells.

CELL INJURY

A person's state of wellness and disease is reflected in the cells. Injury to any of the cell's components can lead to illness. One of the first indications of cell injury is a biochemical lesion that forms on the cell at the point of injury. This lesion changes the chemistry of metabolic reactions inside the cell.

When cell integrity is threatened — by toxins, infection, physical injury, or deficit injury — the cell reacts in one of two ways:
■ by drawing on its reserves to keep functioning
■ by adapting or becoming dysfunctional.

If enough cellular reserve is available and the body doesn't detect abnormalities, the cell adapts. If there isn't enough cellular reserve, cell death (*necrosis*) occurs. Necrosis is usually localized and easily identifiable.

Toxic injury

Toxic injuries may result from factors inside the body (*endogenous factors*) or outside the body (*exogenous factors*). Common endogenous factors include:
■ genetically determined metabolic errors
■ gross malformations
■ hypersensitivity reactions.

Exogenous factors include:

- alcohol
- carbon monoxide
- drugs that alter cellular function, such as chemotherapy drugs and immunosuppressants
- lead.

Infectious injury
Viral, fungal, protozoan, and bacterial agents can cause cell injury or death. These organisms affect cell integrity, usually by interfering with cell synthesis, producing mutant cells. For example, human immunodeficiency virus alters the cell when the virus is replicated in the cell's ribonucleic acid.

Physical injury
Physical injury results from a disruption in the cell or in the relationships of the intracellular organelles. Two major types of physical injury are thermal (electrical or radiation) and mechanical (trauma or surgery). Causes of thermal injury include:
- radiation therapy for cancer
- ultraviolet radiation
- X-rays.
  Causes of mechanical injury include:
- frostbite
- ischemia
- motor vehicle crashes.

Deficit injury
If a cell has insufficient water, oxygen, or nutrients, too wide a temperature fluctuation, or inadequate waste disposal, cellular synthesis can't take place. A lack of just one of these basic requirements can cause cell disruption or death.

CELL DEGENERATION
Nonlethal cell damage known as degeneration typically occurs in the cytoplasm of the cell, leaving the nucleus unaffected. Degeneration usually affects organs with metabolically active cells, such as the liver, heart, and kidneys. It's caused by these problems:
- atrophy
- autophagocytosis, during which the cell absorbs some of its own parts
- calcification
- dysplasia (related to chronic irritation)
- fatty infiltrates
- hyaline infiltration

Factors that affect cell aging

Factors that affect cell aging may be intrinsic or extrinsic, as outlined here.

INTRINSIC FACTORS	EXTRINSIC FACTORS
• Congenital	PHYSICAL AGENTS
• Degenerative	• Chemicals
• Immunologic	• Electricity
• Inherited	• Force
• Metabolic	• Humidity
• Neoplastic	• Radiation
• Nutritional	• Temperature
• Psychogenic	INFECTIOUS AGENTS
	• Bacteria
	• Fungi
	• Insects
	• Protozoa
	• Viruses
	• Worms

■ hyperplasia
■ hypertrophy
■ increased water in the cell or cellular swelling
■ pigmentation changes.

When such changes are found inside the cells, sometimes with an electron microscope, degeneration may be slowed or cell death prevented through prompt treatment. If the disease is diagnosed before the patient complains of symptoms, it's called *subclinical identification.*

Unfortunately, many cell changes remain unidentifiable even under a microscope, making early detection impossible.

CELL AGING

As they age, cells lose structure and function. Lost structure may mean decreased size, or wasting away, a process called *atrophy.* Lost function may involve:
■ hypertrophy, an abnormal thickening or increase in bulk
■ hyperplasia, an increase in the number of cells.

Depending on the number and extent of injuries and the amount of wear and tear on the cell, aging may proceed more quickly or more slowly. Signs of aging occur in all body systems. Examples of the effects of cell aging include:

■ decreased elasticity in blood vessels
■ decreased bowel motility
■ decreased muscle mass
■ decreased subcutaneous fat.

Aging limits the cells' life span. Cells may die because of internal (*intrinsic*) factors that limit the cells' life span or because of external (*extrinsic*) factors that contribute to cell damage and aging. (See *Factors that affect cell aging*.)

Homeostasis

The body works constantly to maintain an internal balance called *homeostasis*. Every cell in the body is involved in maintaining homeostasis, both on the cellular level and as part of an organism.

When an external stressor disrupts homeostasis, the body's internal equilibrium may be disrupted, and illness may occur. Examples of external stressors include:

■ injury
■ invasion by parasites or other organisms
■ lack of nutrients.

Three structures in the brain are responsible for maintaining homeostasis:

■ the medulla oblongata, which controls such vital functions as respiration and circulation
■ the pituitary gland, which influences growth, maturation, and reproduction by regulating the function of other glands
■ the reticular formation, a large network of nerve cells or nuclei that helps control vital reflexes, such as cardiovascular function and respiration.

FEEDBACK MECHANISMS

Homeostasis is maintained by self-regulating feedback mechanisms. These mechanisms have three components:

■ a sensor mechanism that senses disruptions in homeostasis
■ a control center that regulates the body's response to disruptions in homeostasis
■ an effector mechanism that acts to restore homeostasis.

An endocrine (hormone-secreting) gland usually controls the sensor mechanism, which sends a signal to the control center in the CNS, which triggers the effector mechanism.

There are two types of feedback mechanisms:

- a negative feedback mechanism, which works to restore homeostasis by correcting a deficit in the system
- a positive feedback mechanism, which moves the system away from homeostasis.

Negative feedback mechanisms
For a negative feedback mechanism to be effective, it must sense a change in the body — such as a high blood glucose level — and act to return body functions to normal. In the case of a high blood glucose level, for example, the effector mechanism triggers increased insulin production by the pancreas, returning the blood glucose level to normal and restoring homeostasis.

Positive feedback mechanisms
A positive feedback mechanism exaggerates the body's original response. It's said to be positive because the change that occurs proceeds in the same direction as the initial disturbance, causing a further deviation from homeostasis. For example, a positive feedback mechanism is what intensifies labor contractions during childbirth.

Understanding disease

Disease occurs when homeostasis isn't maintained. The patient has findings characteristic of the disease involved, including:
- subjective complaints
- a specific medical history
- signs, symptoms, and laboratory or radiologic findings.

The words *disease* and *illness* are commonly used interchangeably, but they aren't synonymous. Illness refers more to a person's ability to function normally. It's highly individualized and personal. For instance, a person may have a disease — such as coronary artery disease, diabetes, or asthma — but not be "ill" because the body has adapted to the disease and can function normally in daily living.

Diseases are dynamic and may manifest in various ways, depending on the patient and his environment. The course and outcome of a disease may be influenced by:
- genetic factors, such as a tendency toward obesity
- unhealthy behaviors, such as smoking
- stress
- even the patient's perception of the disease, such as acceptance or denial.

CAUSE

One aspect of disease is its cause, or *etiology*. The cause of disease
may be *intrinsic* or *extrinsic*. An intrinsic disease occurs because of a
malfunction or change in the body. Intrinsic causes include:

■ inherited traits
■ the patient's age
■ the patient's gender.

Extrinsic causes of disease come from outside the body. Examples of extrinsic causes include:

■ chemical exposure
■ drug use
■ infectious agents
■ mechanical trauma
■ nutritional problems
■ psychological stress
■ radiation exposure
■ smoking
■ temperature extremes.

Diseases with no known cause are called *idiopathic*.

DEVELOPMENT

A disease's development is called its *pathogenesis*. Unless identified
and successfully treated, most diseases progress according to a typical pattern of symptoms.

Some diseases are self-limiting or resolve quickly with limited
or no intervention; others are chronic and never resolve. Patients
with chronic diseases may undergo periods of remission and exacerbation.

During remission, the patient's symptoms lessen in severity or
disappear. During exacerbation, the patient experiences an aggrava-
tion of symptoms or an increase in the severity of the disease.

Usually, a disease is uncovered because of an increase or decrease in metabolism or cell division. Signs and symptoms may include:

■ hypofunction, such as constipation
■ hyperfunction, such as increased mucus production
■ increased mechanical function, such as a seizure.

STAGES

Typically, diseases progress through these stages:

■ *Exposure* or *injury*. Target tissue is exposed to a causative agent or
is injured.
■ *Latent* or *incubation period*. No signs or symptoms appear.

Physical response to stress

According to Hans Selye's General Adaption Model, the body reacts to stress in the stages depicted below.

Physical or psychological stressor

↓

Alarm reaction
- Arousal of the central nervous system begins.
- Epinephrine, norepinephrine, and other hormones, are released, causing an increase in heart rate, increased force of heart contractions, increased oxygen intake, and increased mental activity.

↓

Resistance
- The body responds to the stressor and attempts to return to homeostasis.
- Coping mechanisms are used.

↓   ↓

Recovery	**Exhaustion**
	- The body can no longer produce hormones as in the alarm stage. - Organ damage begins.

- *Prodromal period.* Signs and symptoms usually are mild and nonspecific.
- *Acute phase.* The disease reaches its full intensity, and complications commonly arise. If the patient can still function normally during this phase, it's called the *subclinical acute phase.*
- *Remission.* Another latent phase occurs in some diseases and is commonly followed by another acute phase.
- *Convalescence.* In this rehabilitation stage, the patient progresses toward recovery after the disease stops.
- *Recovery.* The patient regains health or normal functioning and has no signs or symptoms of the disease.

STRESS AND DISEASE

When a stressor, such as a life change, occurs, a person can respond in one of two ways: by adapting successfully or by failing to adapt. A maladaptive response to stress may result in disease. The underlying stressor may be real or perceived.

Physiologic stressors may elicit a harmful response, leading to an identifiable illness or set of symptoms. Psychological stressors, such as the death of a loved one, may also cause a maladaptive response.

The stress response is controlled by actions taking place in the nervous and endocrine systems. These actions try to redirect energy to the organ most affected by the stress, such as the heart, lungs, or brain.

Hans Selye, a pioneer in the study of stress and disease, described stages of adaptation to a stressful event as:
■ alarm
■ resistance
■ exhaustion or recovery. (See *Physical response to stress.*)

In the alarm stage, the body senses stress. The CNS is aroused. The body releases chemicals to mobilize the fight-or-flight response. This release is the adrenaline rush associated with panic or aggression.

In the resistance stage, the body either adapts and achieves homeostasis, or it fails to adapt and enters the exhaustion stage, resulting in disease.

Stressful events can worsen some chronic diseases, such as diabetes mellitus and multiple sclerosis. Effective coping strategies can prevent or reduce the harmful effects of stress.

2

CANCER

Understanding cancer

Cancer ranks second to cardiovascular disease as the leading cause of death in the United States. Each year, more than 1 million cancer cases are diagnosed in the United States, and 550,000 people die of cancer-related causes (one out of four deaths). Some scientists expect cancer deaths to surpass deaths from cardiovascular disease by 2010.

One-third of cancer deaths stem from nutrition problems, physical inactivity, obesity, and other lifestyle factors and could have been prevented. In most cases, early detection of cancer allows more effective treatment and a better prognosis.

A careful assessment, beginning with an exhaustive history, is critical. In gathering assessment information, ask the patient about risk factors — such as cigarette smoking, a family history of cancer, and exposure to hazards — as well as the extent to which he was exposed.

ABNORMAL CELL GROWTH

Cancer is classified by the tissues or blood cells in which it originates. Most cancers derive from epithelial tissues and are called *carcinomas*. Others arise from these tissues and cells:
- connective, muscle, and bone tissues (sarcomas)
- erythrocytes (erythroleukemia)
- glandular tissues (adenocarcinomas)
- leukocytes (leukemia)
- lymphatic tissue (lymphomas)
- pigment cells (melanomas)
- plasma cells (myelomas)
- tissue of the brain and spinal cord (gliomas).

Cancer begins with a mutation in a single cell. This cell grows without the control that characterizes normal cell growth. At a certain stage of development, the cancer cell fails to mature into the type of normal cell from which it originated.

In addition to this uncontrolled localized growth, cancer cells can spread from the site of origin, a process called *metastasis*. Cancer cells metastasize in three ways:

■ by circulation through the blood and lymphatic system
■ by accidental transplantation during surgery
■ by spreading to adjacent organs and tissues.

CAUSES OF CANCER

All cancers involve the malfunction of genes that control cell growth and division. A cell's transformation from normal to cancerous is called *carcinogenesis*. Carcinogenesis has no single cause but probably results from complex interactions among:

■ dietary factors
■ genetic factors
■ hormonal factors
■ immunologic factors
■ metabolic factors
■ physical and chemical carcinogens
■ viruses.

Viruses

Viruses can transform cells. For instance, the Epstein-Barr virus that causes infectious mononucleosis is linked to Burkitt's lymphoma, Hodgkin's disease, and nasopharyngeal cancer. Human papillomavirus, cytomegalovirus, and herpes simplex virus type 2 are linked to cancer of the cervix. The hepatitis B virus causes hepatocellular carcinoma. The human T-cell lymphotropic virus causes adult T-cell leukemia. And the human immunodeficiency virus is linked to Kaposi's sarcoma.

Ultraviolet radiation

The relationship between excessive exposure to ultraviolet B (UVB) radiation from the sun's rays and skin cancer is well established. UVB radiation damages the deoxyribonucleic acid (DNA) of skin cells.

Exposure to ultraviolet A (UVA) radiation from sunlamps and tanning booths also contributes to skin cancer development. The damaging effects of UVA radiation may be indirect, occurring as a result of energy transferred through reactive oxygen intermediates (free radicals).

The amount of exposure to ultraviolet radiation correlates with the type of cancer that develops. For example, cumulative exposure to ultraviolet radiation is linked to basal and squamous cell skin cancer. Severe episodes of burning and blistering at a young age are linked to melanoma.

Other factors also may contribute to the carcinogenic effect, such as the patient's tissue type, age, and hormonal status.

Environmental exposures
Substances in the environment can cause cancer by damaging DNA in the cells. Examples of common carcinogens and related cancers include:
■ alkylating agents (leukemia).
■ asbestos and airborne aromatic hydrocarbons (lung cancer)
■ tobacco (lung, pancreatic, kidney, bladder, mouth, and esophageal cancer)

Immune system compromise
A severely compromised immune system may lead to the development of certain cancers. For example, transplant recipients receiving immunosuppressants and those with acquired immunodeficiency syndrome have an increased risk of Kaposi's sarcoma, non-Hodgkin's lymphoma, and skin cancer.

Diet
Colorectal cancer is linked to low-fiber, high-fat diets. Food additives, such as nitrates, and food preparation methods, such as charbroiling, also may contribute to the development of cancer.

Specific nutritional guidelines can help prevent cancer. (See *Dietary recommendations for cancer prevention.*)

Genetics
About 5% to 10% of cancers are clearly hereditary in that an inherited faulty gene predisposes the person to be at very high risk for a particular cancer. These cancers may be autosomal recessive, X-linked, or autosomal dominant disorders. (See chapter 5, Genetics.) Such cancers tend to share certain characteristics, including:
■ abnormal chromosome complement in tumor cells
■ early onset
■ increased occurrence of bilateral cancer in paired organs (breasts, adrenal glands, and kidneys)

Dietary recommendations for cancer prevention

The recommendations listed here focus on nutrition and physical activity as prevention measures.

● Eat a variety of healthful foods, emphasizing plant sources.
– Eat five or more servings of a variety of vegetables and fruits each day. Choose whole grains over processed (refined) grains and sugars.
– Limit consumption of red meat, especially processed meats and those high in fat.
– Choose foods that maintain a healthful weight.
● Adopt a physically active lifestyle.
– Adults: Engage in at least moderate activity for 30 minutes or more on 5 or more days of the week; getting 45 minutes or more of moderate to vigorous activity on 5 or more days per week may further reduce the risk of breast and colon cancer.
– Children and adolescents: Engage in at least 60 minutes per day of moderate to vigorous physical activity at least 5 days per week.
● Maintain a healthful weight throughout life.
– Balance calorie intake with physical activity.
– Lose weight if you're overweight or obese.
● If you drink alcoholic beverages, limit consumption.

■ increased occurrence of multiple primary cancers in nonpaired organs
■ two or more family members in the same generation with the same cancer.
■ unique tumor site combinations

Hormones
The role of hormones in the development of cancer is controversial. Excessive intake of hormones, especially estrogen, may contribute to certain forms of cancer while reducing the risk of other forms.

Immunosurveillance failure
One theory suggests that the body develops cancer cells continuously but that the immune system recognizes them as foreign and destroys them. This theoretical defense mechanism, called *immunosurveillance,* promotes antibody production, cellular immunity, and immunologic memory. A disruption of immunosurveillance could lead to the overproduction of cancer cells and, possibly, a tumor.

Cancer types

Types of cancer discussed in this section include:
- breast cancer
- colorectal cancer
- Hodgkin's disease
- leukemia
- lung cancer
- malignant melanoma
- multiple myeloma
- prostate cancer.

BREAST CANCER

Breast cancer is the most common cancer in women. Although the disease may develop any time after puberty, 70% of cases occur in women older than age 50. Breast cancer ranks second among cancer deaths in women, behind cancer of the lung and bronchus.

Pathophysiology

The exact causes of breast cancer remain elusive. Specific genes (called *BRCA1* and *BRCA2*) are linked to about 5% of all cases of breast cancer. Those who inherit either of these genes have an 80% chance of developing breast cancer. (See *Susceptibility to breast cancer*.)

Other significant risk factors have been identified. These include:
- a family history of breast cancer
- radiation exposure
- being a premenopausal woman older than age 45
- obesity
- age
- recent use of hormonal contraceptives
- early onset of menses or late menopause
- being nulligravida (never pregnant)
- first pregnancy after age 30
- high-fat diet
- colon, endometrial, or ovarian cancer
- postmenopausal progestin and estrogen therapy
- alcohol use (one or more alcoholic beverages per day)
- benign breast disease.

Susceptibility to breast cancer

Patients with BRCA1 and BRCA2 genes account for about 5% of all breast cancer cases. General screening of the population for these genes isn't recommended. However, screening women with a strong family history of breast cancer is recommended when genetic counseling is available.

Prophylactic removal of the breasts in women with BRCA1 and BRCA2 greatly decreases their risk of breast cancer, as does removing the ovaries and fallopian tubes in premenopausal women with BRCA1 and BRCA2.

BREAST CANCER CLASSIFICATION

Breast cancer is usually classified by the tissue of origin and the location of the lesion: About half of breast cancers develop in the upper outer quadrant of the breast. (See *Breast tumor sites,* page 18.)

■ Intraductal cancer, the most common form, develops in the ducts.
■ Lobular cancer develops in the lobes.
■ Less than 1% of breast cancers originate in the nonepithelial connective tissue.
■ Inflammatory cancer (rare) grows rapidly and causes the overlying skin to become edematous, inflamed, and indurated.
■ Paget's disease is the growth of cancerous cells within the breast ducts beneath the nipple.

Breast cancer is also classified as invasive or noninvasive. *Invasive tumor cells,* which make up 90% of all breast cancers, break through the duct walls and encroach on other breast tissues. *Noninvasive tumor cells* remain confined to the duct in which they originated.

RED FLAG Breast cancer can spread in lymph and blood, through the right side of the heart to the lungs and, eventually, to the other breast, chest wall, liver, bone, and brain.

Signs and symptoms

Typically, the patient discovers a thickening of the breast tissue or a painless lump or mass in her breast. Breast cancer also may be detected on a mammogram before a lesion becomes palpable.

Inspection may reveal evidence of changes, including:
■ nipple retraction
■ scaly skin around the nipple
■ skin changes

Breast tumor sites

This illustration shows the location and frequency of breast tumors. The upper outer quadrant is the most common site of breast cancer.

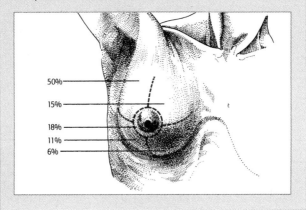

- erythema
- clear, milky, or bloody discharge
- edema in the arm, which indicates advanced nodal involvement.

Palpation may identify a hard lump, mass, or thickening of breast tissue. Palpation of the cervical supraclavicular and axillary nodes may reveal lumps or enlargement. Although growth rates vary, a lump may take up to 8 years to become palpable at 1 cm.

Test results

These tests are used to diagnose breast cancer.

- Breast self-examination (done regularly) with routine breast examination by a clinician detects breast lumps early.
- Mammography — the main test for breast cancer — detects tumors that are too small to palpate.
- Fine-needle aspiration and excisional biopsy provide cells for histologic examination to confirm diagnosis.
- Ultrasonography distinguishes a fluid-filled cyst from a solid mass and a benign from a cancerous tumor.
- Ductoscopy reveals small intraductal lesions that aren't palpable or visible on mammography.

- Ductal lavage identifies cancerous cells in the milk ducts of the breast.
- Chest X-rays pinpoint chest metastasis.
- Scans of bone, brain, liver, and other organs detect distant metastasis.
- Laboratory tests, such as alkaline phosphatase levels and liver function tests, also detect distant metastasis.
- A hormone receptor assay shows whether the tumor is estrogen- or progesterone-dependent and helps determine appropriate treatment.

Treatment

Treatment is based on the disease stage and type, the woman's age and menopausal status, and the disfiguring effects of surgery. It may include a combination of surgery, radiation, chemotherapy, and hormonal therapy. Surgery may involve lumpectomy, partial mastectomy, total mastectomy, or modified radical mastectomy.

LUMPECTOMY

Lumpectomy is used for small, well-defined lesions. Through a small incision, the surgeon removes the tumor, surrounding tissue and, possibly, nearby lymph nodes. The patient usually undergoes radiation therapy afterward.

In early-stage breast cancer, lumpectomy and radiation are as effective as mastectomy.

PARTIAL MASTECTOMY

The surgeon removes the tumor along with a wedge of normal tissue, skin, fascia, and axillary lymph nodes.

Radiation therapy or chemotherapy is usually used after surgery to destroy undetected disease in other breast areas.

TOTAL MASTECTOMY

A total mastectomy removes the breast tissue. This procedure is used if the cancer is confined to breast tissue and no lymph node involvement is detected.

Chemotherapy or radiation therapy may follow. If the patient doesn't have advanced disease, reconstructive surgery can be used to create a breast mound.

MODIFIED RADICAL MASTECTOMY

The surgeon removes the entire breast, axillary lymph nodes, and the lining that covers the chest muscles. Modified radical mastectomy has largely replaced radical mastectomy because the modified approach preserves the pectoral muscles.

If the lymph nodes contain cancer cells, radiation therapy and chemotherapy follow.

RADIATION THERAPY

Before or after tumor removal, radiation therapy may be used to destroy a small, early-stage tumor that has no distant metastasis. Radiation also may be used to prevent or treat local recurrence of the tumor.

Preoperative radiation therapy "sterilizes" the area, making the tumor more manageable surgically, especially in inflammatory breast cancer.

CHEMOTHERAPY

Cytotoxic drugs may be used as primary or adjuvant therapy. Decisions to start chemotherapy are based on several factors, including the stage of the patient's cancer and the hormone receptor assay results.

Chemotherapy may be administered in a hospital, a physician's office, a clinic, or the patient's home. The drugs may be given orally or by I.M., subcutaneous, or I.V. injection.

Chemotherapy commonly involves the use of a combination of drugs. A typical regimen may include:
■ cyclophosphamide (Cytoxan)
■ methotrexate (Trexall)
■ doxorubicin (Adriamycin)
■ fluorouracil (Adrucil).

HORMONE THERAPY

Hormone therapy lowers the levels of estrogen and other hormones that may nourish breast cancer cells.

Anti-estrogen therapy with tamoxifen (Nolvadex) or raloxifene (Evista) is used in women at increased risk for developing breast cancer.

Other commonly used drugs include:
■ the antiandrogen aminoglutethimide (Cytadren)
■ the androgen fluoxymesterone (Halotestin)
■ the estrogen diethylstilbestrol (DES)
■ the progestin megestrol (Megace). (See *Breast cancer teaching topics.*)

Breast cancer teaching topics

To promote early diagnosis and treatment of breast cancer, teach women the importance of breast self-examination, regular examination by a clinician, mammography, and appropriate follow-up care.

If the patient needs chemotherapy or radiation therapy, make sure that she understands the adverse effects that usually occur and the measures she can take to prevent them or decrease their severity.

Before a mastectomy, point out where the incision will be. Show the patient how to ease postsurgical pain by lying on the affected side or placing a hand or pillow on the incision. Explain that a small pillow placed under the arm anteriorly may provide comfort. Reassure the patient that she'll receive analgesics to prevent or relieve pain after surgery.

POSTOPERATIVE TEACHING
Urge the patient to avoid activities that could injure her arm and hand on the side of her surgery. Caution her not to let blood be drawn from or allow injections into that arm. Also, tell her not to have blood pressure taken or I.V. therapy administered in the affected arm.

To help prevent lymphedema, instruct the patient to regularly exercise her hand and arm on the affected side and to avoid activities that might allow infection of this hand or arm. Tell her that infection increases the risk of lymphedema.

Inform the patient that she may experience "phantom breast syndrome," a tingling or pins-and-needles sensation in the area where the breast was removed.

COLORECTAL CANCER

Colorectal cancer accounts for 10% to 15% of all new cancer cases in the United States. It affects both sexes equally and is the third most common cause of cancer death. It arises most commonly in people older than age 50.

Because colorectal cancer progresses slowly and remains localized for a long time, early detection is key to recovery. Unless the tumor metastasizes, the 5-year survival rate is 80% for rectal cancer and 85% for colon cancer.

Pathophysiology

Age is the main risk factor for colorectal cancer. (See *Aging and colorectal cancer,* page 22.) Several disorders are also linked to colorectal cancer, including:

■ familial adenomatous polyposis, such as Gardner's syndrome and Peutz-Jeghers syndrome
■ ulcerative colitis

Aging and colorectal cancer

Age is the main risk factor for colorectal cancer. More than 90% of cases occur in people older than age 50. However, colorectal cancer can also occur in younger people.

■ Crohn's disease
■ Turcot's syndrome
■ hereditary nonpolyposis colorectal carcinoma
■ other pelvic cancers treated with abdominal radiation
■ genetic abnormality.

Colorectal polyps are closely tied to colon cancer. The larger the polyp, the greater the risk.

Colorectal cancer may be related to genetic factors — deletions on chromosomes 17 and 18 — that may promote mutation and malignancy of mucosal cells. (See *Gene alteration and colon cancer*.)

A high-fat, low-fiber diet may contribute to colorectal cancer by slowing the movement of feces through the bowel. This prolongs exposure of the bowel mucosa to digested matter and may encourage mucosal cells to mutate.

Other risk factors include:
■ smoking
■ alcohol consumption
■ obesity
■ physical inactivity.

Estrogen replacement therapy and the use of nonsteroidal anti-inflammatory drugs, such as aspirin, may reduce the risk of colorectal cancer.

Signs and symptoms

In its early stages, colorectal cancer usually causes no symptoms. Rectal bleeding, blood in the stool, a change in bowel habits, and cramping pain in the lower abdomen may signal advanced disease.

RED FLAG As a growing tumor encroaches on abdominal organs, it may cause abdominal distention and intestinal obstruction. Untreated rectal bleeding may lead to anemia.

Test results

Several tests are used to diagnose colorectal cancer.

- A fecal occult blood test detects blood in stool.
- Proctoscopy or sigmoidoscopy visualizes the lower GI tract and helps detect two-thirds of colorectal cancers.
- Colonoscopy is used to visualize and photograph the colon up to the ileocecal valve and provides access for polypectomies and biopsies.
- A barium enema helps locate lesions that aren't visible or palpable.
- About 15% of colorectal cancers, specifically rectal and perianal lesions, are detected by digital rectal examination (DRE).
- Computed tomography (CT) scan helps detect cancer that has spread.
- Carcinoembryonic antigen, a tumor marker that rises in about 70% of patients with colorectal cancer, is used to monitor the patient before and after treatment to detect metastasis or recurrence.
- Liver function studies detect liver metastasis.

Treatment

A combination of surgery and chemotherapy is used to treat colorectal cancer.

SURGERY

The most effective treatment for colorectal cancer is surgical removal of the tumor, adjacent tissues, and cancerous lymph nodes. The surgical site depends on the location of the tumor. If the patient doesn't need extensive surgery involving organs other than the colon, a laparoscopic approach may be a viable option. In rare cases, the pa-

Colorectal cancer teaching topics

• Show the patient a diagram of the intestine before and after surgery, stressing how much of the bowel remains intact.

• If the patient needs a colostomy, explain the procedure and how to care for the colostomy after surgery. Consider referring the patient to an enterostomal therapist before surgery.

• If the patient will have chemotherapy or radiation therapy, explain the adverse effects that usually occur and measures that can prevent them or decrease their severity.

• Because a history of colorectal cancer means an increased risk of other primary cancers, instruct the patient to have close follow-up and screening and to increase his dietary fiber intake. Instruct his family about the familial risks of colorectal cancer, and teach them about dietary modifications to reduce their risk. Also teach them how to recognize early signs and symptoms of colorectal cancer.

tient may need a permanent colostomy. (See *Colorectal cancer teaching topics*.)

CHEMOTHERAPY

If the cancer has deeply perforated the bowel wall or has spread to the lymph nodes, chemotherapy may be given — alone or with radiation therapy — before or after surgery. Common chemotherapy drugs for patients with metastatic carcinoma include oxaliplatin (Eloxatin) with fluorouracil (Adrucil), followed by leucovorin (Wellcovorin).

HODGKIN'S DISEASE

Hodgkin's disease causes painless, progressive enlargement of the lymph nodes, spleen, and other lymphoid tissue. This type of cancer is more common in men, slightly more common in whites, and most common in two age-groups: those ages 15 to 35, and those older than age 50. A family history increases the likelihood of acquiring the disease.

Although Hodgkin's disease is fatal if untreated, recent advances have made it potentially curable, even in advanced stages. With appropriate treatment, about 90% of patients with Hodgkin's disease live at least 5 years.

Pathophysiology

The cause of Hodgkin's disease is unknown. It probably involves a virus. Many patients with Hodgkin's disease have had infectious mononucleosis, so an indirect relationship may exist between the Epstein-Barr virus and Hodgkin's disease.

Another possible risk factor is occupational exposure to herbicides and other chemicals.

Enlargement of the lymph nodes, spleen, and other lymphoid tissues results from proliferation of lymphocytes, histiocytes and, rarely, eosinophils. Patients also have distinct chromosome abnormalities in their lymph node cells. (See *Looking at a Reed-Sternberg cell,* page 26.)

RED FLAG Patients with Hodgkin's disease have an increased risk of bacterial or, less commonly, fungal, viral, or protozoal infection. Death usually results from sepsis or from multiple organ failure.

Signs and symptoms

People with Hodgkin's disease can develop signs and symptoms of whole-body involvement, including:

■ anemia
■ cancerous masses in the spleen, liver, and bones
■ fatigue
■ intermittent fever that can last for several days or weeks
■ jaundice
■ nerve pain
■ night sweats
■ painless swelling of the face and neck
■ painless swelling of the lymph nodes, usually starting in the neck and progressing to the axillary, inguinal, mediastinal, and mesenteric regions
■ pruritus
■ weight loss.

Test results

These tests may be used to rule out disorders that enlarge the lymph nodes.

■ Lymph node biopsy confirms the presence of Reed-Sternberg cells, abnormal histiocyte (macrophage) proliferation, and nodular fibrosis and necrosis. It also determines the extent of lymph node involvement.
■ Bone marrow, liver, mediastinal, and spleen biopsy determine the extent of lymph node involvement.

Looking at a Reed-Sternberg cell

This enlarged, abnormal histiocyte – or Reed-Sternberg cell – from an excised lymph node suggests Hodgkin's disease. Note the large, distinct nucleoli. Reed-Sternberg cells must be present in a patient's blood and lymph tissue to confirm a diagnosis of Hodgkin's disease.

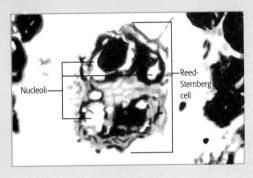

Nucleoli

Reed-Sternberg cell

- Chest X-ray, abdominal CT scan, lung and bone scans, lymphangiography, and laparoscopy determine the extent and stage of the disease.
- Hematologic tests may show:
  - mild to severe normocytic anemia
  - normochromic anemia (in 50% of patients)
  - elevated, normal, or reduced white blood cell (WBC) count and differential with neutrophilia, lymphocytopenia, monocytosis, or eosinophilia (in any combination).
- Elevated serum alkaline phosphatase levels indicate liver or bone involvement.
- Staging laparotomy may be performed for developing a therapeutic plan.

Treatment

Depending on the stage of the disease, the patient may receive chemotherapy, radiation therapy, or both. Other treatments include autologous bone marrow or peripheral stem cell transplantation and immunotherapy used with chemotherapy and radiation therapy. Correct treatment leads to longer survival — in many patients, a cure.

TEACHING FOCUS

Hodgkin's disease teaching topics

- If the patient will have chemotherapy or radiation therapy, make sure that he understands the adverse effects that usually occur and measures to prevent them or decrease their severity.
- Advise the patient to avoid crowds and anyone known to have an infection. Urge him to notify his physician if he develops an infection.
- Because enlarged lymph nodes may indicate disease recurrence, teach the patient the importance of checking his lymph nodes.

CHEMOTHERAPY COMBINATIONS

Chemotherapy consists of various combinations of drugs.

■ The well-known MOPP protocol was the first to result in significant cures and includes:
  – mechlorethamine (Mustargen)
  – vincristine (Oncovin)
  – procarbazine (Matulane)
  – prednisone.
■ Another useful combination is:
  – doxorubicin (Adriamycin)
  – bleomycin (Blenoxane)
  – vinblastine (Velban)
  – dacarbazine (DTIC-Dome).
■ Antiemetics, sedatives, and antidiarrheals may be given with these drugs to prevent adverse GI effects. (See *Hodgkin's disease teaching topics*.)

LEUKEMIA, ACUTE

Leukemia refers to a group of malignant disorders characterized by abnormal proliferation and maturation of lymphocytes and nonlymphocytic cells, leading to the suppression of normal cells.

Acute leukemia is one form of leukemia. If untreated, acute leukemia is fatal, usually from infiltration of leukemic cells into bone marrow or vital organs. With treatment, the prognosis varies. Two types of acute leukemia are:

■ acute lymphocytic leukemia
■ acute myeloid leukemia (also known as *acute nonlymphocytic leukemia* or *acute myeloblastic leukemia*).

Acute lymphocytic leukemia accounts for 80% of childhood leukemias. Treatment leads to remission in 81% of children, who survive an average of 5 years, and in 65% of adults, who survive an average of 2 years. Children ages 2 to 8 who receive intensive therapy have the best survival rate.

Acute myeloid leukemia is one of the most common leukemias in adults. Average survival time is only 1 year after diagnosis, even with aggressive treatment. Remissions lasting 2 to 10 months occur in 50% of children.

The patient's history usually reveals a sudden onset of high fever and abnormal bleeding, such as bruising after minor trauma, nosebleeds, gingival bleeding, and purpura. Fatigue and night sweats also may occur.

Pathophysiology

The exact cause of acute leukemia isn't known. About 40% to 50% of patients have mutations in their chromosomes. People with Down syndrome, trisomy 13, and other hereditary disorders have an increased risk. Certain viruses, such as human T-cell lymphotropic virus, are also linked to an increased risk of leukemia. Other risk factors include:

■ cigarette smoking
■ exposure to certain chemicals, such as benzene, which is present in cigarette smoke and gasoline
■ exposure to large doses of ionizing radiation
■ exposure to drugs that depress the bone marrow.

What probably happens in the development of leukemia is that immature hematopoietic cells undergo an abnormal transformation, giving rise to leukemic cells. Leukemic cells then multiply and accumulate, crowding out other types of cells. Crowding prevents production of normal red and white blood cells and platelets, leading to pancytopenia—a reduction in the number of all cellular elements of the blood.

RED FLAG Acute leukemia increases the risk of infection and, eventually, organ malfunction through encroachment or hemorrhage.

Signs and symptoms

Signs and symptoms of acute lymphocytic and acute myeloid leukemia are similar because they're both related to suppression of bone marrow elements. Signs and symptoms include:

■ anemia
■ bleeding
■ infection
■ fever

■ lethargy
■ malaise
■ night sweats
■ paleness
■ weight loss.

Test results
These tests are used to diagnose acute leukemia.
■ Blood counts show thrombocytopenia and neutropenia; WBC differential determines cell type.
■ Lumbar puncture detects meningeal involvement; cerebrospinal fluid analysis reveals abnormal WBC invasion of the central nervous system (CNS).
■ Bone marrow aspiration and biopsy confirms the disease by showing a proliferation of immature WBCs. It also determines whether the leukemia is lymphocytic or myeloid (important because the treatments and prognoses differ).
■ CT scans show which organs are affected.

Treatment
When less than 5% of blast cells in the bone marrow and peripheral blood are normal, systemic chemotherapy is used to eradicate leukemic cells and induce remission. In addition, treatment also may include:
■ antibiotic, antifungal, and antiviral drugs
■ colony-stimulating factors, such as filgrastim (Neupogen), to spur the growth of granulocytes, red blood cells (RBCs), and platelets
■ platelet transfusion to prevent bleeding
■ RBC transfusion to prevent anemia. (See *Acute leukemia teaching topics,* page 30.)

ACUTE LYMPHOCYTIC LEUKEMIA
Treatment of acute lymphocytic leukemia is divided into three stages:
■ *Induction* usually includes vincristine (Oncovin), prednisone, and an anthracycline given with or without asparaginase (Elspar) for adults.
■ *Consolidation,* in which patients receive high doses of chemotherapy designed to eliminate remaining leukemic cells.
■ *Maintenance,* in which patients receive lower doses of chemotherapy for up to 2 years. The goal is to eliminate stray leukemic cells

TEACHING FOCUS

Acute leukemia teaching topics

● Inform the patient that drug therapy is tailored to his type of leukemia. Explain that he'll probably need a combination of drugs; teach him about the ones he'll receive. Make sure that he understands their adverse effects and measures to prevent them or reduce their severity.
● Review signs and symptoms of infection, such as fever, chills, cough, and sore throat, and abnormal bleeding, such as bruising and small purplish spots, or petechiae, caused by tiny hemorrhages. Also teach the patient and his family how to stop bleeding, such as by applying pressure or ice.
● Instruct the patient to use a soft-bristle toothbrush and to avoid hot, spicy foods and the overuse of commercial mouthwashes.

that have evaded other agents used in the induction and consolidation stages.

ACUTE MYELOID LEUKEMIA
Treatment of acute myeloid leukemia occurs in two stages:
■ *Induction,* which includes cytarabine (Cytosar-U) and an anthracycline.
■ *Postremission,* which includes intensification, maintenance chemotherapy, or bone marrow transplantation.

LEUKEMIA, CHRONIC LYMPHOCYTIC
Chronic lymphocytic leukemia is the most benign and slowest progressing form of leukemia. This type of chronic leukemia occurs commonly in elderly people; more than half of those affected are men. According to the American Cancer Society, this type of leukemia accounts for about one-third of new adult cases annually.

The prognosis is poor if anemia, thrombocytopenia, neutropenia, bulky lymphadenopathy, or severe lymphocytosis develops. Gross bone marrow replacement by abnormal lymphocytes is the most common cause of death, usually 4 to 5 years after diagnosis.

Pathophysiology
Chronic lymphocytic leukemia is a generalized, progressive disease. It causes a proliferation and accumulation of relatively mature looking but immunologically inefficient lymphocytes. After these cells infiltrate, clinical signs appear.

Although the cause of chronic lymphocytic leukemia is unknown, hereditary factors are suspected.

◤ **RED FLAG** *The most common complication of chronic lymphocytic leukemia is infection, which can cause fatal septicemia. In end-stage disease, anemia, progressive splenomegaly, leukemic cell replacement of bone marrow, and profound hypogammaglobulinemia also may occur.*

Signs and symptoms

Signs and symptoms may include:
- fatigue
- fever
- frequent infections
- lymph node enlargement
- splenomegaly.

Test results

These tests are used to diagnose chronic lymphocytic leukemia.
- Lymph node biopsy distinguishes benign tumors from malignant tumors.
- Routine blood tests usually uncover the disease.
  - In early stages, the lymphocyte count is slightly elevated (greater than 20,000/mm^3).
  - Although granulocytopenia is typically seen first, the lymphocyte count climbs (greater than 100,000/mm^3) as the disease progresses.
  - A hemoglobin (Hb) level lower than 11 g/dl, hypogammaglobulinemia, and a depressed serum globulin level also occur.
- Bone marrow aspiration and biopsy can be used to show lymphocytic invasion.

Treatment

If the patient is asymptomatic, treatment may begin with close monitoring. If the patient has autoimmune hemolytic anemia or thrombocytopenia, systemic chemotherapy is administered using the alkylating agents chlorambucil (Leukeran) or cyclophosphamide (Cytoxan). Prednisone may be given if the disease is refractory to treatment.

If the patient develops obstruction or organ impairment or enlargement, local radiation reduces organ size and helps relieve symptoms. Radiation therapy also is used for enlarged lymph nodes, painful bony lesions, and massive splenomegaly.

Allopurinol (Zyloprim) can prevent hyperuricemia. (See *Chronic lymphocytic leukemia teaching topics,* page 32.)

TEACHING FOCUS

Chronic lymphocytic leukemia teaching topics

- Teach the patient and his family how to recognize signs and symptoms of infection, such as fever, chills, cough, and sore throat. Warn the patient to avoid contact with obviously ill people, especially children with common contagious childhood diseases.
- Warn the patient to take measures to prevent bleeding because his blood may not have enough platelets for proper clotting. Tell him to avoid aspirin, and teach him how to recognize products that contain aspirin. Teach him the signs of abnormal bleeding (bruising, petechiae) and

how to apply pressure and ice to the area to stop bleeding. Urge him to report excessive bleeding or bruising to his physician.
- If the patient will have chemotherapy or radiation therapy, make sure that he understands the adverse effects that usually occur and measures to prevent them or reduce their severity.
- Teach the patient the signs of recurrence (swollen lymph nodes in the neck, axilla, and groin; increased abdominal size or discomfort), and tell him to notify his physician immediately if these signs occur.

LEUKEMIA, CHRONIC MYELOID

Also called *chronic myelogenous leukemia,* chronic myeloid leukemia is characterized by myeloproliferation in bone marrow, peripheral blood, and body tissues. It's most common in middle age but may affect those of any age. It affects both sexes equally. In the United States, 4,300 cases are diagnosed annually, accounting for about 20% of all cases of leukemia.

Pathophysiology

Chronic myeloid leukemia is caused by the excessive development of neoplastic granulocytes in the bone marrow. These neoplastic granulocytes circulate into the peripheral circulation, infiltrating the liver and spleen.

These cells contain a distinct abnormality, the *Philadelphia chromosome,* in which the long arm of chromosome 22 translocates to chromosome 9. Radiation exposure may cause this abnormality. Other suspected causes include myeloproliferative diseases or an unidentified virus.

Chronic myeloid leukemia proceeds in two distinct phases:
- the chronic phase, characterized by anemia and bleeding abnormalities

■ the terminal or blastic phase, in which myeloblasts, the most primitive granulocytic precursors, proliferate rapidly.

RED FLAG Chronic myeloid leukemia is a deadly disease. The average survival time is 3 to 4 years after the onset of the chronic phase and 3 to 6 months after the onset of the terminal phase.

Signs and symptoms

Common signs and symptoms of chronic myeloid leukemia include:

■ bruising
■ fatigue
■ fever
■ heat intolerance
■ joint pain
■ splenomegaly with abdominal fullness
■ weakness
■ weight loss.

Test results

These tests are used to diagnose chronic myeloid leukemia.

■ Chromosomal studies of peripheral blood or bone marrow confirm the diagnosis.
■ Serum analysis shows WBC abnormalities, such as:
  – leukocytosis (WBC count greater than 50,000/mm^3 to as high as 250,000/mm^3)
  – leukopenia (WBC count less than 5,000/mm^3)
  – neutropenia (neutrophil count lower than 1,500/mm^3) despite a high WBC count
  – increased circulating myeloblasts.
■ Other possible blood abnormalities include:
  – decreased Hb level (below 10 g/dl)
  – decreased hematocrit (less than 30%)
  – thrombocytosis (more than 1 million thrombocytes/mm^3).
■ The serum uric acid level may exceed 8 mg/dl.
■ Bone marrow biopsy may be hypercellular, showing bone marrow infiltration by many myeloid elements. In the acute phase, myeloblasts predominate.
■ CT scans may identify the affected organs.

Treatment

The treatment goal is to control leukocytosis and thrombocytosis. Imatinib (Gleevec) is a highly specific anticancer drug approved by the Food and Drug Administration for treating chronic myeloid

TEACHING FOCUS

Chronic myeloid leukemia teaching topics

● Teach the patient and his family how to recognize signs and symptoms of infection, such as fever, chills, cough, and sore throat. Warn the patient to avoid contact with obviously ill people, especially children with common contagious childhood diseases.

● Warn the patient to take measures to prevent bleeding because his blood may not have enough platelets for proper clotting. Tell him to avoid aspirin, and teach him how to recognize products that contain aspirin. Teach him the signs of abnormal bleeding (bruising, petechiae) and how to apply pressure and ice to the area to stop bleeding. Urge him to

report excessive bleeding or bruising to his physician.

● If the patient will have chemotherapy or radiation therapy, make sure that he understands the adverse effects that usually occur and measures to prevent them or reduce their severity.

● If the patient will undergo bone marrow transplantation, reinforce the physician's explanation of the procedure, its possible outcome, and potential adverse effects. Make sure that the patient fully understands the therapy. Teach him about total body irradiation, which usually takes place before the procedure, and discuss any planned chemotherapy.

leukemia. Other commonly used drugs are busulfan (Mleran) and hydroxyurea (Hydrea).

Bone marrow transplantation may be effective.

Aspirin may help prevent a stroke if the platelet count exceeds 1 million/mm³. Antibiotics and blood transfusions are supportive treatments. (See *Chronic myeloid leukemia teaching topics.*) Supplemental therapy may include:

- local splenic radiation or splenectomy to increase the platelet count and decrease the effects of splenomegaly
- leukapheresis (selective leukocyte removal) to reduce the WBC count
- allopurinol (Zyloprim) to prevent secondary hyperuricemia
- colchicine to relieve gouty attacks.

LUNG CANCER

Although lung cancer is largely preventable, it remains the most common cause of cancer death in men and women. It's divided into two major classes:

- small-cell lung cancer
- non–small-cell lung cancer.

Non–small-cell cancer is the most common type of lung cancer, accounting for almost 80% of cases. Types of non–small-cell cancer include:

■ adenocarcinoma
■ squamous cell
■ large-cell.

Small-cell lung cancer accounts for 20% of all lung cancers. It starts in the hormonal cells in the lungs. Small-cell lung cancers include:

■ oat cell
■ intermediate
■ combined (small-cell combined with squamous or adenocarcinoma).

The prognosis for lung cancer is, in general, poor, depending on the extent of the cancer and the cells' growth rate. Only about 13% of patients survive 5 years after diagnosis.

Pathophysiology

Lung cancer most commonly results from repeated tissue trauma from inhalation of irritants or carcinogens. These substances include:

■ air pollution
■ arsenic
■ asbestos
■ nickel
■ radon
■ tobacco smoke.

Almost all lung cancers start in the epithelium of the lungs. In normal lungs, the epithelium lines and protects the tissue beneath it. However, when exposed to irritants or carcinogens, the epithelium must continually replace itself, raising the risk that cells will develop chromosomal changes and become dysplastic (altered in size, shape, and organization).

Dysplastic cells don't function well as protectors, so underlying tissue gets exposed to irritants and carcinogens. Eventually, dysplastic cells turn into neoplastic cells and start invading deeper tissues.

RED FLAG If the primary tumor spreads to intrathoracic structures, it may cause tracheal obstruction, esophageal compression with dysphagia, and hypoxemia. Other complications include anorexia and weight loss (sometimes leading to cachexia), finger clubbing, and hypertrophic osteoarthropathy.

Common lung cancers

This table describes the growth rate, metastasis sites, signs and symptoms, and diagnostic tests of four common lung cancers.

TYPE OF CANCER	RATE OF GROWTH	METASTASIS
Adenocarcinoma	Moderate	Early metastasis to hilar nodes, chest wall, and mediastinum
Squamous cell	Slow	Late metastasis mainly to hilar lymph nodes, chest wall, and mediastinum
Large-cell	Fast	Early, extensive metastasis to other thoracic structures and other organs
Small-cell	Very fast	Very early metastasis to mediastinum, hilar lymph nodes, and other organ sites

Signs and symptoms
For signs and symptoms of different types of lung cancers, see *Common lung cancers.*

Test results
These tests are used to diagnose lung cancer.
- Chest X-ray may be used to determine tumor size and location. It usually shows an advanced lesion but can reveal damage 2 years before signs and symptoms appear.
- Cytologic sputum analysis is 80% reliable. It requires a specimen expectorated from the lungs and tracheobronchial tree.
- Bronchoscopy may reveal the tumor site; bronchoscopic washings provide material for cytologic and histologic study.
- Needle biopsy is used to locate peripheral tumors in the lungs and to collect tissue specimens for analysis; it confirms the diagnosis in 80% of patients.
- Tissue biopsy of metastatic sites is used to assess the extent (stage) of the disease and determine prognosis and treatment.

SIGNS AND SYMPTOMS	DIAGNOSTIC TESTS
Pleural effusion	Fiber-optic bronchoscopy, radiography, electron microscopy
Airway obstruction, cough, and sputum production	Sputum analysis, biopsy, immunohistochemistry, electron microscopy, bronchoscopy
Cough, hemoptysis, chest wall pain, pleural effusion, sputum production, and pneumonia-induced airway obstruction	Bronchoscopy, sputum analysis, electron microscopy
Chest pain, cough, hemoptysis, dyspnea, localized wheezing, pneumonia-induced airway obstruction, muscle weakness, facial edema, hypokalemia, hyperglycemia, hypertension, and other signs and symptoms related to excessive hormone secretion	Sputum analysis, immunohistochemistry, electron microscopy, radiography, bronchoscopy

- Thoracentesis allows chemical and cytologic examination of pleural fluid.
- CT scan may show mediastinal and hilar lymph node involvement and the extent of the disease.
- Bone scan, CT brain scan, liver function studies, and gallium scans of the liver and spleen reveal metastasis.

Treatment

Treatment depends on the stage of illness. Various combinations of surgery, radiation therapy, and chemotherapy may improve the patient's prognosis and prolong survival. Unfortunately, lung cancer is usually advanced at diagnosis. (See *Lung cancer teaching topics,* page 38.)

SURGERY

Surgery may involve one of two approaches:
- partial lung removal (wedge resection, segmental resection, lobectomy, or radical lobectomy)

TEACHING FOCUS

Lung cancer teaching topics

● Preoperatively, teach the patient about postoperative procedures and equipment. Teach him how to cough and breathe deeply from the diaphragm and how to perform range-of-motion exercises. Reassure him that analgesics and proper positioning will help to control postoperative pain.

● If the patient will have chemotherapy or radiation therapy, make sure he understands the adverse effects that usually occur and measures to prevent them or reduce their severity.

● To help prevent lung cancer, teach high-risk patients to stop smoking. Refer smokers who want to quit to the local branch of the American Cancer Society or American Lung Association. Explain that nicotine gum or a nicotine patch and an antidepressant may be prescribed in combination with educational and support groups.

■ total lung removal (pneumonectomy). Complete surgical resection is the only chance for a cure, but fewer than 25% of patients have disease that's responsive to surgery.

RADIATION

Preoperative radiation therapy may reduce tumor bulk, allowing surgical resection and improving the patient's response. Radiation typically is recommended for stage I and II lesions (if surgery is contraindicated) and for stage III disease confined to the involved hemithorax and the ipsilateral supraclavicular lymph nodes.

CHEMOTHERAPY

Most types of lung cancer are fairly resistant to chemotherapy, although it may cause dramatic, but temporary, responses in patients with small-cell carcinoma. Unfortunately, patients usually relapse in 7 to 14 months. Drug combinations include:

■ cyclophosphamide (Cytoxan), doxorubicin (Adriamycin), and vincristine (Oncovin)

■ cyclophosphamide, doxorubicin, vincristine, and etoposide (Toposar)

■ etoposide, cisplatin (Platinol), cyclophosphamide, and doxorubicin.

OTHER TREATMENTS

Gefitinib (Iressa), a drug that blocks growth factor receptor activity, may be used as continued treatment for locally advanced or metastatic non–small-cell lung cancer when chemotherapy fails.

MALIGNANT MELANOMA

Malignant melanoma is the most lethal skin cancer. It accounts for 1% to 2% of all malignant tumors, is slightly more common in women, is unusual in children, and occurs most commonly from ages 40 to 50. Occurrence among younger people is increasing because of increased sun exposure or, possibly, a decrease in the ozone layer.

Pathophysiology

Malignant melanoma arises from melanocytes (cells that synthesize the pigment melanin). Melanocytes are found in the skin, meninges, alimentary canal, respiratory tract, and lymph nodes.

RED FLAG Melanoma spreads through the lymphatic and vascular systems and metastasizes to the regional lymph nodes, skin, liver, lungs, and CNS. In most patients, superficial lesions are curable, but deeper lesions are more likely to metastasize.

Up to 70% of malignant melanomas arise from an existing nevus (circumscribed malformation of the skin) or mole. Common sites are the head and neck in men, the legs in women, and the backs of people exposed to excessive sunlight.

Risk factors for developing melanoma are:
■ excessive exposure to sunlight
■ family history of melanoma
■ hormonal factors such as pregnancy
■ increased nevi
■ personal history of melanoma
■ red hair, fair skin, and blue eyes
■ susceptibility to sunburn
■ tendency to freckle from the sun
■ Celtic or Scandinavian ancestry. (Melanoma is rare in Blacks.)
(See *Influences on melanoma development,* page 40.)

An organelle in the melanocyte called a melanosome is responsible for producing melanin. One theory proposes that melanoma arises because the melanosome is abnormal or absent.

Signs and symptoms

Suspect malignant melanoma when a skin lesion or nevus enlarges, changes color, becomes inflamed or sore, itches, ulcerates, bleeds, changes texture, or shows signs of surrounding pigment regression. To assess the malignant potential of a mole, look for asymmetry, an irregular border, color variation, and a diameter larger than 6 mm.

Test results

Diagnostic tests for malignant melanoma include these.

GENETIC CONNECTION

Influences on melanoma development

ULTRAVIOLET LIGHT

During the past few years, scientists have gained an understanding about how ultraviolet light damages deoxyribonucleic acid (DNA) and how the change in DNA causes normal skin to become cancerous. Scientists have also found that DNA damage affecting certain genes causes melanocytes to change into melanoma. Typically, this damage is caused by sun exposure.

INHERITED GENES

On the other hand, some people may inherit mutated genes from their parents. The p16 gene, recently discovered by scientists, causes some melanomas that run in certain families.

POSSIBLE TREATMENTS

These discoveries have led to new treatment options. One approach is to add a specific gene to melanoma cells. This gene makes the melanoma sensitive to oblimersen (Genasense), a gene-blocker drug that's made up of short strands of DNA and neutralizes the melanoma cell's ability to make certain proteins. This drug prevents the cells from making the BCL2 protein, which is found in high levels in most melanoma cells and prevents the cancer cells from dying.

In early studies, combining this drug with chemotherapy and dacarbazine (DTIC-Dome) caused some metastatic melanoma tumors to shrink.

■ Excisional biopsy and full-depth punch biopsy with histologic examination are used to distinguish malignant melanoma from a benign nevus, seborrheic keratosis, or pigmented basal cell epithelioma; they're also used to determine tumor thickness and disease stage.

■ Chest X-ray, gallium scan, bone scan, magnetic resonance imaging (MRI), and CT scans of the chest, abdomen, or brain may detect metastasis, depending on the depth of tumor invasion.

Treatment

Treatment always involves surgical resection of the tumor and a 3- to 5-cm margin. The extent of resection depends on the size and location of the primary lesion. If a skin graft is needed to close a wide resection, plastic surgery provides excellent cosmetic repair.

Surgical treatment may also include regional lymphadenectomy. (See *Malignant melanoma teaching topics*.)

In addition to surgery, other treatments are available:

TEACHING FOCUS

Malignant melanoma teaching topics

● Tell the patient what to expect before and after surgery, what the wound will look like, and what type of dressing he'll have.

● Stress the need for close follow-up care to detect recurrences early. Explain that recurrences and metastases, if they occur, are commonly delayed, so follow-up must continue for years. Teach the patient how to recognize the signs of recurrence.

● To help prevent malignant melanoma, stress the detrimental effects of overexposure to ultraviolet light, especially to fair-skinned, blue-eyed patients. Recommend that they use a sunblock or sunscreen and that they perform monthly skin self-examinations and have yearly screenings by a dermatologist.

● If the patient will have chemotherapy or radiation therapy, make sure he understands the adverse effects that usually occur and measures to prevent them or reduce their severity.

■ For deep primary lesions or metastatic disease, chemotherapy with dacarbazine (DTIC-Dome) may be used.

■ Immunotherapy with bacille Calmette-Guérin vaccine (TICE BCG) is used in advanced melanoma. In theory, this treatment combats cancer by boosting the body's disease-fighting systems.

■ Radiation therapy, usually reserved for metastatic disease, doesn't prolong survival but may reduce pain and tumor size.

■ Gene therapy, although still in early stages of development, may provide a less toxic treatment option.

MULTIPLE MYELOMA

Multiple myeloma is a disseminated cancer of marrow plasma cells that infiltrates bone to produce lesions throughout the flat bones, vertebrae, skull, pelvis, and ribs. In late stages, the cancer infiltrates the liver, spleen, lymph nodes, lungs, adrenal glands, kidneys, skin, and GI tract.

Multiple myeloma affects about 12,300 people yearly, is slightly more common in men, and starts between ages 50 and 80. If the disease is diagnosed early, treatment may prolong life by 3 to 5 years. Usually, however, the prognosis is poor because, by the time of diagnosis, the vertebrae, pelvis, skull, ribs, clavicles, and sternum are infiltrated and skeletal destruction is widespread. More than 50% of patients die within 3 months of diagnosis; 90% die within 2 years.

Pathophysiology

The cause of multiple myeloma isn't known. The disorder has been linked to:

■ genetic factors
■ viral infection
■ occupational exposure to certain chemicals and radiation.

Normally, stem cells in the bone marrow can replicate or differentiate. Lymphoid stem cells can differentiate into T lymphocytes, which take part in cell-mediated immunity, or B lymphocytes, which take part in humoral immunity. B lymphocytes eventually become plasma cells that produce and release immunoglobulins, the most common of which is immunoglobulin (Ig) G.

In multiple myeloma, an unknown factor stimulates B lymphocytes to become malignant plasma cells that produce huge amounts of IgG, IgA, or Bence Jones proteins. This leads to a hyperviscosity syndrome commonly seen in myeloma patients.

Signs and symptoms

Patients with multiple myeloma may have various symptoms, including:

■ cold intolerance
■ confusion
■ frequent infections
■ headaches
■ irritability
■ renal failure
■ skeletal pain
■ somnolence
■ vision disturbances.

RED FLAG Multiple myeloma can cause infections, pyelonephritis, renal calculi, renal failure, hematologic imbalances, fractures, hypercalcemia, hyperuricemia, and dehydration.

Test results

These tests are used to diagnose multiple myeloma.

■ Complete blood count reveals moderate to severe anemia, with 40% to 50% lymphocytes but seldom more than 3% plasma cells.
■ A differential smear also shows rouleau formations (blood cells that stick together, resembling stacks of coins). Commonly the first clue, this results from elevation of the erythrocyte sedimentation rate.

- Urine studies may show proteinuria, Bence Jones protein, and hypercalciuria. Absence of Bence Jones protein doesn't rule out multiple myeloma, but its presence usually confirms the disease.
- Bone marrow aspiration shows an abnormal number of immature plasma cells (10% to 95% instead of 3% to 5%).
- Serum electrophoresis shows the characteristic M band containing paraprotein.
- X-rays during the early stages may reveal only diffuse osteoporosis; later, they show multiple, sharply circumscribed osteolytic (punched out) lesions, particularly on the skull, pelvis, and spine.
- Serum calcium level is elevated because calcium lost from the bone is reabsorbed into the serum.

Treatment

Long-term treatment of multiple myeloma consists mainly of chemotherapy to suppress plasma cell growth and to control pain.

- The most common regimen uses:
  - vincristine (Oncovin)
  - doxorubicin (Adriamycin)
  - dexamethasone (Decadron) for induction.
- Other chemotherapy drugs that may be used but are less suitable for induction include:
  - melphalan (Alkeran)
  - carmustine (BiCNU).
- Interferon may prolong the plateau phase after the initial chemotherapy is completed.
- Survival rates have improved by using high-dose chemotherapy and stem-cell transplantation. However, adverse effects make this option available only to patients who were healthy before acquiring the disease.
- Thalidomide (Thalomid), an immunomodulatory drug, has been effective in treating multiple myeloma, but it causes sleepiness and nerve damage, limiting its use.
- Bortezomib (Velcade), a proteasome 26S inhibitor, may be used in patients who have had two previous courses of therapy with disease progression in the second course.
- Local radiation reduces acute lesions and relieves the pain of collapsed vertebrae.
- Other treatments include:
  - analgesics for pain
  - laminectomy for vertebral compression
  - dialysis for renal complications.

Multiple myeloma teaching topics

● Caution the patient to avoid crowds and people known to have infections.
● If the patient will have stem-cell transplantation, reinforce the physician's explanation of the procedure, its possible outcome, and potential adverse effects. Make sure that the patient fully understands the therapy. Teach him about total body irradiation, which usually takes place before the procedure, and discuss any chemotherapy that he'll undergo.
● If the patient will have chemotherapy or radiation therapy, make sure he understands the adverse effects that usually occur and measures to help prevent them or reduce their severity.

■ Because patients may have bone demineralization and may lose large amounts of calcium into blood and urine, they're prime candidates for renal calculi and renal failure from hypercalcemia. Hypercalcemia is treated with:
 – hydration
 – diuretics
 – corticosteroids
 – pamidronate (Aredia)
 – inorganic phosphates.
■ Plasmapheresis temporarily removes Bence Jones protein from withdrawn blood and retransfuses the cells to the patient. (See *Multiple myeloma teaching topics.*)

PROSTATE CANCER

Prostate cancer is the most common cancer in men and the second leading cause of cancer death. (See *Location of the prostate gland.*) About 85% of prostate cancers originate in the posterior prostate gland; the rest grow near the urethra. Adenocarcinoma is the most common form. Death rates in Black men are more than twice as high as rates in White men.

Pathophysiology

Risk factors for prostate cancer include:
■ age (more than 70% of all prostate cancer cases are diagnosed in men older than age 65)
■ diet high in saturated fats
■ ethnicity. Black men have the highest risk of prostate cancer in the world. The disease is common in North America and northwestern Europe and is rare in Asia and South America.

Location of the prostate gland

This drawing shows the location of the prostate gland. Note that enlargement may occlude the urethra, causing urine retention.

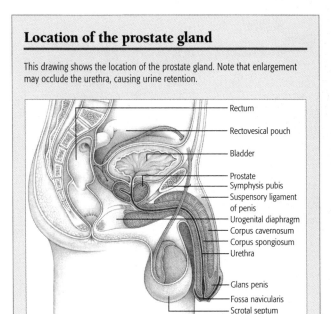

- Rectum
- Rectovesical pouch
- Bladder
- Prostate
- Symphysis pubis
- Suspensory ligament of penis
- Urogenital diaphragm
- Corpus cavernosum
- Corpus spongiosum
- Urethra
- Glans penis
- Fossa navicularis
- Scrotal septum

Prostate cancer grows slowly. When primary lesions spread beyond the prostate gland, they invade the prostatic capsule and then spread along the ejaculatory ducts in the space between the seminal vesicles or perivesicular fascia.

RED FLAG Progressive disease can lead to spinal cord compression, deep vein thrombosis, pulmonary emboli, and myelophthisis.

When prostate cancer is treated in its localized form, the 5-year survival rate is 70%; after metastasis, it's lower than 35%. Fatal prostate cancer usually results from widespread bone metastasis.

Signs and symptoms

Prostate cancer seldom produces signs and symptoms until it's advanced. Evidence of advanced disease stems from obstruction and may include:

- dysuria
- incomplete bladder emptying
- slow urine stream

■ urinary hesitancy.

Test results

These tests and results are common in prostate cancer.

■ Digital rectal examination (DRE) determines the location and size of the prostate and the presence of nodules.

■ Biopsy of the prostate may distinguish a benign from a malignant mass.

■ Blood tests may show elevated levels of prostate-specific antigen (PSA). Although an elevated PSA level occurs with metastasis, it also occurs with other prostate diseases.

■ Transrectal prostatic ultrasonography may be used for patients with abnormal DRE and PSA findings.

■ Bone scan and excretory urography determine the extent of the disease.

■ MRI and CT scans help define the tumor's extent.

Treatment

Depending on the stage of the disease, therapy may include:

■ hormone therapy

■ radiation

■ prostatectomy.

Because most prostate cancers are androgen- or hormone-dependent, the main treatments are:

■ antiandrogens to suppress adrenal function

■ medical castration with estrogen or gonadotropin-releasing hormone analogs.

Radiation therapy may cure locally invasive lesions in early disease and may relieve bone pain from metastatic skeletal involvement. It's also used prophylactically to prevent tumor growth for patients with tumors in regional lymph nodes. Radioactive "seeds" may be implanted into the prostate. This treatment increases radiation to the area while minimizing exposure to surrounding tissues. (See *Prostate cancer teaching topics*.)

Radical prostatectomy usually works for localized lesions that haven't metastasized. Transurethral resection of the prostate may be used to relieve an obstruction.

The chemotherapy drug docetaxel (Taxotere) may be used for men with advanced prostate cancer that doesn't respond to hormone therapy. The drug is given with prednisone. Docetaxel is the first drug to improve the survival rate in men with advanced prostate cancer.

Combination chemotherapy with cyclophosphamide (Cytoxan), doxorubicin (Adriamycin), fluorouracil (Adrucil), methotrexate (Trexall), estramustine (Emcyt), vinblastine (Velban), and cisplatin (Platinol) may reduce pain from metastasis but doesn't lengthen survival.

3

INFECTION

A countless number of harmless microorganisms reside on and in the body. They're found on the skin and in the nose, mouth, pharynx, distal intestine, colon, distal urethra, and vagina. The skin contains 10,000 microorganisms per square centimeter. Trillions of microorganisms are secreted daily from the GI tract alone.

Many of these microorganisms provide useful, protective functions. For example, the intestinal flora help synthesize vitamin K, which is an important part of the blood-clotting mechanism.

Understanding infection

An infection results when tissue-destroying microorganisms enter and multiply in the body. Some pathogens, or infection-causing substances, may cause only minor illness, such as a cold or ear infection. Others may cause life-threatening illness, such as sepsis, which causes widespread vasodilation and multiple organ dysfunction syndrome.

INFECTION-CAUSING MICROBES
Four types of microorganisms can enter the body and cause infection:
- viruses
- bacteria
- fungi
- parasites.

Viruses
Viruses are microscopic genetic parasites. Although they may contain genetic material, such as deoxyribonucleic acid or ribonucleic acid, they have no metabolic capability and need a host cell to replicate.

Viral infections occur when normal inflammatory and immune responses fail. After entering the host cell, the inner capsule of the virus releases genetic material, causing the infection. Some viruses surround the host cell and preserve it; others kill the host cell on contact.

Bacteria

Bacteria are single-celled microorganisms with no true nucleus. They reproduce by cell division. Pathogenic bacteria contain cell-damaging proteins that cause infection. These proteins come in two forms:

■ exotoxins, which are released during cell growth
■ endotoxins, which are released when the bacterial cell wall decomposes. Endotoxins cause fever and aren't affected by antibiotics.

Bacteria are classified in several other ways, including:

■ shape
■ growth requirements
■ motility
■ whether they're aerobic (need oxygen to survive) or anaerobic (don't need oxygen to survive).

Fungi

Fungi are nonphotosynthetic microorganisms that reproduce through asexual (mitotic) and sexual (meiotic) cell division. They're large compared to other microorganisms and contain a true nucleus. Fungi are classified as:

■ yeasts, which are round, single-celled, facultative anaerobes, which can live with or without oxygen
■ molds, which are filament-like, multinucleated, aerobic microorganisms.

Although fungi are present normally on the body, they can overproduce, especially when the normal flora is compromised. For example, vaginal yeast infections may arise when antibiotic treatment kills the normal vaginal flora, allowing yeast to reproduce.

Infections caused by fungi are called *mycotic infections* because pathogenic fungi release mycotoxin. Most of these infections are mild unless they become systemic or if the patient's immune system is compromised.

Parasites

Parasites are single-celled or multicelled organisms that depend on a host for food and a protective environment. Parasitic infections are uncommon except in hot, moist climates. Most common parasitic infections, such as tapeworm infestation, occur in the intestines.

BARRIERS TO INFECTION

In a healthy person, the body's defense mechanisms usually can ward off infections. The body has many built-in infection barriers, including:

■ the skin
■ secretions from the eyes, nasal passages, prostate gland, testicles, stomach, and vagina, most of which contain bacteria-killing particles called lysozymes
■ certain body structures, such as cilia in the pulmonary airways, which sweep foreign material from breathing passages.

THE INFECTION PROCESS

Infection occurs when the body's defense mechanisms break down or when certain properties of microorganisms, such as virulence or toxin production, override the defense system. Other factors that create a climate for infection include:

■ crowded living conditions
■ dust
■ humidity
■ medications
■ pollution
■ poor nutrition
■ poor sanitation
■ stress.

Infection results when a pathogen enters the body through direct contact, inhalation, ingestion, or an insect or animal bite. The pathogen then attaches itself to a cell and releases enzymes that destroy the cell's protective membrane. Next, it spreads through the bloodstream and lymphatic system, finally multiplying and causing infection in the target tissue or organ.

Infections that arise in people who have altered, weak immune systems are called *opportunistic infections*. For example, patients with acquired immunodeficiency syndrome are plagued by opportunistic infections such as *Pneumocystis carinii* pneumonia.

Infectious disorders

The infections discussed in this section include:

■ herpes simplex
■ herpes zoster
■ infectious mononucleosis

- Lyme disease
- rabies
- respiratory syncytial virus
- rubella
- salmonellosis
- toxoplasmosis.

HERPES SIMPLEX

A recurrent viral infection, herpes simplex occurs as two types:

- Type 1 affects mainly skin and mucous membranes and commonly produces cold sores, also known as *fever blisters*.
- Type 2 affects mainly genitals, causing painful clusters of small ulcerations.

Both types of herpes simplex virus (HSV) can infect the eyes and body organs. In addition, both types can result in localized or generalized infection. Although herpes simplex may be latent for years, initial infection makes the patient a carrier susceptible to recurrent attacks. Outbreaks may be provoked by fever, menses, stress, heat, cold, lack of sleep, or sun exposure.

Herpes simplex occurs worldwide and is equally common in men and women. It's most common in lower socioeconomic groups, probably because of crowded living conditions.

Pathophysiology

Herpesvirus hominis, a widespread infectious agent, causes both types of herpes simplex. Type 1 is transmitted by oral and respiratory secretions, and type 2 is transmitted by sexual contact. However, cross-infection may result from orogenital sex. The average incubation for generalized infection is 2 to 12 days; for localized genital infection, 3 to 7 days.

HSV is a linear, double-stranded deoxyribonucleic acid (DNA) molecule with an outer coating of lipid-type membrane. Here's what happens during exposure:

- The virus fuses to the host cell membrane.
- The virus releases proteins, turning off the host cell's protein production or synthesis.
- The virus replicates and synthesizes structural proteins.
- The virus pushes its nucleocapsid (protein coat and nucleic acid) into the cytoplasm of the host cell and releases the viral DNA.
- Complete virus particles capable of surviving and infecting a living cell (called virions) are transported to the cell's surface.

HSV infection doesn't end in cell death. Instead, the virus enters a latent state in which it's maintained by the cell. Viral replication and redevelopment of herpetic lesions is called *reactivation*.

Closer look at a vesicle

A vesicle is a raised, circumscribed, fluid-filled lesion less than 0.6 cm in diameter. It's the typical lesion of chickenpox and herpes simplex.

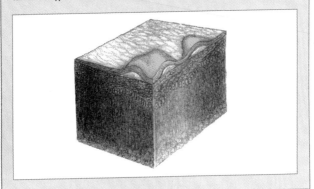

RED FLAG Pregnant women should avoid exposure to herpes simplex because it can cause severe congenital anomalies in neonates. These abnormalities range from localized skin lesions to disseminated infection of major organs. Some examples of common complications in neonates are seizures, mental retardation, blindness, and deafness.

Herpes also may cause severe illness in immunocompromised patients; examples include pneumonia, hepatitis, and neurologic complications. Women with herpes simplex type 2 may have an increased risk of cervical cancer.

Signs and symptoms
TYPE 1 INFECTION

Type 1 herpes simplex may cause generalized or localized infection as the virus invades the cells around the mouth. Generalized infection begins with fever and a sore, red, swollen throat. After a brief prodromal period, primary lesions erupt.

Examination of the mouth may reveal edema and small vesicles (blisters) on a red base. (See *Closer look at a vesicle.*) These vesicles eventually rupture, leaving a painful ulcer and then yellow crusting. Common sites for vesicles are the tongue, gingiva, and cheeks, but they may occur anywhere in or around the mouth.

In addition to characteristic vesicles, the patient may develop submaxillary lymphadenopathy, increased salivation, halitosis, and anorexia. The patient typically reports severe mouth pain.

A generalized infection typically lasts 4 to 10 days.

TYPE 2 INFECTION

With primary genital, or type 2, herpes simplex the patient usually complains first of tingling in the involved area, malaise, dysuria, dyspareunia (painful intercourse) and, in females, leukorrhea (white vaginal discharge containing mucus and pus cells). Next, localized, fluid-filled vesicles appear and may last for weeks.

In women, they occur on the cervix, labia, perianal skin, vulva, and vagina. In men, they develop on the glans penis, foreskin, and penile shaft. Lesions may also occur on the mouth or anus.

After rupture, vesicles become shallow, painful ulcers, red and edematous, with oozing, yellow centers. Inguinal swelling may also be present.

Test results

Confirmation of herpes simplex requires isolating the virus from local lesions and performing a tissue biopsy. In primary infection, an increase in antibodies and a moderate increase in the white blood cell (WBC) count support the diagnosis.

Treatment

A generalized primary herpes infection usually requires drugs to reduce fever and pain.

- ■ Acyclovir (Zovirax), the drug most commonly used to treat herpes, may reduce symptoms, viral shedding, and healing time. It's available in topical, oral, and I.V. forms.
- ■ Valacyclovir (Valtrex), docosanol (Abreva), or famciclovir (Famvir) may also be given.
- ■ Foscarnet (Foscavir) may be used in patients who have shown resistance to acyclovir.
- ■ For oral lesions, an anesthetic mouthwash, such as viscous lidocaine (Xylocaine Viscous), may help the patient eat and drink with less pain. (See *Herpes simplex teaching topics,* page 54.)

HERPES ZOSTER

Also called *shingles,* herpes zoster is an acute inflammation of dorsal root ganglia—nerve cell clusters found on the dorsal root of each spinal nerve. It occurs mainly in people older than age 50. The prognosis is good, and most patients recover completely unless the infection spreads to nerve roots that originate in the brain.

TEACHING FOCUS

Herpes simplex teaching topics

● Teach the patient how to apply topical drugs during a herpes outbreak. If the patient is taking a systemic drug, inform him of potential adverse effects and what to do if they occur.
● Teach the patient how to avoid infecting others. For example, tell a patient with a cold sore to avoid kissing others until the lesion is healed.
● Urge the patient with genital herpes to avoid sexual intercourse during the active disease stage before lesions completely heal, and to inform sexual partners of the condition.
● If the patient is pregnant, explain the risk of infecting the infant during vaginal delivery. Answer her questions about cesarean delivery if she has a herpes outbreak when labor begins and if her membranes haven't ruptured.

Pathophysiology

This disorder is caused by the same virus that causes chickenpox: herpesvirus varicella zoster. Shingles occurs when the varicella zoster virus reactivates after lying dormant in the cerebral ganglia or the ganglia of the posterior nerve roots. What triggers the reactivation is unknown.

Because the infection affects nerves at their roots, localized, vesicular lesions usually appear along an area of skin supplied by branches from a single nerve (called a dermatome). The patient may have severe pain in peripheral areas innervated by the inflamed nerve root. Chronic pain—called postherpetic neuralgia—is the most common persisting adverse effect.

RED FLAG Complications of generalized infection may involve acute urine retention and unilateral paralysis of the diaphragm. In postherpetic neuralgia (most common in elderly patients), intractable neurologic pain may persist for years, and scars may be permanent. Herpes zoster ophthalmicus, which involves the eyes, may cause vision loss.

Signs and symptoms

The first symptom of herpes zoster is pain along a dermatome. Patients also may have fever and malaise. After 2 to 4 days, severe intermittent or continuous deep pain may occur. Pruritus, paresthesia (unusual skin sensations such as prickling), or hyperesthesia (heightened skin sensitivity) in the trunk, arms, or legs may also occur as more nerves are affected.

After the pain starts, small, red, nodular lesions erupt on painful areas and spread unilaterally around the thorax or vertically over the arms or legs. When branches of the trigeminal nerve are involved, lesions appear on the face, in the mouth, or in the eyes. When the sensory branch of the facial nerve is involved, lesions appear in the ear canal and on the tongue.

The lesions change rapidly into pus- or fluid-filled vesicles, which may become infected or even gangrenous. Bacterial infection of the skin is usually caused by *Staphylococcus aureus* or *Streptococcus pyogenes,* and may result from scratching. About 10 to 21 days after the rash appears, the vesicles dry and form scabs.

Test results

Vesicular fluid analysis is used to diagnose herpes zoster. This test differentiates herpes zoster from localized herpes simplex.

Treatment

■ Primary treatment includes:
  – antipruritics, such as calamine lotion (Calamox), to relieve itching
  – analgesics, such as aspirin (Ecotrin), acetaminophen (Tylenol), codeine, or capsaicin (Zostrix), to relieve pain.
■ A systemic corticosteroid, such as cortisone (Cortone Acetate), may also be used to relieve pain and reduce inflammation.
■ Tincture of benzoin applied to unbroken lesions helps prevent a secondary infection.
■ If lesions rupture and become infected with bacteria, systemic antibiotics are given.
■ Other drug treatments may include tranquilizers, sedatives, and tricyclic antidepressants with phenothiazines.
■ Infection that affects the trigeminal nerve and cornea calls for idoxuridine ointment (Herplex Liquifilm) or another antiviral agent.
■ Acyclovir (Zovirax) may be prescribed for immunocompromised patients and those with infections of the ophthalmic branch of the trigeminal nerve. The drug stops the rash from spreading, reduces the duration of viral shedding and acute pain, and prevents visceral complications.
■ Valacyclovir (Valtrex) and famciclovir (Famvir) also are used for the treatment of most herpes infections.
■ If other pain relief measures fail, transcutaneous peripheral nerve stimulation, patient-controlled analgesia, or a small dose of radiotherapy may be effective. (See *Herpes zoster teaching topics,* page 56.)

TEACHING FOCUS

Herpes zoster teaching topics

- To decrease discomfort from oral lesions, tell the patient to use a soft toothbrush, eat soft foods, and use a saline- or bicarbonate-based mouthwash and oral anesthetics.
- Reassure the patient that herpes zoster isn't contagious (except to an immunocompromised patient), but stress the need for meticulous hygiene to prevent spreading infection to other body parts.
- Reassure the patient that herpetic pain eventually will subside. Suggest diversionary or relaxation activities to take his mind off the pain and pruritus.

INFECTIOUS MONONUCLEOSIS

An acute infectious disease, infectious mononucleosis mainly affects young adults and children, although it's usually so mild in children that it's commonly overlooked. It has three hallmarks:

- fever
- sore throat
- swollen cervical lymph nodes.

It's fairly common in the United States, Canada, and Europe, and both sexes are affected equally. About 90% of children older than age 4 have acquired antibodies.

Pathophysiology

Infectious mononucleosis is caused by the Epstein-Barr virus (EBV), a member of the herpesvirus group. Other types of mononucleosis are caused by cytomegalovirus and are benign and self-limiting.

The infection is spread mainly by the oropharyngeal route; however, transmission by blood transfusion and during cardiac surgery is also possible. The disease is contagious before symptoms develop and remains contagious until the fever subsides and oropharyngeal lesions disappear.

The disorder develops this way:

- The virus invades the B cells of the oropharyngeal lymphoid tissues and then replicates.
- As the B cells die, the virus is released into the blood, causing fever and other symptoms.
- During this period, antiviral antibodies appear and the virus disappears from the blood, lodging mainly in the parotid gland, one of the salivary glands. Because it reproduces in the parotid gland, the virus is present in saliva. (See *Glands affected by Epstein-Barr virus*.)

Glands affected by Epstein-Barr virus

These are the glands affected by mononucleosis – the Epstein-Barr virus.

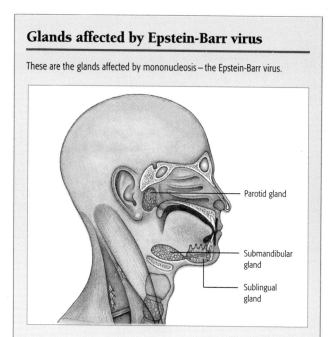

Parotid gland

Submandibular gland

Sublingual gland

The prognosis for patients with infectious mononucleosis is excellent. Major complications are rare but may include splenic rupture, aseptic meningitis, encephalitis, and pericarditis. The disorder also may cause liver dysfunction, increased numbers of lymphocytes and monocytes, and the development and persistence of heterophil antibodies.

Signs and symptoms

After an incubation period of about 10 days in children and 30 to 50 days in adults, the patient experiences headache, malaise, profound fatigue, anorexia, myalgia (muscle tenderness), and abdominal discomfort. Three to 5 days later, he develops an extremely sore throat and dysphagia (difficulty swallowing). Fever usually peaks in the late afternoon or evening, reaching 101° to 102° F (38.3° to 38.9° C).

Inspection of the pharynx reveals exudative tonsillitis and pharyngitis. The patient also may have petechiae on the palate, swollen eyes, a raised and red rash that resembles rubella, and jaun-

TEACHING FOCUS

Infectious mononucleosis teaching topics

- Explain that convalescence may take several weeks, usually until the patient's white blood cell count returns to normal.
- Stress the need for bed rest during acute illness. Warn the patient to avoid excessive activity, which could lead to splenic rupture.
- To minimize throat discomfort, urge the patient to drink milk shakes, fruit juices, and broths and to eat cool, bland foods. Advise using warm saline gargles, analgesics, and antipyretics, as needed.

dice. Cervical lymph nodes swell and are mildly tender when palpated. Inguinal and axillary nodes as well as the spleen and liver also may be swollen.

Test results

These diagnostic tests confirm infectious mononucleosis.

- Monospot test is positive for infectious mononucleosis.
- The WBC count is abnormally high (10,000 to 20,000/mm^3) during the second and third weeks of illness. From 50% to 70% of the total count consists of lymphocytes and monocytes, and 10% of the lymphocytes are atypical.
- Heterophil antibodies in serum drawn during the acute phase and at 3- to 4-week intervals increase to four times normal.
- Indirect immunofluorescence shows antibodies to EBV and cellular antigens. This test is usually more definitive than that for heterophil antibodies.

Treatment

Because mononucleosis is hard to prevent and resists standard antimicrobial treatment, therapy is mainly supportive. It includes:

- relief of symptoms
- bed rest during the acute febrile period
- acetaminophen (Tylenol) or ibuprofen (Motrin) for fever, headache, and sore throat.

Don't give aspirin (Ecotrin) to children because of its link to Reye's syndrome, a serious illness that can lead to death.

In cases of severe inflammation and airway obstruction, steroids can relieve swelling and prevent the need for a tracheotomy.

About 20% of patients also have a streptococcal infection and need antibiotic therapy for at least 10 days.

To avoid splenic rupture, the patient should avoid sports, physical activities, and exercise of any kind for 3 to 4 weeks after the onset of symptoms. (See *Infectious mononucleosis teaching topics*.)

LYME DISEASE

Lyme disease occurs chiefly in the United States and is named for the Connecticut town in which it was first recognized in 1975. It's the most commonly reported (and underreported) insect-borne disease in the United States.

It affects multiple body systems and usually appears in summer or early fall with a skin lesion called *erythema chronicum migrans*. Weeks or months later, cardiac, neurologic, or joint abnormalities may develop, sometimes followed by arthritis.

Pathophysiology

Lyme disease is caused by the spirochete *Borrelia burgdorferi*, which is carried by deer ticks. Here's how the disease develops:

■ The tick injects spirochete-laden saliva into the bloodstream or deposits fecal matter on the skin.
■ After incubating for 3 to 32 days, the spirochetes migrate outward, causing a rash.
■ Spirochetes disseminate to other skin sites or organs through the bloodstream or lymphatic system. They may survive for years in the joints, or they may die after triggering an inflammatory response in the host.

RED FLAG Symptoms of arthritis, including painful joint swelling and stiffness, are the most common complications of untreated disease. Meningitis, focal neurologic problems, and carditis are rare.

Signs and symptoms

Lyme disease occurs in three stages. Signs and symptoms may take years to fully develop.

STAGE 1

A red rash forms at the site of the tick bite — usually the axilla, thigh, or groin — and may expand to more than 20″ (51 cm) in diameter. The rash has a white center and a bright red outer rim, and it may itch, sting, or burn. It usually disappears within 1 month.

A few days after the initial rash forms, a migratory, ringlike rash may form, along with more rashes and conjunctivitis. In 3 to 4 weeks, the rashes fade to small red blotches, which persist for several more weeks.

The rash commonly is accompanied by fatigue, headache, chills, fever, sore throat, stiff neck, nausea, and muscle and joint pain. In children, body temperature may rise to 104° F (40° C) and be accompanied by chills.

At this stage, 10% of patients report such symptoms as palpitations and mild dyspnea. Severe headache and stiff neck, which suggest meningeal irritation, also may occur.

STAGE 2
Weeks to months later, patients who aren't treated may enter the second stage of the disease. Meningitis, cranial nerve palsies, and peripheral neuropathy may occur. With neurologic involvement, neck stiffness usually occurs only with extreme flexion. Fewer than 10% of patients have cardiac signs and symptoms.

STAGE 3
Half of patients who aren't treated progress to this final stage. Six weeks to several years after the tick bite, arthritis develops. Usually, only one or a few joints are affected, especially large ones, such as the knees. Recurrent attacks may lead to chronic arthritis with severe cartilage and bone erosion.

Test results
These tests are used to diagnose Lyme disease.
■ Blood tests may be used to identify *B. burgdorferi,* including:
  – antibody titers
  – enzyme-linked immunosorbent assay
  – Western blot assay.
■ Unfortunately, blood tests don't always confirm Lyme disease, especially in the early stages before the body produces antibodies or seropositivity for *B. burgdorferi.*
■ Mild anemia and elevated erythrocyte sedimentation rate, WBC count, serum immunoglobulin (Ig) M level, and aspartate aminotransferase level support the diagnosis.
■ Cerebrospinal fluid (CSF) analysis shows antibodies to *B. burgdorferi* if the disease has affected the central nervous system (CNS).

Treatment
■ Antibiotics can minimize complications if taken early in the disease.
■ A 3- to 4-week course of oral amoxicillin (Amoxil) or doxycycline (Vibramycin) is the treatment of choice for adults with Lyme disease.

TEACHING FOCUS

Lyme disease teaching topics

- Instruct the patient to take antibiotics as prescribed.
- Urge him to return for follow-up care and to report recurrent or new symptoms to the physician.
- Inform the patient, his family, and other caregivers about ways to prevent Lyme disease. Advise them to avoid tick-infested areas, if possible. If this isn't possible, suggest covering the skin with clothing, using insect repellents, inspecting exposed skin for attached ticks at least every 4 hours, and promptly removing ticks, if present.

- Cefuroxime (Ceftin) or erythromycin (E-Mycin) can be used for patients who are allergic to penicillin or who can't take tetracyclines.
- In later stages of the disease, particularly when neurologic symptoms are present, the patient may need treatment with I.V. ceftriaxone (Rocephin) or penicillin for 4 weeks or more.
- Analgesics and antipyretics reduce inflammation and fever. (See *Lyme disease teaching topics.*)

RABIES

An acute CNS infection, rabies is almost always fatal after symptoms develop. Immunization shortly after infection may prevent death.

Pathophysiology

Rabies is caused by the rabies virus, a rhabdovirus. It's transmitted through the skin or mucous membranes by the bite of an infected animal. Airborne droplets and infected tissue occasionally transmit the virus.

Increased domestic animal control and vaccination in the United States has reduced cases of rabies in humans. Consequently, most human rabies can be traced to dog bites that occurred in other countries or bites from wild animals such as raccoons. Here's how the disease progresses:

- The rabies virus begins replicating in the striated muscle cells at the bite site.
- The virus spreads along the nerve pathways to the spinal cord and brain, where it replicates again.
- The virus moves through the nerves into other tissues, including the salivary glands.
- The incubation period for the rabies virus is hours to weeks.

RED FLAG Untreated rabies can lead to life-threatening complications, including respiratory failure, peripheral vascular collapse, and central brain failure.

Signs and symptoms

Signs and symptoms of rabies begin appearing in 1 to 3 months in patients who don't receive immunization in time.

PRODROMAL SYMPTOMS

At first, the patient complains of local or radiating pain or burning and a sensation of cold, pruritus, and tingling at the bite site. He also may report malaise, headache, anorexia, nausea, sore throat, a persistent loose cough, nervousness, anxiety, irritability, hyperesthesia, sensitivity to light and loud noises, and excessive salivation, tearing, and perspiration. He may have a temperature of 100° to 102° F (37.8° to 38.9° C).

EXCITATION PHASE

About 2 to 10 days after prodromal signs and symptoms begin, the patient enters an excitation phase marked by intermittent hyperactivity, anxiety, apprehension, pupil dilation, shallow respirations, and an altered level of consciousness. Cranial nerve dysfunction may cause ocular palsies, strabismus (deviation of the eye), asymmetrical pupil dilation or constriction, absence of corneal reflexes, facial muscle weakness, and hoarseness. Temperature also rises to about 103° F (39.4° C).

HYDROPHOBIA

About 50% of patients have hydrophobia, which causes forceful, painful pharyngeal muscle spasms that expel fluids from the mouth, resulting in dehydration and, possibly, apnea, cyanosis, and death. Swallowing problems cause frothy drooling, and the sight, sound, or thought of water triggers uncontrollable pharyngeal muscle spasms and excessive salivation.

Nuchal rigidity (rigidity of the neck muscles) and seizures accompanied by cardiac arrhythmias or arrest may occur. Between excitatory and hydrophobic episodes, the patient usually remains cooperative and lucid. After about 3 days, these phases subside, and progressive paralysis leads to coma and death.

Test results

There are no diagnostic tests for rabies before its onset. Histologic examination of brain tissue from human rabies victims shows perivascular inflammation of the gray matter, degeneration of neurons, and characteristic minute bodies, called Negri bodies, in the nerve cells.

Treatment

The wound should immediately be washed with soap and water. Further wound care should be based on the extent of the injury. Postexposure prophylaxis is the most effective treatment. This regimen consists of:

■ one dose of immune globulin and five doses of rabies vaccine during a 28-day period
■ the first dose of vaccine given as soon as possible after exposure
■ additional doses given on days 3, 7, 14, and 28 days after the first vaccine.

There's no treatment for rabies after symptoms appear. If symptoms develop, isolate the patient and wear a gown, gloves, mask, and protective eyewear when handling saliva and articles contaminated with saliva. Take care to avoid being bitten or scratched by the patient during the excitation phase. Provide supportive care. (See *Rabies teaching topics*.)

RESPIRATORY SYNCYTIAL VIRUS INFECTION

Respiratory syncytial virus (RSV) infection occurs almost exclusively in infants and young children. In this group, it's the leading cause of lower respiratory tract infections, pneumonia, tracheobronchitis, bronchiolitis, otitis media, and fatal respiratory diseases.

RSV-related bronchiolitis peaks at age 2 months, making it the only viral disease that has its maximum impact during the first few months after birth. Antibody titers suggest that most children younger than age 4 have contracted some form of RSV infection, although it may be mild. School-age children, adolescents, and young adults with mild reinfections are probably the source of infection for infants and young children.

Pathophysiology

RSV infection is caused by an organism that belongs to a subgroup of a large group of viruses called myxoviruses. Here are the key facts about RSV pathophysiology:

- The organism is transmitted from person to person by respiratory secretions.
- It has an incubation period of 4 to 5 days.
- Bronchiolitis or pneumonia occurs and, in severe cases, may damage the bronchiolar epithelium.
- Interalveolar spaces may thicken, and alveolar spaces may fill with fluid.

 RED FLAG *Acute complications of RSV infection include apnea and respiratory failure.*

Signs and symptoms

Signs and symptoms vary in severity. They include:

- coughing
- dyspnea
- earache
- fever
- malaise
- nasal congestion
- sore throat
- wheezing.

Although uncommon, signs of CNS infection may arise as well, such as:

- weakness
- irritability
- nuchal rigidity.

Along with severe respiratory distress caused by increased mucus production, you may observe nasal flaring, retraction, cyanosis, and tachypnea. With a lower respiratory tract infection, you may auscultate wheezes, rhonchi, and crackles caused by interstitial lung edema and bronchial spasm. Reinfection is common and produces milder symptoms than the primary infection.

TEACHING FOCUS

Respiratory syncytial virus teaching topics

● Describe the ways that respiratory syncytial virus (RSV) infection is transmitted, and caution parents against taking infants into crowds during peak RSV months.
● Teach parents about drugs the child is taking and about adverse effects that should be reported.
● Teach the parents what signs and symptoms of serious complications to watch for and report.

Test results
These tests are used to diagnose RSV infection.
■ Cultures of nasal and pharyngeal secretions may reveal the virus; however, this infection is so labile that cultures aren't always reliable.
■ Serum antibody titers may be elevated, but in infants younger than age 6 months, the presence of maternal antibodies may nullify test results.

Treatment
Treatment aims to support respiratory function, maintain fluid balance, and relieve symptoms.

Ribavirin (Virazole), a broad-spectrum antiviral, is used in infants with severe lower respiratory tract infection. The drug is given in aerosol form by tent, oxygen hood, mask, or ventilator for 2 to 5 days, 12 to 18 hours daily. This therapy reduces the severity of symptoms and improves oxygen saturation.

Preventive therapy may be indicated. Palivizumab (Synagis) is given monthly by I.M. injection for 5 consecutive months during RSV season (November to April). Preventive therapy may be given to high-risk infants or children with congenital heart disease, chronic lung problems, cystic fibrosis, or a history of premature birth. (See *Respiratory syncytial virus teaching topics*.)

RUBELLA
Commonly called *German measles,* rubella is an acute, mildly contagious viral disease that produces a distinctive 3-day rash and enlarged lymph nodes. Worldwide in distribution, rubella flourishes

during the spring, particularly in cities, with epidemics occurring sporadically.

Rubella is most common in children ages 5 to 9, adolescents, and young adults. The disease is self-limiting, and the prognosis is excellent except in congenital rubella, which can cause serious birth defects.

Pathophysiology

The rubella virus is transmitted through contact with the blood, urine, stool, or nasopharyngeal secretions of an infected person. It's communicable from about 10 days before the rash appears until 5 days after.

The virus replicates first in the respiratory tract and then spreads through the bloodstream. It has been detected in blood as early as 8 days before and up to 2 days after the rash appears. Shedding of virus from the oropharynx persists for up to 8 days after the onset of symptoms.

In congenital rubella, the virus is transmitted through the placenta to the fetus by an infected mother. The fetus may have the virus in utero and for 6 to 31 months after birth.

RED FLAG Rubella can cause arthritis (transient and mainly in females), hemorrhagic problems (more common in children) and, less commonly, encephalitis, myocarditis, thrombocytopenia, and hepatitis.

Life-threatening complications of congenital rubella include growth retardation, infiltration of the liver and spleen by hematopoietic tissue (tissue that forms blood cells), interstitial pneumonia, a decreased number of megakaryocytes (giant cells in the bone marrow that produce mature blood platelets), and structural problems in the cardiovascular system and CNS.

Signs and symptoms

The patient's history may reveal inadequate immunization, exposure to someone with a recent rubella infection, or recent travel to an endemic area without reimmunization. Examination reveals a maculopapular, mildly itchy rash that usually begins on the face and then spreads rapidly, commonly covering the trunk and limbs within hours.

Small, red macules on the soft palate (Forschheimer spots) may precede or accompany the rash. By the end of the second day, the rash begins to fade in the opposite order in which it appeared. It usually disappears on the third day, but may persist for 4 or 5 days.

The rapid appearance and disappearance of the rubella rash distinguishes it from rubeola (measles).

A low-grade fever (99° to 101° F [37.2° to 38.3° C]) may occur, but it usually disappears after the first day of the rash. Rarely, a patient's temperature may reach 104° F (40° C).

Children usually don't have prodromal symptoms, but adolescents and adults may have a history of headache, malaise, anorexia, sore throat, and cough before the rash appeared. Palpation reveals suboccipital, postauricular, and postcervical lymph node enlargement, a hallmark sign.

Test results

Signs and symptoms usually are sufficient to make a diagnosis, so laboratory tests are seldom performed. However, these tests may be used:

■ Cell cultures of the throat, blood, urine, and CSF, along with convalescent serum that shows a fourfold rise in antibody titers, confirms the diagnosis.

■ Blood tests confirm rubella-specific IgM antibody. In congenital rubella, rubella-specific IgM antibody appears in umbilical cord blood.

Treatment

Treatment consists of antipyretics and analgesics for fever and joint pain. Bed rest isn't needed, but the patient should be isolated until the rash disappears. Because the rubella rash is self-limiting and only mildly pruritic, it doesn't require topical or systemic medication.

Only hospital workers not at risk for rubella should care for affected patients, and they should use isolation precautions until 5 days after the rash disappears. Infants with congenital rubella need to be isolated for 3 months, until three throat cultures are negative.

Be sure to report confirmed cases of rubella to local public health officials.

PRECAUTIONARY MEASURES

Immunization with the live rubella virus prevents the disease. The vaccine should be given along with measles and mumps vaccines at age 12 to 15 months, followed by a second dose at age 4 to 6 years.

Unimmunized adults can receive rubella vaccine (also along with measles and mumps vaccines) in two doses given 1 month apart if the adult was born after 1957. Immune globulin may be giv-

Rubella teaching topics

- Warn family members and visitors that rubella can be devastating to an un-born baby. Make sure that the patient understands how important it is to avoid exposing pregnant women to this disease.
- Warn women who receive the rubella vaccine to use an effective means of birth control for at least 3 months after immunization.

en I.M. or I.V. to staff and visitors who haven't been immunized. The vaccine is contraindicated in pregnancy, cancer, immunosuppression, and human immunodeficiency virus infection. (See *Rubella teaching topics.*)

Before giving the rubella vaccine:

- make sure that the patient isn't allergic to neomycin
- make sure that the patient isn't pregnant
- advise a woman of childbearing age to avoid pregnancy by using an effective birth control method for at least 3 months after receiving the vaccine.

SALMONELLOSIS

Every year, about 40,000 cases of salmonellosis are reported in the United States. Because many milder cases aren't diagnosed or reported, the actual number may be much greater. About 1,000 people die each year of acute salmonellosis.

Salmonellosis is more common in spring than in winter and tends to be more common in children. Young children, elderly people, and immunocompromised patients are the most likely to contract severe infections.

Salmonellosis occurs as enterocolitis, bacteremia (bacteria in the blood), localized infection, typhoid fever and, rarely, paratyphoid fever. Enterocolitis and bacteremia are especially common and virulent in infants, the elderly, and those already weakened by other infections, especially acquired immunodeficiency syndrome (AIDS).

Typhoid fever, the most severe form of salmonellosis, usually lasts 1 to 4 weeks. Most patients are younger than age 30, but most carriers are women older than age 50. Typhoid fever is on the rise in the United States because of increasing travel to endemic areas.

Pathophysiology

Salmonellosis is caused by gram-negative bacilli of the genus *Salmonella*, a member of the Enterobacteriaceae family. The most common species of *Salmonella* include:

■ *S. typhi*, which causes typhoid fever
■ *S. enteritidis*, which causes enterocolitis
■ *S. choleraesuis*, which causes bacteremia.

Many *Salmonella* bacteria can survive for weeks in water, ice, sewage, and food. Nontyphoidal salmonellosis usually follows ingestion of one of the following contaminated items:

■ dry milk
■ chocolate bars
■ pharmaceuticals of animal origin
■ contaminated or inadequately processed foods, especially eggs, chicken, turkey, and duck. Proper cooking reduces the risk but doesn't eliminate it.

The disease also may spread through contact with infected people or animals and, in young children, through fecal-oral spread. Typhoid fever usually results from drinking water contaminated by the excretions of a carrier.

Typhoid fever progresses this way:

■ After contaminated food is ingested, the bacteria pass the gastric barrier and invade the upper small bowel, causing a transient bacteremia that produces no symptoms.
■ The bacteria are ingested by mononuclear phagocytes and must survive and multiply within them to cause illness.

The mortality rate caused by typhoid fever is about 3% in people who are treated and 10% in those who aren't treated. An attack of typhoid fever confers lifelong immunity.

RED FLAG Salmonellosis may cause such complications as intestinal perforation or hemorrhage, cerebral thrombosis, pneumonia, endocarditis, myocarditis, meningitis, pyelonephritis, osteomyelitis, cholecystitis, hepatitis, septicemia, and acute circulatory failure.

Signs and symptoms

Nontyphoidal forms of salmonellosis usually produce mild to moderate illness, with low mortality. All infections resulting from *Salmonella* bacteria other than *S. typhi* can cause acute diarrhea, septicemic syndrome, focal abscesses, meningitis, osteomyelitis, endocarditis, or mycotic aneurysm (an aneurysm infected by a fungus).

Persistent bacteremia kicks off the clinical phase of infection. The bacteria continue to multiply in the cells and, when the number passes a critical threshold, secondary bacteremia occurs, resulting in invasion of the gallbladder and intestine. Sustained bacteremia causes a persistent fever.

Inflammatory responses to tissue invasion result in cholecystitis, intestinal hemorrhage, or perforation.

Test results
These tests are used to diagnose salmonellosis.
■ Blood cultures isolate the organism in typhoid fever, paratyphoid fever, and bacteremia.
■ Stool cultures isolate the organism in typhoid fever, paratyphoid fever, and enterocolitis.
■ Cultures of urine, bone marrow, pus, and vomitus may show the presence of *Salmonella* organisms.
■ In endemic areas, symptoms of enterocolitis allow a working diagnosis before the cultures are positive. *S. typhi* in stools 1 or more years after treatment indicates that the patient is a carrier (about 3% of patients).

Treatment
■ Drugs used to treat typhoid fever, paratyphoid fever, and bacteremia include:
  - ampicillin
  - amoxicillin (Amoxil)
  - chloramphenicol (Chloromycetin)
  - ciprofloxacin (Cipro)
  - ceftriaxone (Rocephin)
  - cefotaxime (Claforan)
  - co-trimoxazole (Bactrim) for extremely toxemic patients.
■ Localized abscesses may need surgical drainage.
■ To relieve diarrhea and control cramps, patients may try:
  - camphorated opium tincture
  - kaolin and pectin mixtures
  - diphenoxylate and atropine (Lomotil)
  - codeine
  - small doses of morphine.
■ When caring for a patient with salmonellosis, wear gloves and a gown when disposing of feces-contaminated materials, and wash your hands thoroughly after contact with the patient. Continue enteric precautions until three consecutive stool cultures are negative after antibiotic treatment.

Salmonellosis teaching topics

● Advise the patient's close contacts to obtain a medical examination and treatment if cultures are positive.
● Teach the patient and his family measures to prevent salmonellosis, including:
– washing hands after using the bathroom and before eating
– cooking foods thoroughly (especially eggs and chicken)
– refrigerating foods promptly
– cleaning food preparation surfaces with hot, soapy water
– drying food preparation surfaces thoroughly after use.

■ Report all salmonellosis cases to public health officials. (See *Salmonellosis teaching topics*.)

TOXOPLASMOSIS

Seventy percent of people in the United States are infected with *Toxoplasma gondii*. Although it usually causes a localized infection, it may produce a generalized infection in:
■ neonates
■ patients with AIDS or lymphoma
■ patients who have undergone recent organ transplants
■ those on immunosuppressive therapy.

Congenital toxoplasmosis, characterized by CNS lesions, may cause stillbirth or serious birth defects. It's transmitted transplacentally from a mother who acquires primary toxoplasmosis shortly before or during pregnancy. The infection is more severe when it's acquired early in pregnancy.

Pathophysiology

Toxoplasmosis is caused by the intracellular parasite *T. gondii*, which affects birds and mammals. It's transmitted to humans by ingestion of tissue cysts in raw or undercooked meat or by fecal-oral contamination from infected cats. An infected cat may excrete as many as 100 million parasites per day, and a single cyst can cause infection.

Direct transmission can also occur during blood transfusions or organ transplants. The disease also occurs in people who don't eat meat and aren't exposed to cats, so an unknown means of transmission exists.

Here's how the infection develops:

■ When tissue cysts are ingested, parasites are released, which quickly invade and multiply in the GI tract.
■ The parasitic cells rupture the invaded host cell and then disseminate to the CNS, lymphatic tissue, skeletal muscle, myocardium, retina, and placenta.
■ As the parasites replicate and invade adjoining cells, cell death and focal necrosis occur, surrounded by an acute inflammatory response — the hallmarks of this infection.
■ After the cysts mature, the inflammatory process becomes undetectable, and cysts remain latent in the brain until they rupture.

RED FLAG In the normal host, the immune response checks the infection, but this isn't what happens in immunocompromised or fetal hosts. In these patients, focal destruction results in necrotizing encephalitis, pneumonia, myocarditis, and organ failure.

Signs and symptoms
■ Mild, localized toxoplasmosis may cause malaise, myalgia, headache, fatigue, sore throat, and fever.
■ A patient with fulminating, generalized infection may have:
– headache
– vomiting
– cough
– dyspnea
– temperature as high as 106° F (41.1° C)
– delirium
– seizures (signs of encephalitis)
– a maculopapular rash (except on the palms, soles, and scalp)
– cyanosis.
■ An infant with congenital toxoplasmosis may have hydrocephalus or microcephalus, seizures, jaundice, purpura, and rash.
■ Other defects, which may not be apparent until months or years later, include strabismus, blindness, epilepsy, and mental retardation.
■ Once infected with toxoplasmosis, the patient may carry the organism for life. Reactivation of the acute infection is possible.

Test results
■ Testing blood for a specific toxoplasma antibody is the main way to detect active infection.
■ Another test, which isolates *T. gondii* in mice after their inoculation with human body fluids, reveals antibodies for the disease and confirms toxoplasmosis.

TEACHING FOCUS

Toxoplasmosis teaching topics

- Teach the patient about needed drugs and their adverse effects. Stress the importance of regularly scheduled follow-up care.
- Advise all people to do the following to prevent the spread of toxoplasmosis:
- Wash their hands after working with soil because it may be contaminated with cat oocysts.
- Cook meat thoroughly and freeze it promptly if it isn't for immediate use.
- Change cat litter daily (cat oocysts don't become infective until 1 to 4 days after excretion).
- Cover children's sandboxes.
- Keep flies away from food because flies transport oocysts.

Treatment

- Most effective during the acute stage, treatment for toxoplasmosis consists of drug therapy with a sulfonamide and pyrimethamine (Daraprim) for 4 to 6 weeks.
- The patient also may receive folic acid (Folvite) to counteract the drugs' adverse effects, such as anemia and bone marrow toxicity.
- Unfortunately, these drugs don't eliminate cysts that already exist. Therefore, patients with AIDS need toxoplasmosis treatment for life.
- An AIDS patient who can't tolerate sulfonamides may receive clindamycin (Cleocin) instead. This drug is also the primary treatment in ocular toxoplasmosis. (See *Toxoplasmosis teaching topics.*)
- Report all cases of toxoplasmosis to the local public health department.

4

IMMUNE SYSTEM

The body protects itself from infectious organisms and other harmful invaders through a network of safeguards called the host defense system. This system has three lines of defense:
- physical and chemical barriers to infection
- the inflammatory response
- the immune response.

Physical barriers, such as skin and mucous membranes, prevent most organisms from invading the body. Organisms that penetrate this first barrier trigger the inflammatory and immune responses, both of which involve stem cells in bone marrow that develop into blood cells.

Structures of the immune system

Four structures make up the immune system:
- lymph nodes
- thymus
- spleen
- tonsils.

LYMPH NODES
Lymph nodes are distributed along lymphatic vessels throughout the body. They filter lymphatic fluid, which drains from body tissues and later returns to the blood as plasma. They also remove bacteria and toxins from the circulatory system. On occasion, an infectious agent is spread via the lymphatic system.

THYMUS
The thymus is located in the mediastinal area between the lungs. It secretes a group of hormones that allow lymphocytes to develop into mature T cells. T cells attack foreign or abnormal cells and regulate cell-mediated immunity.

SPLEEN
The largest lymphatic organ, the spleen functions as a reservoir for blood. Cells in the splenic tissue, called macrophages, clear cellular debris and process hemoglobin.

TONSILS
The tonsils are made of lymphoid tissue; they produce lymphocytes. The location of the tonsils allows them to guard the body against airborne and ingested pathogens.

Types of immunity

Certain cells have a quality known as immunocompetence; they can distinguish between foreign matter and what belongs to the body. When foreign substances invade the body, two types of immune responses are possible, including:
■ cell-mediated immunity
■ humoral immunity.

CELL-MEDIATED IMMUNITY
In cell-mediated immunity, T cells respond directly to antigens (foreign substances, such as bacteria or toxins that induce antibody formation). Examples of cell-mediated immunity are rejection of transplanted organs and delayed immune responses that fight disease. Target cells — such as virus-infected cells and cancer cells — are destroyed by secretion of lymphokines (lymph proteins).

Among white blood cells (WBCs), 36% are T cells. They probably originate from stem cells in the bone marrow; the thymus gland controls their maturity. In the process, a large number of antigen-specific cells are produced.

T cells may be killer, helper, or suppressor T cells.
■ Killer cells bind to the surface of the invading cell, disrupt the membrane, and destroy it by altering its internal environment.
■ Helper cells stimulate B cells to mature into plasma cells, which produce immunoglobulin (Ig), which are proteins with antibody activity.
■ Suppressor cells reduce the humoral response.

HUMORAL IMMUNITY
In humoral (or Ig-mediated) immunity, B cells recognize and destroy antigens using a mechanism different from that of T cells. B cells originate in bone marrow and mature into plasma cells that produce antibodies (Ig molecules that interact with a specific anti-

gen). The antibodies destroy bacteria and viruses, thereby preventing them from entering host cells.

Immunoglobulins

There are five major Ig classes: IgG, IgM, IgA, IgD, and IgE.

- IgG makes up about 80% of plasma antibodies. It appears in all body fluids and has major antibacterial and antiviral activity.
- IgM is the first Ig produced during an immune response. It's too large to easily cross membrane barriers and usually is present only in the vascular system.
- IgA is found mainly in body secretions, such as saliva, sweat, tears, mucus, bile, and colostrum. It defends against pathogens on body surfaces, especially those that enter the respiratory and GI tracts.
- IgD is present in plasma and is easily broken down. It's the main antibody on the surface of B cells and is mainly an antigen receptor.
- IgE is involved in immediate hypersensitivity reactions (allergic reactions that develop within minutes of exposure to an antigen). It stimulates release of mast cell granules, which contain histamine and heparin.

Complement system

Another part of humoral immunity is the complement system, which is a major mediator of the inflammatory response. It's activated (a process known as the complement cascade) by an antigen-antibody reaction and involves 30 proteins circulating as functionally inactive molecules. It mediates inflammation through increased vascular permeability, chemotaxis (movement of additional WBCs to an area of inflammation), phagocytosis (engulfing of foreign particles by cells called phagocytes), and lysis of foreign cells.

Immune disorders

Disorders of the immune response are of three main types, including:

- immunodeficiency disorders
- hypersensitivity disorders
- autoimmune disorders.

Immunodeficiency disorders result from an absent or depressed immune system and include human immunodeficiency virus (HIV) disease, DiGeorges syndrome, chronic fatigue syndrome, and immune dysfunction syndrome.

Hypersensitivity disorders, which may be immediate or delayed, occur when an allergen (a substance the person is allergic to) enters the body. They're classified as:

■ type I (immunoglobulin [Ig] E-mediated allergic reactions)
■ type II (cytotoxic reactions)
■ type III (immune complex reactions)
■ type IV (cell-mediated reactions).

Autoimmune disorders involve an immunologic response launched by the body against itself. The immune response leads to a sequence of tissue reactions and damage that may produce diffuse systemic signs and symptoms. Examples of autoimmune disorders include rheumatoid arthritis, lupus erythematosus, dermatomyositis, and vasculitis.

Common immune disorders discussed in the rest of the chapter include:

■ allergic rhinitis
■ anaphylaxis
■ HIV infection
■ lupus erythematosus
■ rheumatoid arthritis.

ALLERGIC RHINITIS

Inhaled, airborne allergens may trigger an immune response in the upper airway. This causes two problems:

■ rhinitis, or inflammation of the nasal mucous membrane
■ conjunctivitis, or inflammation of the membrane lining the eyelids and covering the eyeball.

When allergic rhinitis occurs seasonally (spring, summer, and fall), it's called hay fever, even though hay doesn't cause it and no fever occurs. When it occurs year-round, it's called perennial allergic rhinitis.

More than 20 million Americans have allergic rhinitis, making it the most common allergic reaction. Although it can affect anyone at any age, it's most common in young children and adolescents.

Pathophysiology

Allergic rhinitis is a type I, IgE-mediated hypersensitivity response to an environmental allergen in a genetically susceptible person. The seasonal disorder typically results from airborne pollens produced by trees, grass, and weeds. In summer and fall, mold spores may cause it. Major perennial allergens and irritants include house dust and dust mites, feathers, molds, fungi, tobacco smoke, processed materials, industrial chemicals, and animal dander.

Traits of rhinitis

Characteristics of three common disorders of the nasal mucosa are listed here.

CHRONIC VASOMOTOR RHINITIS
● Eyes aren't affected.
● Nasal discharge contains mucus.
● There's no seasonal variation.

INFECTIOUS RHINITIS (COMMON COLD)
● Nasal mucosa is beet red.
● Nasal secretions contain exudate.
● Fever and sore throat occur.

RHINITIS MEDICAMENTOSA
● Disorder is caused by excessive use of nasal sprays or drops.
● Nasal drainage and mucosal redness and swelling subside when the medication is stopped.

RED FLAG Swelling of the nasal and mucous membranes may trigger secondary sinus infections and middle ear infections, especially in perennial allergic rhinitis. Nasal polyps caused by edema and infection may increase nasal obstruction. Bronchitis and pneumonia are also possible complications.

Signs and symptoms

Signs and symptoms vary in severity from year to year and may differ if rhinitis isn't related to allergy. (See *Traits of rhinitis*.) Many patients with allergic rhinitis have dark circles under the eyes (commonly called allergic shiners) from venous congestion in the maxillary sinuses.

HAY FEVER

People with seasonal allergic rhinitis may have signs and symptoms such as these:
■ sneezing attacks
■ rhinorrhea (profuse, watery nasal discharge)
■ nasal obstruction or congestion
■ itching nose and eyes
■ headache or sinus pain
■ itchy throat and malaise.

Allergic rhinitis teaching topics

- Urge the patient to reduce exposure to airborne allergens by:
  - sleeping with the windows closed
  - avoiding the countryside during pollination season
  - using air conditioning and air filtration systems, if possible, to filter allergens and minimize humidity and dust
  - keeping pets outside
  - removing dust-collecting items, such as wool blankets, deep-pile carpets, and heavy draperies, from the home.
- In severe and resistant allergic rhinitis, discuss possible lifestyle changes, such as relocation to a pollen-free area either seasonally or year-round.
- Review drug treatment, teaching proper dosages, administration, and adverse effects.

PERENNIAL ALLERGIC RHINITIS

People with perennial allergic rhinitis may have signs and symptoms such as these:

■ chronic, extensive, nasal obstruction or stuffiness, which can obstruct the eustachian tubes, especially in children

■ conjunctivitis or other extranasal signs and symptoms (rare).

Test results

■ IgE levels may be normal or elevated.

■ Microscopic examination of sputum and nasal secretions shows a high number of eosinophils (granular leukocytes). Although eosinophil activity isn't completely understood, we know that they destroy parasitic organisms and play a role in allergic reactions.

Treatment

Treatment of allergic rhinitis involves:

■ controlling signs and symptoms

■ preventing infection

■ possibly removing the environmental allergen. (See *Allergic rhinitis teaching topics.*)

Nonsedating antihistamines have fewer annoying effects than standard antihistamines and are the treatment of choice. They include:

■ loratadine (Claritin)

- desloratadine (Clarinex)
- fexofenadine (Allegra)
- cetirizine (Zyrtec).

Antihistamines are effective in stopping a runny nose and watery eyes, although they usually produce sedation, dry mouth, nausea, dizziness, blurred vision, and nervousness. Examples of antihistamines include:

- chlorpheniramine (Chlor-Trimeton)
- diphenhydramine (Benadryl)
- promethazine (Phenergan).

Topical intranasal corticosteroids may reduce local inflammation and have minimal systemic adverse effects. Cromolyn sodium (Nasalcrom) is a mast cell stabilizer that may help prevent allergic rhinitis, although it takes 4 weeks to produce a satisfactory effect and must be taken regularly during allergy season.

Immunotherapy or desensitization may be attempted with injections of allergen extracts. They may be given preseasonally, seasonally, or yearly.

ANAPHYLAXIS
Anaphylaxis is an acute type I allergic reaction that causes sudden, rapidly progressive urticaria (hives) and respiratory distress. If severe, anaphylaxis may cause vascular collapse, systemic shock, and death.

Pathophysiology
Anaphylactic reactions result from systemic exposure to sensitizing drugs or other antigens, including:

- serums, such as vaccines
- allergen extracts, such as pollen
- enzymes, such as L-asparaginase
- hormones
- penicillin (the most common cause of anaphylaxis, affecting 4 of every 10,000 patients) and other antibiotics
- local anesthetics
- salicylates
- polysaccharides, such as iron dextran (DexFerrum)
- diagnostic chemicals, such as radiographic contrast media
- foods, such as nuts and seafood
- sulfite-containing food additives
- insect venom, such as that of honeybees, wasps, and certain spiders
- ruptured hydatid cyst (rare).

Reactions typically follow this course. During the first exposure to an antigen, the immune system responds by producing IgE antibodies in the lymph nodes. Helper T cells enhance the process. Antibodies bind to membrane receptors on mast cells in connective tissue and on basophils, a type of leukocyte. If the person is reexposed to the antigen, it binds to adjacent IgE antibodies or cross-linked IgE receptors, activating inflammatory reactions, such as the release of histamine.

RED FLAG Untreated, anaphylaxis causes respiratory obstruction, systemic vascular collapse, and death within hours or even minutes. A delayed or persistent reaction may last up to 24 hours. (See Understanding anaphylaxis, *page 82.)*

Signs and symptoms

Immediately after exposure to an allergen, the patient may report a feeling of impending doom or fright, progressing to a fear of impending death. He also may develop weakness, sweating, sneezing, dyspnea, nasal pruritus, and urticaria. His skin may look cyanotic and pallid. Well-circumscribed, discrete, cutaneous wheals with red, raised wavy or indented borders and blanched centers usually appear and may merge to form giant hives.

The patient may have early signs of potentially fatal respiratory failure. Angioedema may cause the patient to complain of a lump in his throat. Swelling of tongue and larynx also occur. You may hear hoarseness, stridor, or wheezing. Chest tightness signals bronchial obstruction.

The patient may report severe stomach cramps, nausea, diarrhea, urinary urgency, and urinary incontinence.

Cardiovascular effects of anaphylaxis include hypotension, shock, and cardiac arrhythmias, which may precipitate vascular collapse if untreated.

Neurologic signs and symptoms may include dizziness, drowsiness, headache, restlessness, and seizures.

Test results

Diagnosis is based on the patient's history and signs and symptoms. No tests are needed.

Treatment

Anaphylaxis requires emergency treatment. Establish and maintain a patent airway, and watch for early signs of laryngeal edema, such as:
■ stridor
■ hoarseness

Understanding anaphylaxis

This flowchart outlines the sequence of events that occur during anaphylaxis.

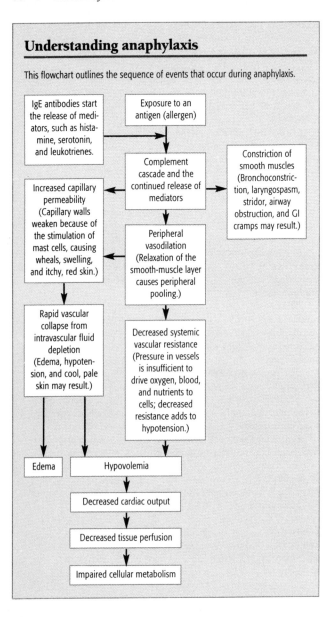

TEACHING FOCUS

Anaphylaxis teaching topics

● After an acute anaphylactic reaction has been controlled, counsel the patient about the risk of delayed symptoms and the need to immediately report any recurrence of shortness of breath, chest tightness, sweating, angioedema, or other symptoms.
● Teach the patient to avoid exposure to known allergens. If he has a food or drug allergy, urge him not to consume the offending food or drug in any of its combinations or forms. If he's allergic to insect stings, he should avoid open fields and wooded areas during the insect season.
● Advise the patient to carry an anaphylaxis kit whenever he's outdoors. Urge him to familiarize himself with the kit and how to use it before the need arises.
● Tell the patient to wear a medical identification bracelet indicating his allergies.

■ dyspnea.

If these occur, the patient will need oxygen and an endotracheal tube or a tracheotomy

Early in anaphylaxis, when the patient is conscious and normotensive, give an immediate injection of epinephrine 1:1,000 aqueous solution (Adrenalin), 0.1 to 0.5 ml, subcutaneously or I.M. Massage the injection site to speed the drug into circulation.

In severe reactions, when the patient is unconscious and hypotensive, give epinephrine 0.1 to 0.25 mg (1 to 2.5 ml of a 1:10,000 solution) I.V. slowly over 5 to 10 minutes. Repeat the dose every 5 to 15 minutes if needed, or follow with an infusion at 1 to 4 mcg/minute. I.V. fluids are needed to prevent vascular collapse after a severe reaction is treated.

Diphenhydramine (Benadryl) may be given I.M. or I.V. for allergic signs and symptoms.

Aminophylline helps relieve bronchospasm. (See *Anaphylaxis teaching topics*.)

HIV DISEASE

Human immunodeficiency virus (HIV) is the infectious agent that causes HIV disease, an immune system disorder that affects up to 950,000 U.S. residents, up to one-fourth of whom don't know they're infected. HIV disease is characterized by progressive immune system impairment and destruction of T cells and the cell-mediated response. It causes immunodeficiency that increases susceptibility to infections and unusual cancers.

The Centers for Disease Control and Prevention (CDC) has set criteria for HIV disease diagnosis. (See *HIV infection classification.*) Although the course of the disease may vary, virtually everyone infected with HIV eventually develops acquired immunodeficiency syndrome (AIDS), which usually results in death from opportunistic infections.

In the United States, the rate of AIDS cases is growing most rapidly among minority populations. For example, AIDS is the leading killer of Black males ages 25 to 44. The CDC estimates that AIDS affects nearly seven times more Blacks and three times more Hispanics than Whites.

Pathophysiology

HIV is an RNA-based retrovirus that requires a human host to replicate. The average time between HIV infection and the development of AIDS is 8 to 10 years.

HIV destroys CD4+ cells — also known as helper T cells — that regulate the normal immune response. The CD4+ antigen serves as a receptor for HIV and allows it to invade the cell. Afterward, virus replicates in the CD4+ cell, causing cell death.

HIV can infect almost any cell that has the CD4+ antigen on its surface, including:

■ monocytes
■ macrophages
■ bone marrow progenitors
■ glial cells
■ gut cells
■ epithelial cells.

RED FLAG HIV infection can cause dementia, wasting syndrome, and blood abnormalities. It also can lead to repeated opportunistic infections. (See Opportunistic diseases in AIDS, *pages 86 to 95.)*

HIV is transmitted three ways, including:

■ contact with infected blood or blood products or by sharing a contaminated needle or during transfusion or tissue transplantation (although routine testing of the blood supply since 1985 has cut the risk of contracting HIV this way)
■ contact with infected body fluids, such as semen and vaginal fluids, during unprotected sex (anal intercourse is especially dangerous because it causes mucosal trauma)

HIV infection classification

The Centers for Disease Control and Prevention's revised classification system for human immunodeficiency virus (HIV)–infected adolescents and adults categorizes patients according to three ranges of CD4+ cell counts and three clinical conditions associated with HIV infection.

The classification system identifies where the patient lies in the progression of the disease and helps to guide treatment.

RANGES OF CD4+ T LYMPHOCYTES
● *Category 1:* CD4+ cell count 500 or greater
● *Category 2:* CD4+ cell count 200 to 499
● *Category 3:* CD4+ cell count less than 200

CLINICAL CATEGORIES
● *Category A* (conditions present in patients with documented HIV infection): asymptomatic HIV infection persistent, generalized lymph node enlargement or acute (primary) HIV infection with accompanying illness or history of acute HIV infection
● *Category B* (conditions present in patients with symptomatic HIV infection): bacillary angiomatosis, oropharyngeal or persistent vulvovaginal candidiasis, fever or diarrhea lasting over 1 month, idiopathic thrombocytopenic purpura, pelvic inflammatory disease (especially with a tubo-ovarian abscess), and peripheral neuropathy
● *Category C* (conditions present in patients with acquired immunodeficiency syndrome): candidiasis of the bronchi, trachea, lungs, or esophagus; invasive cervical cancer; disseminated or extrapulmonary coccidioidomycosis; extrapulmonary cryptococcosis; chronic intestinal cryptosporidiosis; cytomegalovirus (CMV) disease affecting organs other than the liver, spleen, or lymph nodes; CMV retinitis with vision loss; encephalopathy related to HIV; herpes simplex involving chronic ulcers or herpetic bronchitis, pneumonitis, or esophagitis; disseminated or extrapulmonary histoplasmosis; chronic, intestinal isosporiasis; Kaposi's sarcoma; Burkitt's lymphoma or its equivalent; immunoblastic lymphoma or its equivalent; primary brain lymphoma; disseminated or extrapulmonary *Mycobacterium avium* complex or *M. kansasii;* pulmonary or extrapulmonary *M. tuberculosis;* any other species of *Mycobacterium* (disseminated or extrapulmonary); *Pneumocystis carinii* pneumonia; recurrent pneumonia; progressive multifocal leukoencephalopathy; recurrent *Salmonella* septicemia; toxoplasmosis of the brain; wasting syndrome caused by HIV.

■ crossing the placental barrier from an infected mother to a fetus, or from an infected mother to an infant either through cervical or blood contact at delivery or through breast milk.

(Text continues on page 94.)

Opportunistic diseases in AIDS

This table describes some common diseases that occur with acquired immuno-deficiency syndrome (AIDS), their characteristic signs and symptoms, and their treatments.

DISEASE

BACTERIAL INFECTIONS

TUBERCULOSIS
A disease caused by *Mycobacterium tuberculosis*, an aerobic, acid-fast bacillus spread by inhaling droplet nuclei that are aerosolized by coughing, sneezing, or talking

MYCOBACTERIUM AVIUM COMPLEX
A primary infection acquired by oral ingestion or inhalation; may infect the bone marrow, liver, spleen, GI tract, lymph nodes, lungs, skin, brain, adrenal glands, and kidneys; is chronic and may be localized and disseminated in its course of infection; is becoming less common because of changes in treatment of human immunodeficiency virus (HIV)

SALMONELLOSIS
A disease acquired by ingestion of food or water contaminated by *Salmonella* but also linked to snake powders, pet turtles, and domestic turkeys; also can be spread by contaminated medications or diagnostic agents, direct fecal-oral transmission (especially during sexual activity), transfusion of contaminated blood products, and inadequately sterilized fiber-optic instruments used in upper GI endoscopic procedures

FUNGAL INFECTIONS

COCCIDIOIDOMYCOSIS
An infectious disease caused by the fungus *Coccidioides immitis*, which grows in soil in arid regions in the southwestern United States, Mexico, Central America, and South America

SIGNS AND SYMPTOMS	TREATMENT
Fever, weight loss, night sweats, and fatigue, followed by dyspnea, chills, hemoptysis, and chest pain	Isoniazid (Laniazid), rifampin (Rifadin), and ethambutol (Myambutol) or streptomycin are given during the first 2 months of therapy, followed by rifampin and isoniazid for at least 9 months and at least 6 months after culture is negative for bacteria.
Multiple, nonspecific symptoms consistent with systemic illness: fever, fatigue, weight loss, anorexia, night sweats, abdominal pain, and chronic diarrhea; *physical examination findings:* emaciation, generalized lymphadenopathy, diffuse tenderness, jaundice, and hepato-splenomegaly; *laboratory findings:* anemia, leukopenia, and thrombocytopenia	Treatment includes clarithromycin (Biaxin) or azithromycin (Zithromax) and ethambutol. These drugs are given with one or more of the following: amikacin (Amikin), ciprofloxacin (Cipro), rifabutin (Mycobutin), or rifampin.
Nonspecific signs and symptoms, including fever, chills, sweats, weight loss, diarrhea, and anorexia	Although treatment of nontyphoid salmonellosis usually isn't needed by immunocompetent people, it's required in those with HIV. Antibiotic selection depends on drug sensitivities. However, treatment may include co-trimoxazole (Bactrim), amoxicillin (Amoxil), fluoroquinolones, ampicillin (Omnipen), or third-generation cephalosporins.
Flulike illness (malaise, fever, backache, headache, cough, arthralgia), periarticular swelling in knees and ankles, meningitis, bony lesions, skin findings, and pulmonary or genitourinary involvement	Fluconazole (Diflucan), itraconazole (Sporanox), or amphotericin B (Amphocin) is given.

(continued)

Opportunistic diseases in AIDS *(continued)*

DISEASE

FUNGAL INFECTIONS *(continued)*

CANDIDIASIS

A disease caused by the fungus *Candida albicans* that exists on teeth, gingivae, and skin and in the oropharynx, vagina, and large intestine; most infections are endogenous and related to interruption of normal defense mechanisms; possible human-to-human transmission, including congenital transmission in neonates, in whom thrush develops after vaginal delivery

CRYPTOCOCCOSIS

An infectious disease caused by the fungus *Cryptococcus neoformans;* can be found in nature; can be aerosolized and inhaled; settles in the lungs, where it can remain dormant or spread to other parts of the body, particularly the central nervous system (CNS); responsible for three forms of infection: pulmonary, CNS, and disseminated; most pulmonary cases found serendipitously

HISTOPLASMOSIS

A disease caused by the fungus *Histoplasma capsulatum* that exists in nature, is readily airborne, and can reach the bronchioles and alveoli when inhaled

SIGNS AND SYMPTOMS	TREATMENT
Thrush (the most prevalent form in HIV-infected people): creamy, curdlike, white patches, surrounded by an erythematous base, found on any oral mucosal surface; *nail infection:* inflammation and tenderness of tissue surrounding the nails or the nail itself; *vaginitis:* intense pruritus of the vulva and curdlike vaginal discharge	Nystatin suspension (Mycostatin) and clotrimazole troches (Mycelex) are given for thrush; nystatin suspension or pastilles, clotrimazole troches, fluconazole, or itraconazole for esophagitis; topical clotrimazole, miconazole (Micatin), or ketoconazole (Nizoral) for cutaneous candidiasis; oral fluconazole, ketoconazole, or both for candidiasis of nails; and topical clotrimazole, miconazole, or oral fluconazole for vaginitis.
Pulmonary cryptococcosis: fever, cough, dyspnea, and pleuritic chest pain; *CNS cryptococcosis:* fever, malaise, headaches, stiff neck, nausea and vomiting, and altered mentation; *disseminated cryptococcosis:* lymphadenopathy, multifocal cutaneous lesions; *other symptoms:* macules, papules, skin lesions, oral lesions, placental infection, myocarditis, prostatic infection, optic neuropathy, rectal abscess, and lymph node infection	Primary therapy for initial infection is amphotericin B given I.V. for 6 to 8 weeks; sometimes amphotericin B and flucytosine (Ancobon) are used together. Fluconazole and itraconazole are also used. After initial treatment, the patient is typically maintained on lifelong fluconazole therapy.
Most common: fever, weight loss, hepatomegaly, splenomegaly, and pancytopenia; *less common:* diarrhea, cerebritis, chorioretinitis, meningitis, oral and cutaneous lesions, and GI mucosal lesions causing bleeding	Drug of choice is amphotericin B for acute treatment of illness and then for lifelong suppressive therapy. Itraconazole is also used.

(continued)

Opportunistic diseases in AIDS *(continued)*

DISEASE

PROTOZOAN INFECTIONS

PNEUMOCYSTIS CARINII PNEUMONIA
Pneumonia caused by *P. carinii;* also has properties of fungal infection, exists in human lungs, and is transmitted by airborne exposure; the most common life-threatening opportunistic infection in those with AIDS

CRYPTOSPORIDIOSIS
An intestinal infection by the protozoan *Cryptosporidium;* transmitted by person-to-person contact, water, food contaminants, and airborne exposure; most common site: small intestine

TOXOPLASMOSIS
A disease caused by *Toxoplasma gondii;* major means of transmission through ingestion of undercooked meats and vegetables containing oocysts; causes focal or diffuse meningoencephalitis with cellular necrosis and progresses unchecked to the lungs, heart, and skeletal muscle

COCCIDIOSIS
A disease caused by coccidian protozoan parasite *Isospora hominis* or *I. belli;* after ingestion it infects the small intestine and results in malabsorption and diarrhea

VIRAL INFECTIONS

HERPES SIMPLEX VIRUS
Chronic infection caused by a herpes virus; often a reactivation of an earlier herpes infection

SIGNS AND SYMPTOMS	TREATMENT
Fever, fatigue, and weight loss for several weeks to months before respiratory symptoms develop; *respiratory symptoms:* dyspnea, usually noted initially on exertion and later at rest, and cough, usually starting out dry and nonproductive and later becoming productive	Co-trimoxazole may be given orally or I.V., although about 20% of AIDS patients are hypersensitive to sulfa drugs. I.V. pentamidine (Pentam 300) may be given but can cause many adverse effects, including permanent diabetes mellitus. Dapsone with trimethoprim (Trimpex), clindamycin (Cleocin), primaquine, atovaquone (Mepron), or corticosteroids may also be used. Prophylaxis for disease prevention and following treatment includes co-trimoxazole, atovaquone, or dapsone.
Abdominal cramping, flatulence, weight loss, anorexia, malaise, fever, nausea, vomiting, myalgia, and profuse, watery diarrhea	No effective therapy is known. Most is palliative and directed toward symptom control, focusing on fluid replacement, occasionally total parenteral nutrition, correction of electrolyte imbalances, and analgesic, antidiarrheal, and antiperistaltic agents. Paromomycin, spiramycin, and octeotides are used.
Localized neurologic deficits, fever, headache, altered mental status, and seizures	Sulfadiazine or clindamycin with pyrimethamine (Daraprim) may be given; however, about 20% of AIDS patients are hypersensitive to sulfa drugs. Folinic acid (Wellcovorin) may be given to prevent marrow toxicity from pyrimethamine. Patients must receive maintenance combination therapy in lower doses to prevent relapse.
Watery, nonbloody diarrhea; crampy abdominal pain; nausea; anorexia; weight loss; weakness; occasional vomiting; and a low-grade fever	Fluconazole, itraconazole, or amphotericin B is used.
Red, blisterlike lesions occurring in oral, anal, and genital areas; also found on the esophageal and tracheobronchial mucosa; pain, bleeding, and discharge	Acyclovir (Zovirax), famciclovir (Famvir), or valacyclovir (Valtrex) is given I.V. or by mouth. Lower maintenance doses may be given to prevent recurrence of symptoms. *(continued)*

Opportunistic diseases in AIDS (continued)

DISEASE

VIRAL INFECTIONS (continued)

CYTOMEGALOVIRUS (CMV)
A viral infection of the herpesvirus that may result in serious, widespread infection; most common sites: lungs, adrenal glands, eyes, CNS, GI tract, male genitourinary tract, and blood

PROGRESSIVE MULTIFOCAL LEUKOENCEPHALOPATHY
Progressive demyelinating disorder caused by hyperactivation of a papovavirus that leads to gradual brain degeneration

HERPES ZOSTER
A disease also known as *acute posterior ganglionitis, shingles, zona,* and *zoster;* acute infection caused by reactivation of the chickenpox virus

NEOPLASMS

KAPOSI'S SARCOMA
A generalized disease with characteristic lesions involving all skin surfaces, including the face (tip of the nose, eyelids), head, upper and lower limbs, soles of the feet, palms of the hands, conjunctivae, sclerae, pharynx, larynx, trachea, hard palate, stomach, liver, small and large intestines, and glans penis

SIGNS AND SYMPTOMS	TREATMENT
Unexplained fever, malaise, GI ulcers, diarrhea, weight loss, swollen lymph nodes, hepatomegaly, splenomegaly, blurred vision, floaters, dyspnea (especially on exertion), dry nonproductive cough, and vision changes leading to blindness in patients with ocular infection	Ganciclovir (Cytovene) or foscarnet (Foscavir) is used to treat CMV. Ganciclovir has shown some anti-HIV properties. Foscarnet or intraocular ganciclovir implants (Vitrasert) may be used to treat CMV retinitis.
Progressive dementia, memory loss, headache, confusion, weakness, and other possible neurologic complications such as seizures	No form of therapy has been effective, but attempted therapies include prednisone, acyclovir, and adenine arabinoside administered both I.V. and intrathecally.
Small clusters of painful, reddened papules that follow the route of inflamed nerves; may be disseminated, involving two or more dermatomes	Herpes zoster is most often treated with oral acyclovir capsules until healed. Treatment may have to continue at lower doses indefinitely to prevent recurrence. I.V. acyclovir is effective in disseminated varicella zoster lesions in some patients. Medications, such as capsaicin (Zostrix), may relieve pain from infection and postherpetic neuropathies. Famciclovir and valacyclovir also may be used.
Cutaneous and subcutaneous; usually painless, nonpruritic tumor nodules that are pigmented and violaceous (red to blue), nonblanching and palpable; patchy lesions appearing early and possibly mistaken for bruises, purpura, or diffuse cutaneous hemorrhages	Treatment isn't indicated for everyone. Indications include painful, obstructive, or cosmetically offensive lesions or rapidly progressing disease. Systemic chemotherapy using single or multiple drugs may be given to alleviate symptoms. Radiation therapy may be used to treat lesions. Intralesional therapy with vinblastine may be given for cosmetic purposes with small cutaneous lesions. Laser therapy and cryotherapy may be used to treat small isolated lesions. Interferon alfa-2a (Roferon-A) and interferon alfa-2b (Intron A) are also used.

(continued)

Opportunistic diseases in AIDS *(continued)*

DISEASE

NEOPLASMS *(continued)*

MALIGNANT LYMPHOMAS
Immune system cancer in which lymph tissue cells begin growing abnormally and spread to other organs; incidence in people with AIDS: about 4% to 10%; diagnosed in HIV-infected individuals as widespread disease involving extranodal sites, most commonly in the GI tract, CNS, bone marrow, and liver

CERVICAL NEOPLASM
Emerging as a significant gynecologic complication of HIV infection as more women become infected with HIV and live longer with illness because of antiretroviral therapy

Blood, semen, vaginal secretions, and breast milk are the body fluids that most readily transmit HIV. The virus also has been found in saliva, urine, tears, and feces, but there's no evidence of transmission through these fluids.

Signs and symptoms
ADULTS
After initial exposure, the infected person may have no signs or symptoms, or he may have a flulike illness (primary infection) and then remain asymptomatic for years. As the syndrome progresses, neurologic symptoms may develop from HIV encephalopathy or symptoms of an opportunistic infection, such as *Pneumocystis carinii* pneumonia, cytomegalovirus, or cancer. Eventually, repeated opportunistic infections overwhelm the patient's weakened immune defenses, invading every body system.

Signs and symptoms	Treatment
Unexplained fever, night sweats, or weight loss greater than 10% of patient's total body weight; signs and symptoms commonly confined to one body system: CNS (confusion, lethargy, and memory loss) or GI tract (pain, obstruction, changes in bowel habits, bleeding, and fever)	Individualized therapy may include a modified combination of methotrexate (Folex), bleomycin (Blenoxane). Doxorubicin (Doxil), cyclophosphamide (Cytoxan), vincristine (Oncovin), and dexamethasone (Decadron). Radiation therapy rather than chemotherapy is used to treat primary CNS lymphoma.
Possible indicators of early invasive disease: abnormal vaginal bleeding, persistent vaginal discharge, or postcoital pain and bleeding; *possible indicators of advanced disease:* pelvic pain, vaginal leakage of urine and feces from a fistula, anorexia, weight loss, and fatigue	Treatment is tailored to the disease stage. Preinvasive lesions may require total excisional biopsy, cryosurgery, laser destruction, conization (and frequent Papanicolaou test follow-up) and, rarely, hysterectomy. Invasive squamous cell carcinoma may require radical hysterectomy and radiation therapy.

CHILDREN

In general, signs and symptoms in children resemble those in adults, although the incubation period in children averages only 17 months. Children also are more likely to have a history of bacterial infection, such as otitis media or lymphoid interstitial pneumonia, as well as types of pneumonia not caused by *P. carinii*, sepsis, and chronic salivary gland enlargement.

Test results

The CDC recommends testing for HIV 1 month after a possible exposure — the approximate length of time before antibodies can be detected in the blood. However, an infected patient can test negative for as long as 35 months. Antibody tests in neonates also may be unreliable because transferred maternal antibodies persist for up to 10 months, causing a false-positive result.

Standard HIV testing typically consists of the enzyme immunoassay, Western blot, or immunofluorescence assay. If results are positive, they're confirmed at the next health care visit, typically in 1 to 2 weeks. Other blood tests support the diagnosis and are used to evaluate the severity of immunosuppression. They include:

■ CD4+ and CD8+ cell (killer T cell) subset counts
■ erythrocyte sedimentation rate (ESR)
■ complete blood count (CBC)
■ serum beta (sub 2) microglobulin test
■ p24 antigen test
■ neopterin levels
■ anergy testing.

Many opportunistic infections in AIDS patients are reactivations of previous infections. Therefore, patients may be tested for certain other disorders, including:

■ syphilis
■ hepatitis B
■ histoplasmosis
■ toxoplasmosis
■ tuberculosis.

Treatment

There's no cure for HIV disease, but several types of drugs are used to manage the disease and prolong life.

ANTIRETROVIRALS

Antiretrovirals are used to control viral reproduction and to slow progression of HIV-related disease. The recommended treatment is known as highly active antiretroviral therapy, commonly called HAART. It combines three or more antiretrovirals in a daily regimen. The Food and Drug Administration has approved four classes of antiretroviral drugs.

Nonnucleoside reverse transcriptase inhibitors bind to and disable reverse transcriptase, a protein that HIV needs to make copies of itself. Examples of this drug class include:

■ delavirdine (Rescriptor)
■ efavirenz (Sustiva)
■ nevirapine (Viramune).

Nucleoside reverse transcriptase inhibitors provide faulty versions of building blocks that HIV needs to make copies of itself, which halts viral production. Examples of this drug class include:

■ abacavir (Ziagen)
■ didanosine (Videx)

TEACHING FOCUS

Human immunodeficiency virus teaching topics

- Poor drug compliance may lead to resistance and treatment failure. Stress that the drug regimen must be followed closely, possibly for many years, possibly for life.
- Teach the patient how to identify the signs of impending infection and explain the importance of seeking immediate medical attention.
- Discuss ways to prevent the spread of human immunodeficiency virus, such as wearing a condom during vaginal or anal intercourse; not sharing needles or syringes; and not donating blood, body organs or tissue, or sperm.
- Provide information on support groups and other community resources.

- emtricitabine (Emtriva)
- lamivudine (Epivir)
- stavudine (Zerit)
- tenofovir DF (Viread)
- zalcitabine (HIVID)
- zidovudine (Retrovir).

Protease inhibitors disable protease, a protein that HIV needs to make copies of itself. Examples of this drug class include:

- amprenavir (Agenerase)
- atazanavir (Reyataz)
- fosamprenavir (LEXIVA)
- indinavir (Crixivan)
- lopinavir (Kaletra)
- nelfinavir (Viracept)
- ritonavir (Norvir)
- saquinavir (Fortovase).

Fusion inhibitors block HIV entry into cells. An example of this drug class is:

- enfuvirtide (Fuzeon).

ANTI-INFECTIVES AND ANTINEOPLASTICS

Anti-infectives are used to treat opportunistic infections. Antineoplastics are used to treat associated cancers. (See *Human immunodeficiency virus teaching topics.*)

LUPUS ERYTHEMATOSUS

A chronic, inflammatory, autoimmune disorder, lupus erythematosus affects connective tissue. There's no cure, but the prognosis improves with early detection and treatment. Lupus erythematosus has two forms: discoid and systemic.

■ The discoid form affects only the skin. It causes superficial lesions — typically over the cheeks and bridge of the nose — that leave scars after healing.

■ The systemic form affects multiple organs, is characterized by recurrent remissions and exacerbations, and may be fatal. About 16,000 new cases are diagnosed yearly. It's about 8 times more common in women than men and about 15 times more common during the childbearing years. It's also more common among Asians and Blacks. The prognosis is worse for those who develop cardiovascular, renal, or neurologic complications or severe bacterial infection.

Pathophysiology

The exact cause of lupus isn't known, although autoimmunity probably is the main cause. It also may involve environmental, hormonal, genetic, and possibly viral factors. (See *Theories about lupus.*)

In autoimmunity, the body produces antibodies against its own cells. People with systemic lupus erythematosus (SLE) produce antibodies against many different tissue components, such as red blood cells, neutrophils, platelets, lymphocytes, and almost any organ or tissue in the body. Formed antigen-antibody complexes can suppress the body's normal immunity and damage tissues.

Most people with SLE have a genetic predisposition. Other predisposing factors include:

■ stress
■ streptococcal or viral infection
■ exposure to sunlight or ultraviolet light
■ immunization
■ pregnancy
■ abnormal estrogen metabolism.

Drugs also may trigger or aggravate the disease. They include:

■ procainamide (Procanbid)
■ hydralazine (Apresoline)
■ isoniazid (Laniazid)
■ methyldopa (Aldomet)
■ anticonvulsants
■ penicillins, sulfa drugs, and hormonal contraceptives (less common).

RED FLAG Lupus can affect almost every major body system, resulting in pulmonary abnormalities, cardiac involvement,

GENETIC CONNECTION

Theories about lupus

APOPTOSIS
Researchers looking for genes that influence the development of lupus suspect that a genetic defect in apoptosis may be the culprit. Apoptosis is a cellular process that lets the body eliminate and replace cells that have fulfilled their function. A problem with apoptosis could allow harmful cells to linger and damage the body's tissue.

COMPLEMENT
Researchers are also studying genes for complement, a series of blood proteins that play an important role in the immune system. Complement acts as a backup for antibodies, helping them destroy foreign substances that invade the body. A decrease in the amount of complement makes the body less able to fight or destroy foreign substances. If they aren't removed, the immune system may become overactive and make autoantibodies.

renal disease that can progress to renal failure, and neurologic effects, such as seizures and mental dysfunction.

Signs and symptoms
SLE has no characteristic clinical pattern, and the onset may be acute or insidious. The patient may complain of:
■ abdominal pain
■ anorexia
■ diarrhea or constipation
■ fatigue
■ fever
■ malaise
■ nausea and vomiting
■ pain in joints
■ rash
■ weight loss.

Blood disorders may result from circulating antibodies. They include:
■ anemia
■ elevated ESR
■ leukopenia
■ lymphopenia
■ thrombocytopenia

TEACHING FOCUS

Lupus erythematosus teaching topics

Make sure the patient understands how to avoid infection. Direct her to avoid crowds and people with known infections.
● Teach the importance of good skin care, avoiding dryness and the use of irritating soaps, hair dryers, hair coloring, and permanent wave solutions.
● Encourage exercise, such as aerobics, yoga, swimming, walking, bicycling, and range-of-motion exercises.
● Instruct a photosensitive patient to wear protective clothing (hat, sunglasses, long-sleeved shirts or sweaters, and pants) and to use a sunscreen when outdoors.
● Teach the patient to perform meticulous mouth care to relieve discomfort and prevent infection.

Women may report irregular menstruation or amenorrhea, especially during exacerbations.

Nearly all patients have joint involvement that resembles rheumatoid arthritis.

Nearly 50% of patients have Raynaud's phenomenon — intermittent, severe pallor of the fingers, toes, ears, or nose. About 50% of patients have a "butterfly" rash. Rash also occurs on other areas exposed to light and may vary in severity from red areas to disc-shaped plaque. Patchy alopecia is common.

About 50% of patients have cardiopulmonary signs and symptoms, which may signal pulmonary embolism, such as:
▪ chest pain, indicating pleuritis
▪ dyspnea, which suggests parenchymal infiltrates and pneumonitis
▪ tachycardia
▪ central cyanosis
▪ hypotension.

Seizure disorders and confusion may indicate that the patient has neurologic damage. Other central nervous system signs and symptoms include:
▪ emotional lability
▪ psychosis
▪ headaches
▪ irritability
▪ stroke
▪ depression.

Be especially alert for infrequent urination, which may signal renal failure, and urinary frequency, painful urination, and bladder spasms, which are signs and symptoms of urinary tract infection (UTI).

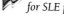 **RED FLAG** *UTIs and renal failure are the leading causes of death for SLE patients.*

Test results
These tests are used to diagnose lupus erythematosus.
- CBC with differential may show anemia and a reduced WBC count.
- Serum electrophoresis may show hypergammaglobulinemia.
- Other blood tests may show a decreased platelet count and an elevated ESR.
- Active disease is diagnosed by decreased serum complement levels, leukopenia, mild thrombocytopenia, and anemia.
- Chest X-rays may reveal pleurisy or lupus pneumonitis.
- Antinuclear antibodies are elevated.

Treatment
Drugs are the mainstay of treatment for SLE. In mild disease, nonsteroidal anti-inflammatory drugs such as ibuprofen (Motrin) usually control arthritis and arthralgia.

Skin lesions require sun protection and topical corticosteroid cream, such as triamcinolone (Aristocort) and hydrocortisone (Westcort). (See *Lupus erythematosus teaching topics*.)

Fluorinated steroids may control acute or discoid lesions. Stubborn lesions may respond to intralesional or systemic corticosteroids or antimalarials, such as hydroxychloroquine (Plaquenil), chloroquine (Aralen), and dapsone (DDS). Because hydroxychloroquine and chloroquine can cause retinal damage, patients receiving them should have an ophthalmologic examination every 6 months.

Corticosteroids are the treatment of choice for systemic symptoms, acute generalized exacerbations, and injury to vital organs from pleuritis, pericarditis, nephritis, vasculitis, and central nervous system involvement. With initial prednisone doses of 60 mg or more, the patient's condition usually improves noticeably within 48 hours. After symptoms are controlled, the dosage is gradually reduced and the drug is stopped.

If the kidneys or central nervous system are affected, immunosuppressive drugs may be given, such as cyclophosphamide (Cytoxan) and mycophenolate (CellCept).

Methotrexate (Rheumatrex) is sometimes effective in controlling the disease.

RHEUMATOID ARTHRITIS

A chronic, systemic, potentially crippling inflammatory disease, rheumatoid arthritis usually attacks peripheral joints and surrounding muscles, tendons, ligaments, and blood vessels. It currently affects 2.1 million U.S. residents — 1.5 million women and 600,000 men. It occurs in all age-groups, with peak onset between ages 20 and 50. (See *Effects of aging on immune function.*)

This disease is marked by spontaneous remissions and unpredictable exacerbations, and it usually requires lifelong treatment and sometimes surgery. Its intermittent effects usually allow periods of normal activity, although 10% of patients have total disability from severe joint deformity, related symptoms, or both. The prognosis worsens with development of nodules, vasculitis (inflammation of a blood or lymph vessel), and high titers of rheumatoid factor.

Pathophysiology

The cause of rheumatoid arthritis isn't known. Infections, genetics, and endocrine factors may play a part. (See *Rheumatoid arthritis marker,* page 104.)

When exposed to an antigen, a person susceptible to rheumatoid arthritis may develop abnormal or altered IgG antibodies. The body doesn't recognize these antibodies as "self," so it forms an antibody known as rheumatoid factor against them. By aggregating into complexes, rheumatoid factor causes inflammation.

Eventually inflammation causes cartilage damage. Immune responses continue, including complement system activation, which attracts leukocytes and stimulates release of inflammatory mediators, which then worsen joint destruction. If unarrested, joint inflammation occurs in four stages.

■ Synovitis develops from congestion and edema of the synovial membrane and joint capsule.

■ Pannus (thickened layers of granulation tissue) forms. It covers and invades cartilage and eventually destroys the joint capsule and bone.

■ The third stage is characterized by fibrous ankylosis (fibrous invasion of the pannus and scar formation that occludes the joint space). Bone atrophy and misalignment cause visible deformities and restrict movement, causing muscle atrophy, imbalance, and, possibly, partial dislocations.

■ Fibrous tissue calcifies, resulting in bony ankylosis (fixation of a joint) and total immobility. Painful movement may restrict active

Effects of aging on immune function

The ability of the immune system to fight off infections and other immune system disorders decreases with age. The configuration of lymphocytes and their reaction to infection changes. Lymphocytes are also decreased in number and are less responsive to invasion of the body by infection and other antigens. In addition, autoantibodies are more likely to be produced during the aging process. Autoantibodies are factors in causing such diseases as rheumatoid arthritis and atherosclerosis.

joint use and cause fibrous or bony ankylosis, soft-tissue contractures, and joint deformities.

RED FLAG Complications of rheumatoid arthritis include pain, impaired movement, vasculitis, recurrent infections, necrosis of the hip joint, cardiac and pulmonary disorders, renal insufficiency, GI disturbances, and pleural effusions. Vasculitis can lead to skin lesions, leg ulcers, and multisystem complications.

Signs and symptoms
At first the patient may complain of nonspecific symptoms, including:

■ anorexia
■ fatigue
■ malaise
■ persistent low-grade fever
■ vague articular symptoms
■ weight loss.

As inflammation progresses through the four stages, specific symptoms develop, typically in the fingers. These symptoms usually occur bilaterally and symmetrically. They may extend to the wrists, elbows, knees, and ankles.

Test results
No test can be used to definitively diagnose rheumatoid arthritis, but these tests are useful.

■ X-rays may show bone demineralization and soft-tissue swelling and help determine the extent of cartilage and bone destruction, erosion, subluxations, and deformities.
■ Rheumatoid factor test is positive in 75% to 80% of patients, as indicated by a titer of 1:160 or higher. Rheumatoid factor doesn't

GENETIC CONNECTION

Rheumatoid arthritis marker

Many people with rheumatoid arthritis have a genetic marker called HLA-DR4. Researchers suspect that a virus may trigger rheumatoid arthritis in some people who have this inherited tendency for the disease. They suspect that other genes may be implicated in rheumatoid arthritis as well.

confirm the disease, but it helps determine the prognosis. A patient with a high titer usually has more severe and progressive disease with extra-articular signs and symptoms.
■ Synovial fluid analysis shows increased volume and turbidity but decreased viscosity and complement levels. WBC count usually exceeds 10,000/mm^3.
■ Serum protein electrophoresis may show elevated serum globulin levels.
■ ESR is elevated in 85% to 90% of patients. Because an elevated rate often parallels disease activity, this test helps monitor the patient's response to therapy.

Treatment
Treatment aims to reduce pain and inflammation and preserve the patient's functional capacity and quality of life. (See *Rheumatoid arthritis teaching topics.*)

DRUG THERAPY
Nonsteroidal anti-inflammatory drugs (NSAIDs) are the mainstay of treatment because they decrease inflammation and relieve joint pain. They may include:
■ traditional NSAIDs such as ibuprofen (Motrin)
■ salicylates such as aspirin
■ the COX-2 inhibitor celecoxib (Celebrex).
    Disease-modifying antirheumatic drugs (DMARDs) are started immediately after diagnosis to delay joint destruction. They may include:
■ methotrexate (Rheumatrex), the most commonly used DMARD
■ auranofin (Ridaura).
    Tumor necrosis factor (TNF) inhibitors slow or halt the damage caused by rheumatoid arthritis. They may include:
■ etanercept (Enbrel)
■ infliximab (Remicade)

TEACHING FOCUS

Rheumatoid arthritis teaching topics

● Explain the nature of rheumatoid arthritis. Make sure the patient and his family understand that it's a chronic disease with spontaneous remissions and exacerbations.
● Urge the patient to eat a balanced diet. Stress the need for weight control because obesity further stresses the joints.
● Teach the patient how to use correct posture when standing, sitting, and walking. Teach proper body mechanics.
● Suggest that the patient take a hot shower or bath before bed or in the morning to help relieve pain.
● Provide information about adaptive devices, such as dressing aids (long-handled shoehorn, reacher, elastic shoelaces, zipper pull, and button hook) and eating utensils.

■ adalimumab (Humira).
   Other drugs may include:
■ anakinra (Kineret), an injectable drug that blocks the inflammatory protein interleukin-1
■ hydroxychloroquine (Plaquenil)
■ gold salts
■ penicillamine (Cuprimine)
■ corticosteroids such as prednisone
■ immunosuppressants — cyclophosphamide (Cytoxan) and azathioprine (Imuran) — after other treatments have failed.

PROTEIN-A IMMUNOADSORPTION THERAPY

Patients with moderate to severe rheumatoid arthritis who haven't responded well to drug therapy may opt for protein-A immuno-adsorption therapy. In it, blood is drawn from a vein in the patient's arm and pumped into an apheresis machine, which separates plasma from blood cells. Plasma then passes through a Prosorba column, which is a plastic cylinder about the size of a coffee mug that contains a sandlike substance coated with protein A. Protein A in the cylinder binds with the antibodies produced in rheumatoid arthritis.

After plasma passes through the column, it's returned to the body through a vein in the patient's other arm. This procedure typically lasts 2 hours, and the recommended regimen is one treatment weekly for 12 weeks.

PHYSICAL AND OTHER THERAPIES

Joint function can be preserved through range-of-motion exercises and a carefully individualized physical and occupational therapy program. For joints that are damaged or painful, surgery may be available.

5

GENETICS

Understanding genetics

Genetics is the study of heredity, the passing of traits from parents to their children. Physical traits, such as eye color, are inherited as well as biochemical and physiologic traits, including the tendency to develop certain diseases. Inherited traits are transmitted from parents to offspring through genes in germ cells (gametes). Human gametes are eggs (ova), and sperm. A person's genetic makeup is determined at fertilization, when ovum and sperm are united.

CHROMOSOMES

In the nucleus of each germ cell are chromosomes. Each chromosome contains a strand of genetic material called deoxyribonucleic acid (DNA). DNA is a long molecule that's made up of thousands of segments called genes. Each of the traits a person inherits — from blood type to toe shape and a myriad of others in between — is coded in the genes.

A human ovum contains 23 chromosomes. A sperm also contains 23 chromosomes, each similar in size and shape to a chromosome in the ovum. When ovum and sperm unite, the corresponding chromosomes pair up. The result is a fertilized cell with 46 chromosomes (23 pairs) in the nucleus.

CELL DIVISION

The fertilized cell soon undergoes cell division (mitosis). In mitosis, each of the 46 chromosomes produces an exact duplicate of itself. The cell then divides and each new cell receives one set of 46 chromosomes. Each of the two cells that result likewise divides, and so on, eventually forming a many-celled human body. Therefore, each cell in a person's body (except the ova or sperm) contains 46 identical chromosomes.

The ova and sperm are formed by a different cell-division process called meiosis. In meiosis, there are two cell divisions. Each new cell (an ovum or sperm) receives one set of 23 chromosomes. The location of a gene on a chromosome is called a locus. The locus of each gene is specific and doesn't vary from person to person. This allows each of the thousands of genes in an ovum to join the corresponding genes from a sperm when the chromosomes pair up at fertilization.

INHERITANCE

A person receives one set of chromosomes and genes from each parent, two genes for each trait inherited. One gene may be more influential than the other in developing a specific trait. The more influential gene is said to be dominant and the less influential gene is recessive. For example, a child may receive a gene for brown eyes (which is dominant) from one parent and a gene for blue eyes (which is recessive) from the other parent. The dominant gene is more likely to be expressed. Therefore, the child is more likely to have brown eyes.

A variation of a gene and the trait it controls — such as brown, green, or blue eye color — is called an allele. When two different alleles are inherited, they're said to be heterozygous. When the alleles are identical, they're termed homozygous. A dominant allele may be expressed when it's carried by only one of the chromosomes in a pair. A recessive allele is incapable of expression unless recessive alleles are carried by both chromosomes in a pair.

Of the 23 pairs of chromosomes in each living human cell, 22 pairs are not involved in controlling a person's gender; they're called autosomes. The two sex chromosomes of the 23rd pair determine a person's gender. In a female, both chromosomes are relatively large and each is designated by the letter X; females have two X chromosomes. In a male, one sex chromosome is an X chromosome and one is a smaller chromosome, designated by the letter Y.

Each gamete produced by a male contains either an X or a Y chromosome. When a sperm with an X chromosome fertilizes an ovum, the offspring is female. When a sperm with a Y chromosome fertilizes an ovum, the offspring is male.

MUTATIONS

A mutation is a permanent change in genetic material. When a gene mutates, it may produce a trait that's different from its original trait. Gene mutations in a gamete may be transmitted during reproduction. Some mutations cause serious or deadly disorders that occur in three different forms, including:

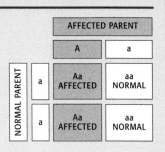

Understanding autosomal dominant inheritance

This diagram shows the possible offspring of a parent with recessive normal genes (aa) and a parent with an altered dominant gene (Aa). Note that with each pregnancy there's a 50% chance that the offspring will be affected.

		AFFECTED PARENT	
		A	a
NORMAL PARENT	a	Aa AFFECTED	aa NORMAL
	a	Aa AFFECTED	aa NORMAL

■ single-gene disorders
■ chromosomal disorders
■ multifactorial disorders.

Single-gene disorders

Single-gene disorders are inherited in clearly identifiable patterns. Two important inheritance patterns are called autosomal dominant and autosomal recessive. A third pattern is called sex-linked inheritance. Because there are 22 pairs of autosomes and only 1 pair of sex chromosomes, most hereditary disorders are caused by autosomal defects.

AUTOSOMAL DOMINANT INHERITANCE

Dominant genes produce abnormal traits in offspring even if only one parent has the gene. The autosomal dominant inheritance pattern has these characteristics:
■ Male and female offspring are affected equally.
■ One of the parents is also usually affected.
■ If one parent is affected, the children have a 50% chance of being affected.
■ If both parents are affected, all of their children will be affected.

Marfan syndrome is an example of an autosomal dominant disorder. (See *Understanding autosomal dominant inheritance*.)

AUTOSOMAL RECESSIVE INHERITANCE

Recessive genes don't produce abnormal traits unless both parents have the gene and pass them to their offspring. The autosomal recessive inheritance pattern has these characteristics:

Understanding autosomal recessive inheritance

This diagram shows the possible offspring of two unaffected parents, each with an altered recessive gene (a) on an autosome. Each offspring will have a one in four chance of being affected and a two in four chance of being a carrier.

		HETEROZYGOUS PARENT Aa	
		A	a
HETEROZYGOUS PARENT Aa	A	AA NORMAL	Aa CARRIER
	a	Aa CARRIER	aa AFFECTED

- Male and female offspring are affected equally.
- If both parents are unaffected but heterozygous for the trait (carriers), each of their offspring has a one in four chance of being affected.
- If both parents are affected, all of their offspring will be affected.
- If one parent is affected and the other is not a carrier, all of the parents' offspring will be unaffected but will carry the altered gene.
- If one parent is affected and the other is a carrier, each of the offspring will have a one in two chance of being affected.

Certain autosomal recessive conditions are more common in specific ethnic groups; for example, cystic fibrosis is more common in Whites and sickle cell anemia is more common in Blacks. In many cases no evidence of the trait appears in past generations. (See *Understanding autosomal recessive inheritance*.)

SEX-LINKED INHERITANCE

Some genetic disorders are caused by genes located on the sex chromosomes and are termed sex-linked. Because the Y chromosome isn't known to carry disease-causing genes, the terms X-linked and sex-linked are interchangeable.

Because females receive two X chromosomes (one from the father and one from the mother), they can be homozygous for a dis-

Understanding X-linked dominant inheritance

This diagram shows the possible offspring of a normal parent and a parent with an X-linked dominant gene on the X chromosome (shown by a dot). When the father is affected, only his daughters have the abnormal gene. When the mother is affected, both male and female offspring may be affected.

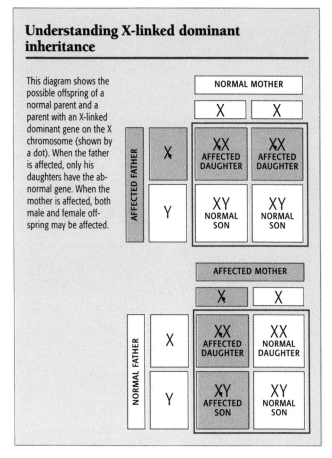

ease allele, homozygous for a normal allele, or heterozygous. Because males have only one X chromosome, a single X-linked recessive gene can cause disease in a male. In comparison, a female needs two copies of the diseased gene. Therefore, males are more commonly affected by X-linked recessive diseases than females. (See *Understanding X-linked dominant inheritance* and *Understanding X-linked recessive inheritance,* page 112.)

Characteristics of the X-linked *dominant* inheritance pattern include the following:

Understanding X-linked recessive inheritance

This diagram shows the possible offspring of a normal parent and a parent with a recessive gene on the X chromosome (shown by an open dot). All of the female offspring of an affected male will be carriers. The son of a female carrier may inherit a recessive gene on the X chromosome and be affected by the disease.

NORMAL MOTHER		
	X	X
AFFECTED FATHER X	XX CARRIER DAUGHTER	XX CARRIER DAUGHTER
Y	XY NORMAL SON	XY NORMAL SON

CARRIER MOTHER		
	X	X
NORMAL FATHER X	XX CARRIER DAUGHTER	XX NORMAL DAUGHTER
Y	XY AFFECTED SON	XY NORMAL SON

- A person with the abnormal trait typically will have one affected parent.
- If a father has an X-linked dominant disorder, all of his daughters and none of his sons will be affected.
- If a mother has an X-linked dominant disorder, there's a 50% chance that each of her children will be affected.
- Evidence of the inherited trait most commonly appears in the family history.

X-linked dominant disorders are commonly lethal in males (prenatal or neonatal deaths). The family history may show miscarriages and the predominance of female offspring.

Characteristics of the X-linked *recessive* inheritance pattern include the following:

- In most cases, affected people are males with unaffected parents. In rare cases, the father is affected and the mother is a carrier.
- All of the daughters of an affected male will be carriers.
- Sons of an affected male are unaffected. Unaffected sons can't transmit the disorder.
- Unaffected male children of a female carrier don't transmit the disorder.
- Hemophilia is an example of an X-linked recessive inheritance disorder.

Chromosomal disorders

Disorders also may be caused by chromosomal aberrations — deviations in either the structure or the number of chromosomes. Deviations involve the loss, addition, rearrangement, or exchange of genes. If the remaining genetic material is sufficient to maintain life, an endless variety of clinical manifestations may occur. These disorders may involve nondisjunction or translocation, or they may be multifactorial.

NONDISJUNCTION

During cell division chromosomes normally separate in a process called disjunction. Failure to do so — called nondisjunction — causes an unequal distribution of chromosomes between the two resulting cells. Nondisjunction may occur during very early cell divisions after fertilization and may involve all the resulting cells. The risk of nondisjunction increases with parental age.

A mixture of cells, some with a specific chromosome aberration and some with normal cells, results in mosaicism. The effect on the offspring depends on the percentage of normal cells. Miscarriages can also result from chromosomal aberrations. Fertilization of an ovum with a chromosome aberration by a sperm with a chromosome aberration usually doesn't occur.

Gain or loss of chromosomes is usually from nondisjunction of autosomes or sex chromosomes during meiosis. When chromosomes are gained or lost, the name of the affected cell contains the suffix "-somy."

A cell that contains one fewer than the normal number of chromosomes is called a monosomy. If the monosomy involves an auto-

Understanding nondisjunction of chromosomes

This illustration shows normal disjunction and nondisjunction of an ovum. Nondisjunction produces one trisomic cell and one monosomic (nonviable) cell.

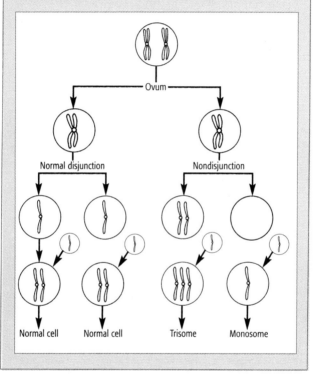

some the cell will be nonviable. Monosomy X can be viable and result in a female who has Turner's syndrome. A cell that contains one extra chromosome is called a trisomy. (See *Understanding nondisjunction of chromosomes*.)

TRANSLOCATION

Another aberration, translocation, is the shifting or moving of a chromosome. Translocation occurs when chromosomes break and rejoin in an abnormal arrangement.

When the rearrangements preserve the normal amount of genetic material (balanced translocations), there are usually no visible abnormalities. When the rearrangements alter the amount of genetic material, typically, there are visible or measurable abnormalities.

The children of parents with balanced translocations may have serious chromosomal aberration, such as partial monosomies or partial trisomies. Parental age doesn't seem to be a factor.

MULTIFACTORIAL DISORDERS
Disorders caused by both genetic and environmental factors are classified as multifactorial. Examples include:
- cleft lip
- cleft palate
- myelomeningocele (spina bifida with a portion of the spinal cord and membranes protruding).

 Environmental factors that contribute include:
- maternal age
- use of chemicals (drugs, alcohol, hormones) by mother or father
- maternal infections during pregnancy or maternal diseases
- maternal or paternal exposure to radiation
- maternal nutritional factors
- general maternal or paternal health
- other factors, including high altitude, maternal-fetal blood incompatibility, maternal smoking, and poor prenatal care.

Genetic disorders

This section describes the following:
- a multifactorial disorder
  - cleft lip and cleft palate
- single-gene disorders
  - cystic fibrosis
  - hemophilia
  - Marfan syndrome
  - phenylketonuria [PKU]
  - sickle cell anemia
  - Tay-Sachs disease
- a chromosomal disorder
  - Down syndrome.

CLEFT LIP AND CLEFT PALATE
Cleft lip and cleft palate malformations occur in about 1 in 800 births. Cleft lip, with or without cleft palate, is more common in males. Cleft palate alone is more common in females.

Types of cleft lip and cleft palate

These illustrations show four variations of cleft lip and cleft palate.

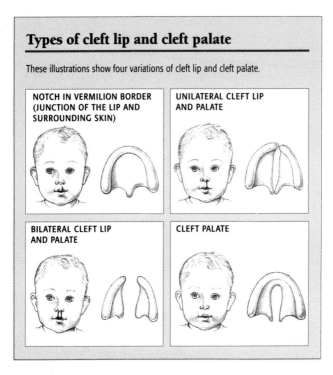

NOTCH IN VERMILION BORDER (JUNCTION OF THE LIP AND SURROUNDING SKIN)

UNILATERAL CLEFT LIP AND PALATE

BILATERAL CLEFT LIP AND PALATE

CLEFT PALATE

Nutritional intake is affected by an abnormal lip and palate. Also, children with cleft palates commonly have hearing problems caused by middle ear damage or infection.

Pathophysiology

Cleft lip and palate is a multifactorial genetic disorder. It originates in the second month of gestation when the front and sides of the face and the shelves of the palate fuse imperfectly. These malformations fall into four categories:

■ clefts of the lip (unilateral or bilateral)

■ clefts of the palate (along the midline)

■ unilateral clefts of the lip, alveolus (gum pad), and palate

■ bilateral clefts of the lip, alveolus, and palate. (See *Types of cleft lip and cleft palate.*)

RED FLAG *An unrepaired cleft may lead to failure to thrive (from poor oral intake), speech trouble. dentition problems, increased risk of otitis media, hearing defects, and an altered appearance.*

TEACHING FOCUS

Cleft lip and cleft palate teaching topics

● Stress to the parents that surgery can repair the cleft. Provide instructions so they can take proper care of the infant at home.

● Urge the mother of an infant with cleft lip to breast-feed if the cleft doesn't impede effective sucking. Tell the mother of an infant who has a cleft palate or has just had corrective surgery that breast-feeding is most likely impossible for up to 6 weeks.

However, if the mother desires, suggest that she use a breast pump to express her milk for bottle feedings.

● Teach the mother to hold the infant in a near-sitting position when feeding to prevent choking and aspiration, with the flow directed to the side or back of the infant's tongue. Tell her to burp the infant often because he may tend to swallow excess air.

Signs and symptoms

The malformation may range from a simple notch to a complete cleft that extends from the lip through the floor of the nostril on either side of the midline. A complete cleft palate may involve the soft palate, the bones of the maxilla (upper jawbone), and the cavity on one or both sides of the premaxilla (front of the upper jawbone).

In a bilateral cleft, the most severe of all cleft malformations, the cleft runs from the soft palate forward to either side of the nose, separating the maxilla and the premaxilla into free-moving segments. The tongue and other muscles can displace these segments, enlarging the cleft.

Another cleft malformation, Pierre Robin malformation sequence, involves a cleft palate plus an abnormally small jaw (micrognathia) and downward dropping of the tongue (glossoptosis).

Because the palate is essential to speech, structural changes can permanently affect speech, even after surgical repair.

Test results

Cleft lip may be detected prenatally using a level 2 ultrasound.

Treatment

Cleft malformations must be treated with speech therapy and surgery. The timing of surgery varies. Special bottles and nipples designed for infants with cleft palate should be used for feedings. (See *Cleft lip and cleft palate teaching topics*.) Infants with Pierre Robin malformation sequence should never be placed on their backs because the tongue can fall back and obstruct the airway.

CYSTIC FIBROSIS

A chronic, progressive, inherited disease, cystic fibrosis is the most common fatal genetic disease in white children. When both parents carry the recessive gene, each pregnancy brings a 25% chance that the offspring will inherit the disease. There's a 50% chance that the child will be a carrier and a 25% chance the child won't carry the gene.

Cystic fibrosis affects about 30,000 children and adults in the United States. It's most common in Whites (1 in 3,300 births) and less common in Blacks (1 in 15,300 births), Native Americans, and Asians. It occurs equally in both sexes.

Pathophysiology

Cystic fibrosis is inherited as an autosomal recessive trait. One implicated gene, the cystic fibrosis transmembrane conductance regulator (CFTR) gene, is located on chromosome 7. Research now suggests that there may be more than 900 CFTR mutations that code for cystic fibrosis.

Most cases of cystic fibrosis arise from a mutation that affects the genetic coding for a single amino acid, resulting in a protein that doesn't function properly. The abnormal protein resembles other transmembrane transport proteins. It lacks a phenylalanine (an essential amino acid) that's usually produced by normal genes.

This abnormal protein may interfere with chloride transport by preventing adenosine triphosphate from binding to the protein or by interfering with activation by protein kinase. The lack of an essential amino acid leads to dehydration and mucosal thickening in the respiratory and intestinal tracts.

RED FLAG Cystic fibrosis increases the viscosity of bronchial, pancreatic, and other mucous gland secretions, obstructing glandular ducts. As the disease progresses, complications include hepatic disease, diabetes, arthritis, pancreatitis, clotting problems, retarded bone growth, and delayed sexual development.

Signs and symptoms

The clinical effects of cystic fibrosis may become apparent soon after birth, or they may take years to develop. Signs and symptoms stem from major aberrations in sweat gland, respiratory, GI, and reproductive functions.

RESPIRATORY EFFECTS

Accumulation of thick secretions in the bronchioles and alveoli causes these respiratory changes:

■ frequent upper respiratory tract infections
■ dyspnea
■ paroxysmal (sudden) cough
■ frequent bouts of pneumonia.
   Respiratory effects may eventually lead to collapsed lungs (atelectasis) or emphysema.
   A child with cystic fibrosis may have:
■ a barrel chest
■ cyanosis
■ clubbing of the fingers and toes
■ a distended abdomen
■ coughing with tenacious, yellow-green sputum
■ wheezy respirations and crackles on auscultation.

GASTROINTESTINAL EFFECTS
Cystic fibrosis also affects the intestines, pancreas, and liver.
■ Diabetes mellitus and pancreatitis may result from insult to the pancreas.
■ Hepatic failure and cholecystitis may result from blockage of pancreatic ducts.
■ Deficiency of the enzymes trypsin, amylase, and lipase (also a result of obstruction of pancreatic ducts) may prevent the conversion and absorption of fat and protein in the intestinal tract, which interferes with food digestion and absorption of the fat-soluble vitamins A, D, E, and K.
■ Patients typically have greasy, bulky stools and poor weight gain (despite an excessive appetite).

REPRODUCTIVE EFFECTS
■ Males may have no sperm in their semen (azoospermia).
■ Females may have secondary amenorrhea and increased mucus in the reproductive tract, which blocks normal passage of the ovum.

Test results
According to the Cystic Fibrosis Foundation, a diagnosis of cystic fibrosis should be based on:
■ the presence of one or more of the clinical findings typically associated with cystic fibrosis
■ a history of cystic fibrosis in a sibling
■ two elevated sweat chloride tests obtained on separate days
■ identification of mutations in each CFTR gene.
   Several tests may support the diagnosis.

GENETIC CONNECTION

Gene therapy and cystic fibrosis

Researchers think gene therapy can correct the basic defect that causes cystic fibrosis. Therapy would include adding enough normal genes to the patient's airway to correct the defective cells, with the goal of retaining existing lung function and preventing further damage.

Clinical trials have shown that normal genes can be safely transferred to an airway affected by cystic fibrosis. Scientists are now working on developing efficient delivery methods.

- If a patient's sweat chloride levels are normal or borderline, a nasal potential difference measurement is obtained. This test measures salt transport in the nasal cavity; an abnormality obtained on two separate days indicates cystic fibrosis.
- Chest X-rays show early signs of lung obstruction.
- Stool specimen analysis shows the absence of trypsin, suggesting pancreatic insufficiency.
- DNA testing can detect CFTR mutations that cause cystic fibrosis. This test can also be used to detect carriers and for prenatal diagnosis in families with an affected child.

Treatment

There's no cure for cystic fibrosis, but treatment can greatly increase life expectancy and can allow the patient to lead as normal a life as possible. (See *Gene therapy and cystic fibrosis*.) Specific treatments depend on the organ systems involved.

- Salt supplements are used to combat electrolyte loss through sweat.
- Oral pancreatic enzymes taken with meals and snacks offset deficiencies.
- Broad-spectrum antibiotics and oxygen therapy are administered as needed.
- To manage pulmonary dysfunction, chest physiotherapy, including postural drainage and chest percussion over all lobes, is usually performed several times daily.
- Dornase alfa (Pulmozyme), a mucus-thinning drug, is given to improve lung function and reduce the number of lung infections.
- Lung transplantation may also be needed. (See *Cystic fibrosis teaching topics.*)

TEACHING FOCUS

Cystic fibrosis teaching topics

● Tell the patient and his family members about the disease and thoroughly explain all treatment measures. Make sure they know about tests to determine whether family members carry the cystic fibrosis gene.

● Explain aerosol therapy, including intermittent nebulizer treatments before postural drainage. Tell the patient and his family that these treatments

help loosen secretions and dilate bronchi.

● Instruct family members in proper methods of chest physiotherapy.

● Teach the patient and his family signs of infection and sudden changes in the patient's condition that they should report to the physician. These include increased coughing, decreased appetite, sputum that thickens or contains blood, shortness of breath, and chest pain.

DOWN SYNDROME

Down syndrome results from a chromosomal aberration that occurs in 1 per 800 to 1,000 births. The disorder produces:

■ mental retardation
■ characteristic facial features
■ distinctive physical abnormalities
■ heart defects
■ other congenital disorders.

The risk of having a child with Down syndrome increases with maternal age. At age 20, a mother has about 1 chance in 2,000 of having a child with Down syndrome. By age 49, she has 1 chance in 12. Although women older than age 35 account for fewer than 8% of all births, they bear 20% of all children who have Down syndrome.

Life expectancy and quality of life for patients with Down syndrome have increased significantly because of improved treatment of related complications and better developmental education programs. Nevertheless, up to 44% of patients with congenital heart disease die before they reach age 1.

Pathophysiology

Also called trisomy 21, Down syndrome is caused by an aberration in which chromosome 21 has three copies instead of two. Most patients with Down syndrome have 47 chromosomes instead of the normal 46.

Understanding Down syndrome

Chromosomes are arranged in seven groups designated by the letters A through G. These illustrations show the arrangement of chromosomes (karyotype) in a normal person and a person with Down syndrome. Most people with Down syndrome have an extra chromosome known as trisomy 21.

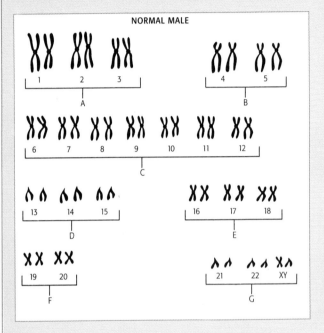

The most common cause of this extra chromosome 21 is nondisjunction. The extra chromosome originates from the mother more than 90% of the time. About 4% of the time, Down syndrome results from translocation and infusion of the long arm of chromosome 21 and 14, an event known as robertsonian translocation. In some cases, the abnormality results from deterioration of the oocyte (primitive egg), which may result from age or the cumulative effects of radiation, viruses, and other environmental factors. (See *Understanding Down syndrome*.)

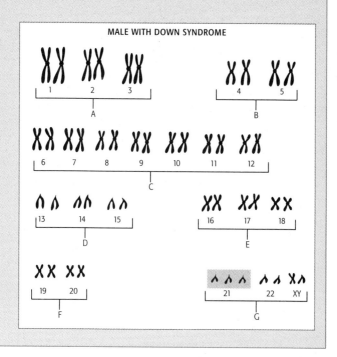

MALE WITH DOWN SYNDROME

Signs and symptoms

The physical signs of Down syndrome are apparent at birth. The infant is lethargic and has one or more of these problems:

- slanting, almond-shaped eyes
- protruding tongue
- small, open mouth
- single, transverse crease on the palm (called a simian crease)
- small white spots on the iris (Brushfield's spots)
- small skull
- flat nose bridge
- flattened face
- small ears
- short neck with excess skin.
    Other characteristic findings include:
- dry, sensitive skin with decreased elasticity
- umbilical hernia
- short stature
- short limbs
- broad, flat, and squarish hands and feet
- a wide space between the first and second toes
- decreased muscle tone in limbs with impaired reflex development.
    Many infants have:
- congenital heart disease
- duodenal obstruction
- clubfoot
- imperforate anus
- cleft lip and cleft palate
- Hirschsprung's disease (congenital colon enlargement)
- myelomeningocele
- pelvic bone abnormalities.
    Dental development is slow with abnormal or absent teeth. Strabismus and, occasionally, cataracts occur.

    The genitals develop poorly, and puberty is delayed. A female with Down syndrome may menstruate and be fertile. The male is infertile with low serum testosterone levels and, in many cases, undescended testes.

    Patients may have an IQ as low as 30, although most can be educated. Some have IQs approaching 80. Intellectual development slows with age. Social performance is usually beyond that expected for their mental age.

Test results
- A karyotype showing the chromosomal abnormality confirms the diagnosis of Down syndrome.

Down syndrome teaching topics

● Stress the need for adequate exercise and maximal environmental stimulation. Refer the parents to infant stimulation classes, which may start shortly after birth.

● Help the parents set realistic goals for their child. Although his mental development may seem normal at first, dissuade them from viewing this early development as a sign of future progress. By the time the child reaches age 1 his development clearly will lag behind that of unaffected children. Help the parents view their child's achievements in a positive light.

● Teach parents the importance of a balanced diet. Stress the need for patience while feeding their child, who may have more trouble sucking, be less demanding, and seem less eager to eat than other babies.

■ Certain tests reveal Down syndrome before birth.
  – Prenatal ultrasonography that shows a duodenal obstruction or an atrioventricular canal defect suggests Down syndrome.
  – Maternal blood tests during pregnancy show low unconjugated estriol levels, low alpha-fetoprotein levels, and high human chorionic gonadotropin levels, all indicative of Down syndrome.
  – Amniocentesis or chorionic villi sampling is recommended for pregnant women older than age 35 and for a pregnant woman of any age when she or the father is a carrier of a translocated chromosome.

Treatment

Treatment for Down syndrome includes:
■ surgery to correct cardiac defects and other congenital abnormalities
■ antibiotic therapy for recurrent infections
■ thyroid hormone replacement for hypothyroidism.

Cosmetic surgery is performed to correct protruding tongue, cleft lip, and cleft palate, improving the patient's appearance and speech and reducing the risk of cavities and orthodontic problems. (See *Down syndrome teaching topics*.)

Special education programs, mandated in most communities, promote self-esteem and help children reach their potential.

HEMOPHILIA

Hemophilia is the most common X-linked genetic disease, occurring in about 125 of 1 million male births. A hereditary bleeding disorder, hemophilia is extremely rare in females.

Two types of hemophilia may occur:

■ hemophilia A, or classic hemophilia, which affects more than 80% of all hemophiliacs
■ hemophilia B, or Christmas disease (named for Stephen Christmas, in whom it was discovered in 1952), which affects 15% of all hemophiliacs.

Severity and prognosis vary with the degree of deficiency or nonfunction and the site of bleeding. Advances in treatment have greatly improved the prognosis, and many patients have a normal life span.

Pathophysiology

Hemophilia A is caused by deficiency or nonfunction of factor VIII. Hemophilia B is caused by deficiency or nonfunction of factor IX. Both are inherited as X-linked recessive traits. In other words, female carriers have a 50% chance of transmitting the gene to each daughter, making her a carrier, and a 50% chance of transmitting the gene to each son, who would be born with hemophilia.

Hemophilia produces mild to severe abnormal bleeding. After a platelet plug develops at a bleeding site, the lack of clotting factor prevents a stable fibrin clot from forming. Although hemorrhaging doesn't usually happen immediately, delayed bleeding is common.

RED FLAG Bleeding into joints and muscles causes pain, swelling, extreme tenderness, limited range of motion and, sometimes, permanent deformity.

Bleeding near peripheral nerves may cause peripheral neuropathies, pain, paresthesia, and muscle atrophy. If bleeding impairs blood flow through a major vessel, it can cause ischemia and gangrene.

Signs and symptoms

Signs and symptoms vary with severity. Severe hemophilia causes spontaneous bleeding, with the first evidence commonly being excessive bleeding after circumcision. Later, spontaneous or severe bleeding after minor trauma may produce large subcutaneous and deep intramuscular hematomas.

Moderate hemophilia causes symptoms similar to severe hemophilia, but spontaneous bleeding occurs only occasionally.

Mild hemophilia commonly goes undiagnosed until adulthood because the patient doesn't bleed spontaneously or after minor trauma. Major trauma or surgery can cause prolonged bleeding; blood may ooze slowly or stop and start for up to 8 days after surgery. Patients with mild hemophilia have the best prognosis.

Patients with undiagnosed hemophilia usually complain of pain and swelling in a weight-bearing joint, such as the hip, knee, or ankle. The history may reveal prolonged bleeding after surgery, dental extractions, or injury. The patient also may have signs and symptoms of internal bleeding, such as:

▪ abdominal, chest, or flank pain
▪ hematuria (bloody urine) or hematemesis (bloody vomit)
▪ tarry stools.

Inspection may reveal hematomas on the limbs, torso, or both, and joint swelling if bleeding has occurred there.

The patient also may have evidence of decreased tissue perfusion, including:

▪ anxiety
▪ chest pain
▪ confusion
▪ cool, clammy skin
▪ decreased urine output
▪ hypotension
▪ pallor
▪ restlessness
▪ tachycardia.

Test results

Specific coagulation factor assays can be used to diagnose the type and severity of hemophilia. A family history can also aid in diagnosis. These test results help diagnose hemophilia A:

▪ Factor VIII assay reveals 0% to 25% of normal factor VIII.
▪ Partial thromboplastin time is prolonged.
▪ Platelet count and function, bleeding time, prothrombin time, and International Normalized Ratio are normal.

These test results help diagnose hemophilia B:

▪ Factor IX assay shows deficiency.
▪ Baseline coagulation result is similar to that of hemophilia A, with normal factor VIII.

Treatment

Hemophilia isn't curable but treatment can prevent crippling deformities and prolong life. Increasing plasma levels of deficient clotting

Hemophilia teaching topics

● Urge parents to protect their child from injury while avoiding restrictions that impair his normal development. For example, for a toddler, padded patches can be sewn into the knees and elbows of clothing to protect these joints during frequent falls. An older child must not participate in contact sports, such as football, but he can be encouraged to swim or play golf.
● If an injury occurs, direct the parents to apply cold compresses or ice bags and to elevate the injured part or apply light pressure to the bleeding. To prevent recurrence of bleeding after treatment, instruct parents to

restrict the child's activity for 48 hours after bleeding is under control.
● Tell parents to watch for signs of internal bleeding, such as severe pain and swelling in joints or muscles, stiffness, decreased joint movement, severe abdominal pain, blood in urine, tarry stools, and severe headache.
● Refer new patients to a hemophilia treatment center for evaluation. This center will devise a treatment plan for the patient's primary physician and is a resource for other medical and school personnel, dentists, and others involved in the patient's care. Explain that these centers also offer carrier testing, prenatal diagnosis, and other genetic counseling services.

factors helps prevent disabling deformities caused by repeated bleeding into muscles, joints, and organs.

CLOTTING FACTOR

In hemophilia A, normal hemostasis (arrest of bleeding) is obtained by giving cryoprecipitate antihemophilic factor (AHF) and lyophilized AHF (AHF that's been frozen and dehydrated under high vacuum). In hemophilia B, administration of recombinant factor VIII and purified factor IX promotes hemostasis. Doses should be large enough to raise clotting factor levels, which must be kept within the desired range until the wound heals.

Fresh frozen plasma can also be given but it has drawbacks, such as the potential for volume overload and a transfusion reaction.

A hemophiliac who undergoes surgery needs factor replacement before and after the procedure. This may be needed even for minor surgery such as a dental extraction.

OTHER TREATMENTS

Joint pain may be controlled with an analgesic. Don't give the drug by I.M. injection because a hematoma may form at the site. Never give aspirin or aspirin-containing drugs because they decrease platelet adherence and may increase bleeding.

To help avoid injury, young children should wear clothing with padded patches on the knees and elbows. Older children should avoid contact sports such as football. Warn parents to notify the physician immediately after even a minor injury, especially to the head, neck, or abdomen. Early recognition is the key to stopping bleeding. (See *Hemophilia teaching topics.*)

MARFAN SYNDROME

Marfan syndrome is an inherited disease of connective tissue that causes mainly ocular, skeletal, and cardiovascular anomalies. Signs and symptoms range from mild to severe. The disorder affects about 1 in 5,000 people in the United States, men and women equally.

Pathophysiology

This disorder is inherited as an autosomal dominant trait. Patients are heterozygous for the mutation, which means that they have one gene with the mutation and one normal gene.

Marfan syndrome has been mapped to a specific chromosome location: chromosome 15 (of the 22 autosomes in the human cell). On this chromosome, more than 20 mutations have been identified that can occur in a gene that codes for fibrillin, a component of connective tissue. These small fibers are abundant in the large blood vessels and the suspensory ligaments of the ocular lenses. The exact function of fibrillin is unknown.

 RED FLAG *Possible complications of Marfan syndrome include:*

■ *weak joints and ligaments (predisposing to injury)*
■ *cataracts caused by lens displacement*
■ *retinal detachments and tears*
■ *severe mitral valve regurgitation caused by mitral valve prolapse*
■ *spontaneous pneumothorax caused by chest wall instability*
■ *inguinal and incisional hernias*
■ *dilation of the dural sac (portion of the dura mater beyond the caudal end of the spinal cord).*

Signs and symptoms

Genetic mutations in Marfan syndrome may cause functional and structural changes. Skeletal malformations include:

■ increased height (patients are usually taller than family members)
■ unusually long limbs
■ arachnodactyly—a spiderlike appearance of the hands and fingers

- chest depression (pectus excavatum)
- chest protrusion (pectus carinatum)
- chest asymmetry
- scoliosis and kyphosis
- arched palate
- joint hypermobility.

Lens displacement usually isn't progressive but it may contribute to cataract formation. An elongated ocular globe causes nearsightedness in most patients. Retinal detachments and retinal tears also may develop. Most patients have adequate vision with corrective lenses.

Cardiovascular abnormalities are the most serious consequences of Marfan syndrome. They may involve valves and aorta. Valvular abnormalities result from anatomic defects, such as redundancy to the leaflets, stretching of the chordae tendineae, and calcification of the mitral annulus.

Mitral valve prolapse (dropping down of the cusps of the mitral valve into the left atrium during systole) develops early in life. It can progress to severe mitral valve regurgitation (backflow of blood from the left ventricle into the left atrium).

Dilation of the aortic root and ascending aorta may cause aortic regurgitation (backflow of blood into the left ventricle), dissection (separation of the layers of the aortic wall), and rupture. In adults, dilation may be accelerated by physical and emotional stress as well as by pregnancy.

Marfan syndrome also may cause:
- a thin body build with little subcutaneous fat
- striae over the shoulders and buttocks
- spontaneous pneumothorax
- inguinal and incisional hernias
- dilation of the dural sac.

Test results
- No laboratory tests can be used to diagnose Marfan syndrome.
- Diagnostic tests based on detection of fibrillin defects in cultured skin fibroblasts or DNA analysis of the gene may be available in the near future.
- Diagnosis may be made through physical examination if the patient has skeletal involvement and at least two other systems are affected.
- Diagnosis also may be made if only two body systems are involved and there's a documented family history of Marfan syndrome.

TEACHING FOCUS

Marfan syndrome teaching topics

● Instruct high school and college athletes (particularly basketball players) who fit the criteria for Marfan syndrome to undergo a careful clinical and cardiac examination before participating in sports. Those who don't do so may have a risk of sudden death from dissecting aortic aneurysm or other cardiac complications.

● Refer a female patient with Marfan syndrome to genetic counseling because pregnancy and the increased cardiovascular workload it causes can produce aortic rupture.

■ Diagnosis of ectopia lentis is made by pupillary dilation and slit lamp examination.

■ Cardiac problems may be discovered by an echocardiogram.

Treatment

No established treatment exists for Marfan syndrome.

Propranolol (Inderal) or other beta blockers may delay or prevent aortic dilation. Surgery to repair the aorta may be needed. Surgical replacement of the aortic and mitral valves has been successful in some patients. (See *Marfan syndrome teaching topics*.)

Scoliosis is progressive and should be treated accordingly. If the curvature is greater than 20 degrees, treatment includes mechanical bracing and physical therapy. If the curvature progresses beyond 45 degrees, the patient may need surgery.

PHENYLKETONURIA

Phenylketonuria (PKU) is an inborn error in metabolism of the amino acid phenylalanine. It causes high serum levels of phenylalanine and increased urine levels of phenylalanine and its by-products. It results in cerebral damage and mental retardation.

The disorder occurs in about 1 of 14,000 births in the United States. About 1 person in 60 is an asymptomatic carrier. PKU is less common among Blacks and Ashkenazic Jews and more common among Whites and Native Americans.

Pathophysiology

PKU is transmitted through an autosomal recessive gene. People with classic PKU have almost no activity of phenylalanine hydroxylase, an enzyme that helps convert phenylalanine to tyrosine. As a result, phenylalanine accumulates in blood and urine, and tyrosine levels are low.

Patients may have a family history of PKU. Usually, no abnormalities are apparent at birth, when blood phenylalanine levels are essentially normal. Within a few days, levels begin to rise. By the time they reach about 30 mg/dl, cerebral damage has begun. Irreversible damage is probably complete by age 2 or 3, although early detection and treatment can minimize it.

 RED FLAG *Phenylalanine accumulation causes mental retardation.*

Signs and symptoms

By age 4 months, the untreated child begins to show signs of arrested brain development, including mental retardation. Later, personality disturbances occur, such as:
■ schizoid and antisocial behavior
■ an uncontrollable temper.

About one-third of patients have seizures, which usually begin between ages 6 and 12 months. Many patients also show a marked decrease in IQ.

Other signs include:
■ macrocephaly
■ eczematous skin lesions or dry, rough skin
■ hyperactivity
■ irritability
■ purposeless
■ repetitive motions
■ an awkward gait
■ possibly a musty odor caused by skin and urine excretion of phenylacetic acid.

Test results

Several tests are used to diagnose PKU.
■ The Guthrie screening test on a capillary blood sample reliably detects PKU and is required by most states at birth. However, because phenylalanine levels may be normal at birth, infants should be reevaluated 24 to 48 hours after they begin protein feedings.
■ Fluorometric or chromatographic assays provide additional diagnostic information.
■ EEG is abnormal in about 80% of untreated affected children.
■ DNA-based tests are used in prenatal diagnosis of PKU.

TEACHING FOCUS

Phenylketonuria teaching topics

● Teach the child and his parents about the critical importance of sticking to his diet. Encourage compliance with the frequent blood tests needed to evaluate the effectiveness of the prescribed diet.

● Teach parents about normal physical and mental growth and development to help them recognize any developmental delay from excessive phenylalanine intake.

● As the child grows older and is supervised less closely, his parents have less control over what he eats. As a result, deviation from the restricted diet becomes more likely, as does the risk of further brain damage. Encourage parents to give the child some choices in the kinds of low-protein foods he eats; this will help make him feel trusted and more responsible.

Treatment

To prevent or minimize brain damage from PKU, phenylalanine blood levels should be kept between 3 and 15 mg/dl by restricting dietary intake of phenylalanine. Dietary restrictions with supplementation will be needed for life. A special, low-phenylalanine amino acid mixture is substituted for most dietary protein, supplemented with a small amount of natural foods. (See *Phenylketonuria teaching topics*.)

DIETARY RESTRICTIONS

Patients must avoid:
■ aspartame
■ bread
■ cheese
■ eggs
■ fish
■ flour
■ legumes
■ meat
■ milk
■ nuts
■ poultry.

Even with this diet, central nervous system dysfunction may occur. Frequent tests for urine phenylpyruvic acid and blood phenylalanine levels evaluate the diet's effectiveness. Patients also need careful monitoring because overzealous dietary restrictions can induce phenylalanine deficiency, which causes:

■ lethargy
■ anorexia
■ anemia
■ rashes
■ diarrhea
■ death.

SICKLE CELL ANEMIA

Sickle cell anemia is a congenital hematologic disease that causes impaired circulation, chronic ill health, and premature death. It's most common in people of African descent, but it also occurs in Puerto Rico, Turkey, India, the Middle East, and the Mediterranean.

If two carriers have offspring, each child has a one in four chance of developing the disease. In the United States, more than 70,000 people have sickle cell disease. About 1 in 10 Blacks carries the abnormal gene, and 1 in every 400 to 600 black children has sickle cell anemia.

In the past, many people with this disease died in their early 20s. Today, the average life expectancy is age 45, with 40% to 50% of patients living into their 40s and 50s.

Pathophysiology

Sickle cell anemia results from homozygous inheritance of an autosomal recessive gene mutation that encodes the beta chain of hemoglobin and produces a defective hemoglobin molecule (hemoglobin S). Hemoglobin S causes red blood cells (RBCs) to become sickle shaped. A single amino acid change from glutamic acid to valine occurs in the sixth position of the beta-hemoglobin chain. (See *Distinguishing sickled and normal cells.*)

Sickle cell trait, which results from heterozygous inheritance of this gene mutation, causes few or no symptoms. Those who have sickle cell trait are carriers and can pass the gene to their children. This gene mutation may have persisted because the heterozygous sickle cell trait provides resistance to malaria.

In sickle cell anemia, when hypoxia (oxygen deficiency) occurs, several things happen:

■ Hemoglobin S in the RBCs becomes insoluble.
■ As a result, blood cells become rigid and rough, forming an elongated crescent, or sickle, shape. Sickling can cause hemolysis (cell destruction).

Distinguishing sickled and normal cells

Normal red blood cells (RBCs) and sickled cells vary in more ways than shape. They also differ in life span, oxygen-carrying capacity, and the rate at which they're destroyed.

NORMAL RBCS

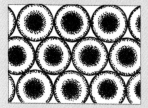

SICKLED RBCS

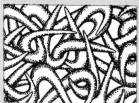

- 120-day life span
- Normal oxygen-carrying capacity
- 12 to 14 g of hemoglobin (Hb) per milliliter
- Destroyed at a normal rate

- 30- to 40-day life span
- Decreased oxygen-carrying capacity
- 6 to 9 g of Hb per milliliter
- Destroyed at an accelerated rate

■ Sickle cells also accumulate in capillaries and smaller blood vessels, causing occlusions and increasing blood viscosity.

■ This impairs circulation, causing pain, tissue death, swelling, and anoxic changes that lead to further sickling and obstruction.

Each patient with sickle cell anemia has a different hypoxic threshold and different factors that trigger a sickle cell crisis. In most patients, they include:

■ illness

■ cold exposure

■ stress

■ anything that induces an acidotic state

■ any pathophysiologic process that pulls water out of sickle cells. (See *Understanding sickle cell crisis*, page 136.)

 RED FLAG *Complications of sickle cell anemia may include:*

■ *retinopathy, nephropathy, and cerebral vessel occlusion caused by organ infarction*

■ *hypovolemic shock and death from massive entrapment of cells*

■ *necrosis*

■ *infection and gangrene.*

Understanding sickle cell crisis

Sickle cell crisis is triggered by infection, cold exposure, high altitudes, overexertion, and other conditions that cause cellular oxygen deprivation. Here's what happens:

● Deoxygenated, sickle-shaped erythrocytes stick to the capillary wall and to one another, blocking blood flow and causing cellular hypoxia.

● The crisis worsens as tissue hypoxia and acidic waste products cause more sickling and cell damage.

● With each new crisis, organs and tissues are destroyed and areas of tissue die slowly – especially in the spleen and kidneys.

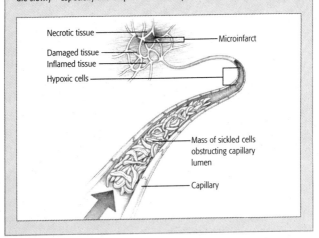

Signs and symptoms

Signs and symptoms of sickle cell anemia usually don't develop until after age 6 months because large amounts of fetal hemoglobin protect infants until then. Fetal hemoglobin has a higher oxygen concentration and inhibits sickling.

The patient's history includes:
▪ chronic fatigue
▪ unexplained dyspnea or dyspnea on exertion
▪ joint swelling
▪ aching bones
▪ severe localized and generalized pain
▪ leg ulcers (especially on the ankles)
▪ frequent infections

■ priapism (unexplained, painful erections) in men.

In sickle cell crisis, symptoms include:

■ severe pain
■ hematuria
■ lethargy
■ irritability
■ pale lips, tongue, palms, and nail beds.

Various types of sickle cell crises can occur, including painful crisis, aplastic crisis, acute sequestration crisis, and hemolytic crisis. Painful crisis is the hallmark of sickle cell anemia, appearing periodically after age 5. It results from blood vessel obstruction by rigid, tangled sickle cells, leading to tissue anoxia and, possibly, necrosis. It's characterized by severe abdominal, thoracic, muscle, or bone pain and, possibly, worsened jaundice, dark urine, and a low-grade fever.

Aplastic crisis results from bone marrow depression and is linked to infection (usually viral). It's characterized by pallor, lethargy, sleepiness, dyspnea, possible coma, markedly decreased bone marrow activity, and RBC hemolysis (destruction).

Acute sequestration crisis (rare) occurs in infants between ages 8 months and 2 years and may cause sudden, massive entrapment of RBCs in the spleen and liver. Lethargy and pallor progress to hypovolemic shock and death if untreated.

Hemolytic crisis (rare) usually affects patients who have glucose-6-phosphate dehydrogenase deficiency along with sickle cell anemia. It probably results from complications of sickle cell anemia, such as infection, rather than from the disease itself. In this crisis, degenerative changes cause liver congestion and enlargement, and chronic jaundice worsens.

Test results

■ A family history and typical clinical features suggest sickle cell anemia.
■ These tests confirm the disease:
  – Stained blood smear shows sickle cells.
  – Hemoglobin electrophoresis shows hemoglobin S.
■ Additional blood tests show:
  – low RBC counts
  – increased white blood cell and platelet counts
  – decreased erythrocyte sedimentation rate
  – increased serum iron levels
  – decreased RBC survival
  – reticulocytosis

TEACHING FOCUS

Sickle cell anemia teaching topics

- Urge the patient to avoid strenuous exercise, vasoconstricting drugs, cold temperatures, unpressurized aircraft, high altitudes, and conditions that provoke hypoxia.
- Stress the importance of meticulous wound care, good oral hygiene, regular dental and eye checkups, and a balanced diet as safeguards against infection.
- Advise the patient to maintain a high fluid intake to prevent dehydration.

- Recommend that family members be screened to find out if they're heterozygous carriers of the sickle cell trait.
- Warn a female patient that both pregnancy and hormonal contraceptives can pose risks for her. Refer her to a gynecologist for birth control counseling.
- Inform a male patient that he may experience sudden, painful episodes of priapism (abnormal erection of the penis). Frequent or severe episodes may lead to impotence.

  – low or normal hemoglobin levels.
■ Lateral chest X-ray detects the "Lincoln log" deformity in the vertebrae of many adults and some adolescents.

Treatment

Treatment aims to alleviate symptoms and prevent painful crises. Warm compresses and analgesics, such as hydromorphone (Dilaudid) or morphine may help relieve the pain from vaso-occlusive crises.

Hydroxyurea (Hydrea), an antitumor drug, may help reduce painful episodes in adults with severe sickle cell anemia (at least three painful crises in the previous year). It works by inducing formation of fetal hemoglobin — a hemoglobin normally found in the fetus or neonate. When present in patients with sickle cell anemia, fetal hemoglobin prevents sickling. Patients receiving hydroxyurea must be monitored closely to make sure their blood count isn't depressed to a level that places them at risk for bleeding or infection.

I.V. therapy may be needed to prevent dehydration and vessel occlusion. Encourage the patient to drink plenty of fluids.

Iron and folic acid supplements may help prevent anemia. If the patient's hemoglobin level drops, blood transfusions may be needed. (See *Sickle cell anemia teaching topics.*)

Complications resulting from the disease and from transfusion therapy may be reduced using:

■ certain vaccines
■ anti-infectives such as low-dose penicillin (Bicillin)
■ chelating agents such as deferoxamine (Desferal).

TAY-SACHS DISEASE

Tay-Sachs disease results from a congenital enzyme deficiency. It causes progressive mental and motor deterioration and is always fatal, usually before age 5.

This disorder occurs in fewer than 100 infants born each year in the United States. It strikes people of Ashkenazic Jewish ancestry about 100 times more often than the general population. In this ethnic group, it occurs in about 1 of 3,600 live births. About 1 in 30 are heterozygous carriers of the defective gene. If two carriers have children, each of their offspring has a 25% chance of having Tay-Sachs disease.

Pathophysiology

Tay-Sachs disease is an autosomal recessive disorder in which the enzyme hexosaminidase A is deficient. Hexosaminidase A is needed for metabolism of gangliosides — water-soluble glycolipids found mainly in tissues of the central nervous system (CNS). Without hexosaminidase A, accumulating lipid pigments distend and progressively demyelinate (remove the protective myelin sheath) and destroy CNS cells.

RED FLAG Complications of Tay-Sachs disease may include blindness, generalized paralysis, and recurrent bronchopneumonia (usually fatal by age 5).

Signs and symptoms

The child usually looks normal at birth. Abnormal clinical signs appear between ages 5 and 6 months, when progressive weakness of the neck, trunk, arm, and leg muscles prevents him from sitting up or lifting his head. He has trouble turning over, can't grasp objects, and has vision loss progressing to blindness. He's easily startled by loud sounds.

By age 18 months the patient may have seizures, generalized paralysis, and spasticity. His pupils are always dilated. Although blind, he may hold his eyes wide open and roll his eyeballs. Decerebrate rigidity and a complete vegetative state follow.

Around age 2, the patient contracts recurrent bronchopneumonia, caused by diminished protective reflexes. Other findings include an enlarged head circumference, optic nerve atrophy, and a distinctive cherry red spot on the retina.

TEACHING FOCUS

Tay-Sachs disease teaching topics

● If parents plan to care for their child at home, teach them how to do suctioning, postural drainage, and tube feedings. Refer them to home health agencies and for hospice care as appropriate.
● Teach parents how to provide skin care to prevent pressure ulcers.

Test results

■ Serum analysis shows deficient hexosaminidase A in affected infants.
■ A simple blood test can identify carriers.
■ Carrier screening is offered to all couples in which one or both are of Ashkenazic Jewish ancestry and for others with a family history of the disease.

Treatment

Tay-Sachs disease has no cure; treatment is supportive. (See *Tay-Sachs disease teaching topics*.) Most children with Tay-Sachs disease are treated at home with the aid of hospice care. Anticonvulsants usually don't prevent seizures. Care includes:
■ tube feedings with nutritional supplements
■ suctioning and postural drainage to remove secretions
■ skin care to prevent pressure ulcers when the child becomes bedridden
■ mild laxatives to relieve neurogenic constipation.

6

ENDOCRINE SYSTEM

Understanding the endocrine system

The endocrine system consists of glands, specialized cell clusters, and hormones, which are chemical transmitters secreted by the glands in response to stimulation. Together with the central nervous system (CNS), the endocrine system regulates and integrates the body's metabolic activities and maintains homeostasis.

The hypothalamus is the integrative center for the endocrine and autonomic (involuntary) nervous systems. It helps control some endocrine glands by neural and hormonal pathways. Neural pathways connect the hypothalamus to the posterior pituitary gland; stimulation of this gland causes secretion of two effector hormones: antidiuretic hormone (ADH) and oxytocin. When ADH is secreted, the body retains water. Oxytocin stimulates uterine contractions during labor and milk secretion in lactating women..

Hormonal pathways allow the hypothalamus to affect the anterior pituitary gland. Hypothalamic hormones stimulate the anterior pituitary gland to release four types of trophic (gland-stimulating) hormones:

- adrenocorticotropic hormone (ACTH), also called corticotropin
- thyroid-stimulating hormone (TSH)
- luteinizing hormone (LH)
- follicle-stimulating hormone (FSH).

Secretion of trophic hormones stimulates their respective target glands, such as the adrenal cortex, thyroid gland, and gonads.

Hypothalamic hormones also control the release of hormones from the pituitary gland. Examples are growth hormone (GH) and prolactin. A negative feedback system regulates the endocrine system by inhibiting hormone overproduction. This system may be simple or complex.

Simple feedback occurs when the level of one substance regulates secretion of hormones. For example, a low serum calcium level

141

stimulates the parathyroid gland to release parathyroid hormone (PTH). PTH, in turn, promotes resorption of calcium. A high serum calcium level inhibits PTH secretion.

Complex feedback occurs when the hypothalamus receives feedback from the target glands in a more complicated mechanism. It works through an axis established between the hypothalamus, pituitary, and target organ. For example, secretion of the hypothalamic corticotropin-releasing hormone stimulates release of pituitary corticotropin, which in turn stimulates cortisol secretion by the adrenal gland (the target organ). A rise in serum cortisol level inhibits corticotropin secretion by decreasing the level of corticotropin-releasing hormone.

A patient with a possible endocrine disorder needs careful assessment to identify the cause of the dysfunction. Dysfunction may result from defects in:

■ the gland
■ release of trophic or effector hormones
■ hormone transport
■ the target tissue.

Endocrine disorders may be caused by:

■ hypersecretion or hyposecretion of hormones
■ hyporesponsiveness of hormone receptors
■ inflammation of glands
■ gland tumors.

Hypersecretion or hyposecretion may originate in the hypothalamus, the pituitary effector glands, or the target gland. Regardless of origin, the result is abnormal hormone concentrations in the blood. Hypersecretion leads to elevated levels. Hyposecretion leads to deficient levels.

In hyporesponsiveness, the cells of the target organ don't have appropriate receptors for a hormone. This means the effects of the hormone aren't detected. Because receptors don't detect the hormone, there's no feedback mechanism to turn the hormone off, and blood levels of the hormone are normal or high. Hyporesponsiveness causes the same clinical symptoms as hyposecretion.

Inflammation is usually chronic, commonly resulting in glandular secretion of hormones. However, it may be acute or subacute, as in thyroiditis.

Tumors can occur within a gland, as in thyroid carcinoma. In addition, tumors occurring in other areas of the body can cause abnormal hormone production (ectopic hormone production). For example, certain lung tumors secrete ADH or PTH.

GLANDS

The endocrine glands release hormones into the circulatory system, which distributes them throughout the body. (See *Endocrine system components,* page 144.) Glands discussed here include:

▪ adrenal glands
▪ pancreas
▪ pituitary gland
▪ thyroid gland
▪ parathyroid glands.

Adrenal glands

The adrenal glands produce steroids, amines, epinephrine, and norepinephrine. Hyposecretion or hypersecretion of these substances causes a variety of disorders and complications that range from psychiatric and sexual problems to coma and death. The adrenal cortex is the outer layer of the adrenal gland. It secretes three types of steroidal hormones:

▪ mineralocorticoids such as aldosterone
▪ glucocorticoids such as cortisol
▪ adrenal androgens and estrogens.

Aldosterone maintains extracellular fluid volume by regulating reabsorption of sodium and excretion of potassium by the kidneys. It may be involved with other hormones in the development of hypertension.

Cortisol carries out five important functions, including:

▪ stimulation of gluconeogenesis (formation of glycogen from non-carbohydrate sources), which occurs in the liver in response to low carbohydrate intake or starvation
▪ breakdown of increased protein and mobilization of free fatty-acid
▪ suppression of immune response
▪ assistance with stress response
▪ assistance with maintenance of blood pressure and cardiovascular function.

Androgens (male sex hormones) promote male traits, especially secondary sex characteristics. Examples of such characteristics are facial hair and a low-pitched voice. Estrogens promote female traits. They are also thought to be responsible for sex drive.

The adrenal medulla is the inner portion of the adrenal gland. It's an aggregate of nerve tissue that produces the catecholamine hormones epinephrine and norepinephrine that cause vasoconstriction. Epinephrine causes the response to physical or emotional stress called the fight-or-flight response. This response produces

Endocrine system components

Endocrine glands secrete hormones directly into the bloodstream to regulate body function. This illustration shows the location of all major endocrine glands except the gonads.

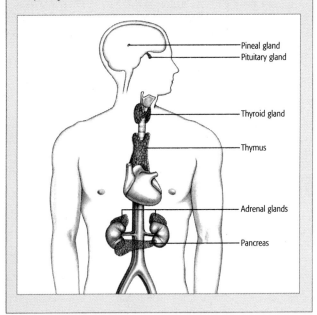

Pineal gland
Pituitary gland
Thyroid gland
Thymus
Adrenal glands
Pancreas

marked dilation of bronchioles and increased blood pressure, blood glucose level, and heart rate.

Pancreas

The pancreas produces the hormones glucagon and insulin. Glucagon is released during a fasting state. It stimulates release of stored glucose from the liver to raise blood glucose levels.

Insulin is released during a postprandial (fed) state. It aids glucose transport into the cells and promotes glucose storage. It also stimulates protein synthesis and enhances free fatty acid uptake and storage. Insulin deficiency or resistance causes diabetes mellitus.

Pituitary gland

The posterior pituitary gland, located at the base of the brain, secretes two effector hormones:

■ oxytocin, which stimulates uterine contractions during labor and causes the milk letdown reflex in lactating women

■ ADH, which controls the concentration of body fluids by altering the permeability of the distal renal tubules and collecting ducts in the kidneys, thereby conserving water.

ADH secretion depends on plasma osmolality (concentration), which is monitored by hypothalamic neurons. Hypovolemia and hypotension are the most powerful stimulators of ADH release. Other stimulators include pain, stress, trauma, nausea, and the use of morphine, tranquilizers, certain anesthetics, and a positive-pressure breathing apparatus.

The anterior pituitary gland secretes trophic hormones, prolactin, and GH. Trophic hormones include ACTH, TSH, LH, and FSH. Prolactin stimulates milk secretion in lactating women. GH triggers growth in most body tissues by increasing protein production and fat mobilization and decreasing carbohydrate use.

Thyroid gland

The thyroid gland, located in the anterior neck, secretes the iodine-containing hormones thyroxine (T_4) and triiodothyronine (T_3). Thyroid hormones are needed for normal growth and development. They also act on many tissues by increasing metabolic activity and protein synthesis.

Diseases of the thyroid are caused by thyroid hormone overproduction or deficiency and gland inflammation and enlargement. Most patients have a good prognosis with treatment. Untreated, thyroid disease may progress to an emergency known as thyroid crisis or storm. It also can cause irreversible disabilities such as vision loss.

Parathyroid glands

Four parathyroid glands are located behind the thyroid gland. These glands secrete PTH, which helps regulate calcium levels and control bone formation.

Disorders of the parathyroid gland involve hyposecretion or hypersecretion of PTH. Hyposecretion of PTH results in decreased serum calcium levels that may lead to tetany and seizures. Hypersecretion of PTH results in increased serum calcium levels that may lead to cardiac arrhythmias, muscle and bone weakness, and renal calculi.

Endocrine disorders

Endocrine disorders discussed in this chapter include:
▪ two adrenal disorders
  – Addison's disease
  – Cushing's syndrome
▪ a pituitary disorder of water metabolism
  – diabetes insipidus
▪ a pancreatic disorder
  – diabetes mellitus
▪ three thyroid gland disorders
  – goiter
  – hyperthyroidism
  – hypothyroidism.

ADDISON'S DISEASE

This relatively uncommon disorder, also called adrenal hypofunction or adrenal insufficiency, occurs in people of all ages and both sexes. It occurs in two forms: primary and secondary. Either form may progress to adrenal crisis.

The primary form of Addison's disease originates in the adrenal glands. It's characterized by decreased mineralocorticoid, glucocorticoid, and androgen secretion. The secondary form of Addison's disease is caused by a disorder outside the gland, such as a pituitary tumor with corticotropin deficiency. In secondary forms of the disorder, aldosterone secretion may be unaffected.

Adrenal crisis, also known as addisonian crisis, is a critical deficiency of mineralocorticoids and glucocorticoids. It's a medical emergency that requires immediate, vigorous treatment. (See *Understanding adrenal crisis,* pages 148 and 149.)

Pathophysiology

PRIMARY ADDISON'S DISEASE

In this form of the disease, more than 90% of both adrenal glands are destroyed. This massive destruction usually results from an autoimmune process in which circulating antibodies attack adrenal tissue. Destruction of the gland also may be idiopathic (no known cause). Other causes of primary Addison's disease include:
▪ tuberculosis
▪ removal of both adrenal glands
▪ hemorrhage into the adrenal gland
▪ neoplasms

■ infections, such as human immunodeficiency virus infection, histoplasmosis, meningococcal pneumonia, and cytomegalovirus (CMV).

Rarely, a familial tendency toward autoimmune disease predisposes a patient to Addison's disease and other endocrine disorders. Signs and symptoms result from decreased glucocorticoid production. They may develop slowly and stay unrecognized if production is adequate for the normal demands of life. They may progress to adrenal crisis if trauma, surgery, or other severe physical stress exhausts the body's store of glucocorticoids.

SECONDARY ADDISON'S DISEASE

This form of Addison's disease may result from:

■ hypopituitarism, which may lead to decreased corticotropin secretion (Usually it occurs when long-term corticosteroid therapy is abruptly stopped, because such therapy suppresses pituitary corticotropin secretion and causes adrenal gland atrophy.)

■ removal of a nonendocrine corticotropin-secreting tumor

■ disorders of hypothalamic-pituitary function that decrease corticotropin production.

RED FLAG *Possible complications of Addison's disease include:*

■ *hyperpyrexia*

■ *psychotic reactions*

■ *shock*

■ *profound hypoglycemia*

■ *if left untreated, vascular collapse, renal shutdown, coma, and death.*

Signs and symptoms

These signs and symptoms may indicate Addison's disease:

■ confusion

■ fatigue

■ GI disturbances and weight loss

■ hyperkalemia

■ hyperpigmentation

■ hypoglycemia

■ hyponatremia

■ hypotension

■ muscle weakness.

The patient's history may reveal:

■ synthetic steroid use

■ adrenal surgery

Understanding adrenal crisis

Adrenal crisis (acute adrenal insufficiency) is the most serious complication of Addison's disease. It may occur gradually or suddenly.

WHO'S AT RISK
This potentially lethal condition usually develops in patients who:
● don't respond to hormone replacement therapy
● undergo extreme stress without adequate glucocorticoid replacement
● stop hormone therapy abruptly
● undergo trauma
● undergo bilateral adrenalectomy
● develop adrenal gland thrombosis after a severe infection (Waterhouse-Friderichsen syndrome).

WHAT HAPPENS
In adrenal crisis, destruction of the adrenal cortex leads to a rapid decline in the steroid hormones cortisol and aldosterone. This directly affects the liver, stomach, and kidneys. This flowchart illustrates what happens in adrenal crisis.

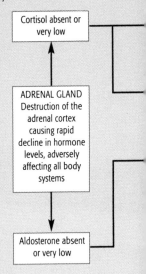

Cortisol absent or very low

ADRENAL GLAND
Destruction of the adrenal cortex causing rapid decline in hormone levels, adversely affecting all body systems

Aldosterone absent or very low

■ recent infection.

The patient may complain of:
■ fatigue
■ light-headedness when rising from a chair or bed
■ cravings for salty food
■ decreased tolerance for even minor stress
■ anxiety and irritability
■ various GI disturbances, such as nausea, vomiting, anorexia, and chronic diarrhea.

The patient also may have reduced urine output and other symptoms of dehydration.

Women may have decreased libido from reduced androgen production and amenorrhea.

Examination may reveal:
■ poor coordination
■ dry skin and mucous membranes

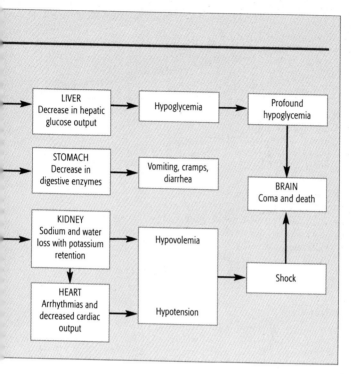

- sparse axillary and pubic hair in women
- deep bronze skin, especially in the creases of the hands and on the knuckles, elbows, and knees
- darkening of scars
- areas of vitiligo (an absence of pigmentation)
- increased pigmentation of the mucous membranes, especially in the mouth.

Abnormal coloration results from decreased secretion of cortisol, which causes the pituitary gland to secrete excessive amounts of melanocyte-stimulating hormone (MSH) and corticotropin. Secondary adrenal hypofunction doesn't cause hyperpigmentation because corticotropin and MSH levels are low.

Test results

These laboratory tests are used in diagnosing adrenal hypofunction:

■ Plasma and urine tests detect decreased corticosteroid concentrations.

■ Measurement of corticotropin levels classifies the disease as primary or secondary. A high level indicates the primary disorder, and a low level points to the secondary disorder.

■ Rapid corticotropin test (ACTH stimulation test) shows plasma cortisol response to corticotropin. After obtaining plasma cortisol samples, an I.V. infusion of cosyntropin is given. Plasma samples are taken 30 and 60 minutes later. If the cortisol level doesn't increase, adrenal insufficiency is suspected.

In a patient with typical symptoms of Addison's disease, these laboratory findings strongly suggest adrenal crisis:

■ reduced serum sodium levels

■ increased serum potassium, serum calcium, and blood urea nitrogen levels

■ increased hematocrit and lymphocyte and eosinophil counts

■ X-rays showing a small heart and adrenal calcification

■ decreased plasma cortisol levels — less than 10 mcg/dl in the morning with lower levels at night. (Because this test is time-consuming, crisis therapy shouldn't be delayed while waiting for results.)

Treatment

With early diagnosis and treatment, the prognosis is good for either form of Addison's disease. Lifelong corticosteroid replacement is the main treatment for patients with primary or secondary Addison's disease.

■ In general, cortisone (Cortone) or hydrocortisone (Hydrocortone) is given because they have a mineralocorticoid effect.

■ Fludrocortisone (Florinef), a synthetic drug that acts as a mineralocorticoid, also may be given to prevent dehydration and hypotension.

■ Women with muscle weakness and decreased libido may benefit from testosterone injections but they risk masculinizing effects.

■ In stressful situations, the patient may need to double or triple the usual corticosteroid dose. These situations include acute illness (because a fever increases the basal metabolic rate), injury, or psychologically stressful times. (See *Addison's disease teaching topics.*)

CRISIS CONTROL

Treatment for adrenal crisis involves prompt I.V. bolus administration of hydrocortisone followed by hydrocortisone diluted with dex-

TEACHING FOCUS

Addison's disease teaching topics

- Explain that the patient will need lifelong steroid therapy. Teach the patient and family members to identify and report evidence of overdose (weight gain and edema) or underdose (fatigue, weakness, and dizziness).
- Caution against stopping the drug suddenly because doing so can cause adrenal crisis.
- Advise the patient to increase the dosage during times of stress (when

he has a cold, for example), as prescribed.
- Warn that infection, injury, or profuse sweating in hot weather can cause adrenal crisis.
- Instruct the patient to take steroids with antacids or meals to minimize gastric irritation. Suggest taking two-thirds of the dosage in the morning and the remaining one-third in the early afternoon to mimic diurnal adrenal gland secretion.

trose in normal saline solution until the patient's condition stabilizes. Up to 300 mg/day of hydrocortisone and 3 to 5 L of I.V. normal saline solution may be required during the acute stage.

If the patient has hyperkalemia, treatment may include I.V. administration of insulin with dextrose in normal saline solution to shift potassium back into the cells, reducing the serum level.

With proper treatment, the crisis usually subsides quickly, with blood pressure stabilizing and water and sodium levels returning to normal. Afterward, maintenance doses of hydrocortisone keep the patient's condition stable.

CUSHING'S SYNDROME

Cushing's syndrome is a cluster of physical abnormalities caused by excess glucocorticoid secretion by the adrenal glands. It also may be caused by excessive androgen secretion. When glucocorticoid excess is caused by pituitary-dependent conditions, it's called Cushing's syndrome.

Pathophysiology

Cushing's syndrome appears in three forms:
- primary, caused by a disease of the adrenal cortex
- secondary, caused by hyperfunction of corticotropin-secreting cells of the anterior pituitary gland
- tertiary, caused by hypothalamic dysfunction or injury.

In about 70% of patients, Cushing's syndrome results from an excess of corticotropin. This leads to hyperplasia (excessive cell proliferation) of the adrenal cortex. Corticotropin overproduction may stem from:

■ pituitary hypersecretion (Cushing's disease)
■ a corticotropin-producing tumor in another organ, especially a malignant tumor of the pancreas or bronchus
■ administration of synthetic glucocorticoids.

In the remaining 30% of patients, Cushing's syndrome results from a cortisol-secreting adrenal tumor, which is usually benign. In infants, the usual cause is adrenal carcinoma. Giving steroids during treatment can also lead to Cushing's syndrome.

RED FLAG Complications of Cushing's syndrome are caused by the effects of cortisol, the principal glucocorticoid. These complications may include:

■ *osteoporosis and pathologic fractures from increased calcium resorption from bone*
■ *peptic ulcer from increased gastric secretions, pepsin production, and decreased gastric mucus*
■ *lipidosis (a disorder of fat metabolism)*
■ *impaired glucose tolerance from increased hepatic gluconeogenesis and insulin resistance*
■ *frequent infections or slow wound healing from decreased lymphocyte production and suppressed antibody formation, which may mask infection*
■ *hypertension from sodium and water retention, which may lead to ischemic heart disease and heart failure*
■ *menstrual disturbances and sexual dysfunction from increased adrenal androgen secretion*
■ *decreased ability to handle stress, which may lead to mental problems ranging from mood swings to psychosis.*

Signs and symptoms

A patient with some or all of these signs may have Cushing's syndrome:

■ broad purple striae
■ bruising
■ buffalo hump
■ fatigue
■ hirsutism
■ impaired wound healing
■ moon face and ruddy complexion
■ muscle weakness and atrophy

- thin, fragile skin
- thinning limbs with muscle wasting and fat mobilization
- thinning scalp hair
- truncal obesity
- weight gain.

Test results
- Diagnosis of Cushing's syndrome depends on a demonstrated increase in cortisol production and failure to suppress endogenous cortisol secretion after dexamethasone is given.
- Plasma ACTH level determines whether Cushing's syndrome is ACTH-dependent.
- A low-dose dexamethasone suppression test or 24-hour urine test determines the free cortisol excretion rate. Failure to suppress plasma and urine cortisol levels confirms the diagnosis.
- A high-dose dexamethasone suppression test determines whether Cushing's syndrome results from pituitary dysfunction. If dexamethasone suppresses plasma cortisol levels, the test result is positive. Failure to suppress plasma cortisol levels indicates an adrenal tumor or a nonendocrine, corticotropin-secreting tumor. This test can produce false-positive results.
- Radiologic evaluation may locate a tumor in the pituitary or adrenal glands. Tests include:
  - ultrasonography
  - computed tomography (CT) scan
  - magnetic resonance imaging (MRI) enhanced with gadolinium.
- Petrosal sinus sampling is the most accurate way to determine whether Cushing's syndrome is from a pituitary tumor or some other cause. ACTH levels that are higher in the petrosal sinuses than in a forearm vein indicate the presence of a pituitary adenoma.

Treatment
Treatment depends on the cause of the disease. Restoring hormone balance and reversing Cushing's syndrome may require drug therapy, radiation, or surgery.

A patient with a nonendocrine corticotropin-producing tumor will need excision of the tumor, followed by drug therapy that may include:

- mitotane (Lysodren), metyrapone (Metopirone), or aminoglutethimide (Cytadren)

TEACHING FOCUS

Cushing's syndrome teaching topics

● Explain that the patient will need lifelong steroid therapy. Teach the patient and his family to identify and report evidence of overdose (weight gain and edema) or underdose (fatigue, weakness, and dizziness).
● Caution against stopping the drug suddenly because doing so can cause adrenal crisis.
● Instruct the patient to take steroids with antacids or meals to minimize gastric irritation. Suggest taking two-thirds of the dosage in the morning and the remaining one-third in the early afternoon to mimic diurnal adrenal gland secretion.

■ a combination of aminoglutethimide, cyproheptadine (Periactin), and ketoconazole (Nizoral) to decrease cortisol levels
■ aminoglutethimide, alone or with metyrapone, in metastatic adrenal carcinoma.

A patient with pituitary-dependent Cushing's disease and adrenal hyperplasia may need hypophysectomy (removal of the pituitary gland) or pituitary irradiation. If these treatments are unsuccessful or impractical, bilateral adrenalectomy may be performed. (See *Cushing's syndrome teaching topics.*)

PREVENTIVE MEASURES
■ Before surgery, the patient needs to control edema, diabetes, hypertension, and other cardiovascular problems and prevent infection.
■ Glucocorticoids given before surgery can help prevent acute adrenal insufficiency during surgery.
■ Cortisol therapy is essential during and after surgery to combat the physiologic stress of removing the pituitary or adrenal glands.
■ If normal cortisol production resumes, steroid therapy may gradually be tapered and eventually stopped. A patient with bilateral adrenalectomy or a total hypophysectomy will need lifelong steroid replacement.

DIABETES INSIPIDUS
This disorder of water metabolism is caused by a deficiency of ADH, also called vasopressin. The absence of ADH allows filtered water to be excreted in the urine instead of reabsorbed. The disease causes excessive urination (polyuria) and excessive thirst (polydipsia) and

fluid intake. It may first appear in childhood or early adulthood and is more common in men than in women.

Pathophysiology

Some drugs as well as injury to the posterior pituitary gland can cause abnormalities in ADH secretion. A less common cause is a failure of the kidneys to respond to ADH. Also, lesions of the hypothalamus, infundibular stem, and posterior pituitary gland can interfere with ADH synthesis, transport, or release. Lesions may be caused by:

■ brain tumor
■ removal of the pituitary gland (hypophysectomy)
■ aneurysm
■ thrombus
■ immunologic disorder
■ infection.

Normally, ADH is synthesized in the hypothalamus and then stored by the posterior pituitary gland. When it's released into the general circulation, ADH increases the water permeability of the distal and collecting tubules of the kidneys, causing water reabsorption. If ADH is absent, the filtered water is excreted in the urine instead of being reabsorbed, and the patient then excretes large quantities of dilute urine. (See *Understanding antidiuretic hormone,* page 156.)

With adequate water replacement, the prognosis is good for uncomplicated diabetes insipidus, and patients usually lead normal lives. If the disease is complicated by an underlying disorder, such as cancer, the prognosis varies.

RED FLAG Untreated diabetes insipidus can produce hypovolemia, hyperosmolality, circulatory collapse, loss of consciousness, and CNS damage. These complications are most likely to occur if the patient has an impaired or absent thirst mechanism. A prolonged urine flow may produce chronic complications, such as bladder distention, enlarged calyces, hydroureter (distention of the ureter with fluid), and hydronephrosis (collection of urine in the kidney). Complications also may result from certain underlying conditions, such as metastatic brain lesions, head trauma, and infections.

Signs and symptoms

The patient's history shows:

■ abrupt onset of extreme polyuria (usually 4 to 16 L/day of dilute urine, but sometimes as much as 30 L/day)

Understanding antidiuretic hormone

In response to increased serum osmolality and reduced circulating volume, the posterior pituitary gland releases antidiuretic hormone (ADH). Circulating ADH alters permeability of the distal renal tubules and collecting ducts in the kidney, increasing reabsorption of water. This decreases serum osmolality and increases circulating volume. Through a negative feedback mechanism, decreased osmolality and increased volume halt the release of ADH.

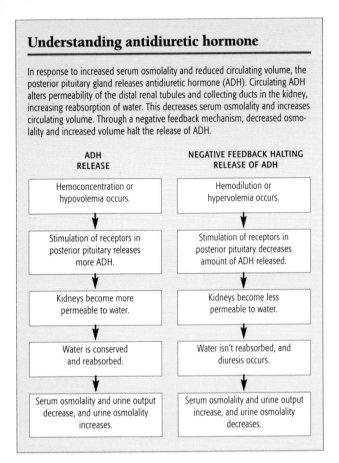

ADH RELEASE

Hemoconcentration or hypovolemia occurs.

↓

Stimulation of receptors in posterior pituitary releases more ADH.

↓

Kidneys become more permeable to water.

↓

Water is conserved and reabsorbed.

↓

Serum osmolality and urine output decrease, and urine osmolality increases.

NEGATIVE FEEDBACK HALTING RELEASE OF ADH

Hemodilution or hypervolemia occurs.

↓

Stimulation of receptors in posterior pituitary decreases amount of ADH released.

↓

Kidneys become less permeable to water.

↓

Water isn't reabsorbed, and diuresis occurs.

↓

Serum osmolality and urine output increase, and urine osmolality decreases.

■ polydipsia (extreme thirst) and consumption of very large volumes of fluid.

In severe cases, fatigue occurs because sleep is interrupted by the need to void and drink fluids.

Children typically have enuresis (involuntary urination), sleep disturbances, irritability, anorexia, and decreased weight gain and linear growth.

Additional signs and symptoms may include:

■ constipation

- dizziness
- hypertension
- increased serum sodium and osmolality
- tachycardia
- weakness
- weight loss.

Test results

- These tests distinguish diabetes insipidus from other disorders that cause polyuria:
  - Urinalysis reveals almost colorless urine of low osmolality (50 to 200 mOsm/kg of water, less than that of plasma) and low specific gravity (less than 1.005).
  - Dehydration test differentiates ADH deficiency from other forms of polyuria by comparing urine osmolality after dehydration and after ADH administration. If the increase in urine osmolality after ADH administration exceeds 9%, the patient has diabetes insipidus. Patients with neurogenic diabetes insipidus (from damage to the posterior pituitary gland) have decreased urine output and increased urine specific gravity. Those with nephrogenic diabetes insipidus (failure of the kidneys to respond to ADH) show no response to ADH. ADH levels are decreased in neurogenic diabetes insipidus and elevated in the nephrogenic type.
- If the patient is critically ill, diagnosis may be based on these laboratory values alone:
  - urine osmolality of 200 mOsm/kg
  - urine specific gravity of 1.005
  - serum osmolality of 300 mOsm/kg
  - serum sodium of 147 mEq/L.

Treatment

Until the cause of diabetes insipidus is identified and eliminated, patients are given various forms of vasopressin to control fluid balance and prevent dehydration. (See *Diabetes insipidus teaching topics,* page 158.)

Aqueous vasopressin (Pitressin) is a replacement agent given by subcutaneous injection. It's used in the initial management of diabetes insipidus after a person has head trauma or a neurosurgical procedure.

Desmopressin acetate, a synthetic vasopressin analogue, affects prolonged antidiuretic activity and has no pressor effects. A long-acting drug, desmopressin acetate is given intranasally.

DIABETES MELLITUS

In this disorder, the body doesn't produce or properly use insulin, leading to hyperglycemia. The disease occurs in two primary forms:
■ type 1 (once known as insulin-dependent diabetes mellitus)
■ type 2 (once known as non–insulin-dependent diabetes mellitus), the more prevalent form.
Several secondary forms also exist, caused by such conditions as pancreatic disease, pregnancy (gestational diabetes mellitus), hormonal or genetic problems, and certain drugs or chemicals.

Diabetes mellitus affects about 6.3% of the U.S. population (18.2 million people); 5.2 million people are unaware that they have the disease. The risk increases with age. Diabetes is the fifth leading cause of death in the United States.

Pathophysiology

Normally, insulin allows glucose to travel into cells. There it's used for energy and stored as glycogen. It also stimulates protein synthesis and free fatty acid storage in adipose tissue.

Insulin deficiency blocks tissue access to essential nutrients for fuel and storage.

TYPE 1 DIABETES

In type 1 diabetes, beta cells in the pancreas are destroyed or suppressed. This form of the disease has idiopathic and immune-mediated types.
■ In the idiopathic type, patients have a permanent insulin deficiency with no evidence of autoimmunity.
■ In the immune-mediated type, a local or organ-specific deficit may induce an autoimmune attack on beta cells. This attack, in

Diabetes screening guidelines

These guidelines from the American Diabetes Association are also endorsed by the National Institutes of Health.

● Adults should be tested for diabetes every 3 years starting at age 45. Those with a high blood glucose level should have the test repeated on another day.

● People at increased risk of diabetes may need to be tested earlier or more often. Higher-risk groups include Native Americans, Blacks, Asians, Hispanics, and anyone who is overweight or has high blood pressure, high cholesterol, or a strong family history of diabetes.

● Diabetes is diagnosed if the person has a fasting plasma glucose level of 126 mg/dl or above on at least two occasions, a random blood glucose level of 200 mg/dl or above, or a blood glucose level above 200 mg/dl on the second hour of a glucose tolerance test.

turn, causes an inflammatory response in the pancreas called insulitis.

Islet cell antibodies may be present long before symptoms become apparent. These immune markers also precede evidence of beta cell deficiency. Autoantibodies against insulin have also been noted. Some experts believe that the beta cells aren't destroyed but rather are disabled by the antibodies and might later be reactivated. By the time the disease becomes apparent, 80% of the beta cells are gone.

TYPE 2 DIABETES
Type 2 diabetes may be caused by:
■ resistance to insulin action in target tissues
■ abnormal insulin secretion
■ inappropriate hepatic gluconeogenesis (overproduction of glucose)
■ obesity. (See *Diabetes screening guidelines.*)

SECONDARY DIABETES
Three common causes of secondary diabetes are:
■ physical or emotional stress, which may cause prolonged elevation in levels of the stress hormones cortisol, epinephrine, glucagon, and GH (which, in turn, raises the blood glucose level and increases demands on the pancreas)
■ pregnancy, which causes weight gain and high levels of estrogen and placental hormones

Understanding diabetic ketoacidosis and hyperosmolar hyperglycemic nonketotic syndrome

Diabetic ketoacidosis (DKA) and hyperosmolar hyperglycemic nonketotic syndrome (HHNS) are acute complications of hyperglycemic crisis that may occur with diabetes. If not treated properly, either may result in coma or death.

DKA occurs most commonly in patients with type 1 diabetes and may be the first evidence of the disease. HHNS occurs most commonly in patients with type 2 diabetes, but it also occurs in anyone whose insulin tolerance is stressed and in patients who have undergone certain therapeutic procedures, such as peritoneal dialysis, hemodialysis, tube feedings, or total parenteral nutrition.

Acute insulin deficiency (absolute in DKA; relative in HHNS) precipitates both conditions. Causes include illness, stress, infection and, in patients with DKA, failure to take insulin.

BUILDUP OF GLUCOSE

Inadequate insulin hinders glucose uptake by fat and muscle cells. Because the cells can't take in glucose to convert to energy, glucose accumulates in the blood. At the same time, the liver responds to the demands of the energy-starved cells by converting glycogen to glucose and releasing glucose into the blood, further increasing the blood glucose level. When this level exceeds the renal threshold, excess glucose is excreted in urine.

The insulin-deprived cells can't use glucose. Their response is rapid metabolism of protein, which results in loss of intracellular potassium and phosphorus and excessive liberation of amino acids. The liver converts these amino acids into urea and glucose.

As a result of these processes, blood glucose levels become grossly

---

■ use of adrenal corticosteroids, hormonal contraceptives, and other drugs that antagonize the effects of insulin.

Some viral infections have been implicated, such as CMV, adenovirus, rubella, and mumps.

RED FLAG Two acute complications of diabetes are diabetic keto-acidosis (DKA) and hyperosmolar hyperglycemic nonketotic syndrome. These life-threatening conditions require immediate intervention. (See Understanding diabetic ketoacidosis and hyperosmolar hyperglycemic nonketotic syndrome.) What's more, chronic complications may occur in virtually all body systems. The most common are cardiovascular disease, peripheral vascular disease, eye disease (retinopathy), kidney disease, skin disease (diabetic dermopathy), and peripheral and autonomic neuropathy. Glucose levels don't have to be as high as once thought for complications to develop.

elevated. The aftermath is increased serum osmolarity and glycosuria (high amounts of glucose in the urine), leading to osmotic diuresis. Glycosuria is higher in HHNS than in DKA because blood glucose levels are higher in HHNS.

A DEADLY CYCLE
The massive fluid loss from osmotic diuresis causes fluid and electrolyte imbalances and dehydration. Water loss exceeds glucose and electrolyte loss, contributing to hyperosmolarity. This, in turn, perpetuates dehydration, decreasing the glomerular filtration rate and reducing the amount of glucose excreted in the urine. This leads to a deadly cycle: Diminished glucose excretion further raises blood glucose levels, producing hyperosmolarity and

dehydration and finally causing shock, coma, and death.

DKA COMPLICATION
All of these steps hold true for DKA and HHNS, but DKA involves an additional, simultaneous process that leads to metabolic acidosis. The absolute insulin deficiency causes cells to convert fats into glycerol and fatty acids for energy. The fatty acids can't be metabolized as quickly as they're released, so they accumulate in the liver where they're converted into ketones (ketoacids). These ketones accumulate in the blood and urine and cause acidosis. Acidosis leads to more tissue breakdown, more ketosis, more acidosis and, eventually, shock, coma, and death.

Meticulous blood glucose control is essential to help prevent acute and chronic complications.

Signs and symptoms
Patients with type 1 diabetes usually report rapidly developing symptoms, including muscle wasting and loss of subcutaneous fat.

In type 2 diabetes, symptoms typically are vague, long-standing, and develop gradually. Most patients have:
■ a family history of diabetes mellitus
■ gestational diabetes
■ delivery of an infant weighing more than 9 lb (4 kg)
■ severe viral infection
■ another endocrine disease
■ recent stress or trauma
■ use of drugs that increase blood glucose levels

■ obesity, especially in the abdominal area.

Patients with either type of diabetes may report symptoms related to hyperglycemia, such as:
■ excessive urination (polyuria)
■ excessive thirst (polydipsia)
■ excessive eating (polyphagia)
■ weight loss
■ fatigue
■ weakness
■ vision changes
■ frequent skin infections
■ dry, itchy skin
■ vaginal discomfort.

Patients with either type of diabetes also may have:
■ poor skin turgor
■ dry mucous membranes related to dehydration
■ decreased peripheral pulses
■ cool skin temperature
■ decreased reflexes.

Patients in crisis with DKA may have a fruity breath odor because of increased acetone production.

Test results

■ In nonpregnant adults, a diagnosis of diabetes mellitus may be confirmed by one of two blood tests that evaluate plasma glucose levels.
■ The fasting plasma glucose test may have these results:
  – normal—< 100 mg/dl
  – pre-diabetes— 100 to 126 mg/dl
  – diabetes—≥ 126 mg/dl on two occasions
■ The oral glucose tolerance test may have these results:
  – normal—< 140 mg/dl
  – pre-diabetes— 140 to 200 mg/dl
  – diabetes—≥ 200 mg/dl.
■ Three other tests may be done:
  – An eye examination may show diabetic retinopathy.
  – Urinalysis shows the presence of acetone.
  – Blood tests for glycosylated hemoglobin level are used to monitor the long-term effectiveness of diabetes therapy. These tests show variants in hemoglobin levels that reflect average blood glucose levels during the preceding 2 to 3 months. The goal is to achieve a glycosylated hemoglobin level of 7%.

Treatment

Effective treatment optimizes blood glucose levels and decreases complications. Type 1 diabetes treatment includes insulin replacement, meal planning, and exercise. Type 2 diabetes treatment may include meal planning, weight reduction if the patient is obese, and an oral antidiabetic drug.

INSULIN

■ Current forms of insulin replacement include single-dose, mixed-dose, split-mixed-dose, and multiple-dose regimens.
■ Insulin may be:
  – rapid-acting (Humalog)
  – fast-acting (regular)
  – intermediate-acting (NPH and Lente)
  – long-acting (insulin glargine [Lantus])
  – a premixed combination of fast-acting and intermediate-acting.
■ Purified human insulin is used commonly today.
■ Patients may inject insulin subcutaneously throughout the day or receive insulin through an insulin pump. Multiple-dose regimens are most likely to use an insulin pump.
■ Patients with type 1 or type 2 diabetes may benefit from inhaled insulin.

ANTIDIABETIC DRUG THERAPY

Patients with type 2 diabetes who can't achieve their target blood glucose levels with meal planning and exercise may need oral antidiabetic drugs to help maintain normal blood glucose levels by stimulating endogenous insulin production and increasing insulin sensitivity at the cellular level. These drugs comprise several different classes.

■ Insulin secretagogues enhance pancreatic insulin secretion. Examples include:
  – first-generation sulfonylureas, such as acetohexamide (Dymelor), chlorpropamide (Diabinese), tolazamide (Tolinase), and tolbutamide (Orinase)
  – second-generation sulfonylureas, such as glyburide (Micronase), glipizide (Glucotrol), and glimepiride (Amaryl)
  – repaglinide (Prandin), which enhances insulin secretion but acts more quickly.
■ Biguanides prevent inappropriate hepatic gluconeogenesis. Examples include:
  – metformin (Glucophage).

TEACHING FOCUS

Diabetes mellitus teaching topics

- Teach the patient about insulin if prescribed, including type, peak times, dosage, drawing up, mixing (if applicable), administration technique, and site rotation.
- Teach the patient about oral antidiabetic therapy if prescribed.
- Review the prescribed meal plan and teach the patient how to adjust his diet during periods of increased activity. Teach him how to select restaurant meals and how to obtain nutrient composition lists from fast-food restaurants.
- Advise the patient about aerobic exercise programs. Explain how exercise affects blood glucose levels, and provide safety guidelines.

■ Alpha-glucosidase inhibitors delay intestinal absorption of carbohydrates. Examples include:
  – acarbose (Precose)
  – miglitol (Glyset).
■ Thiazolidinedione insulin sensitizers enhance the sensitivity of peripheral cells to insulin. Examples include:
  – pioglitazone (Actos)
  – rosiglitazone (Avandia).

PERSONALIZED MEAL PLAN

Patients with either type of diabetes need a meal plan to meet nutritional needs, control blood glucose levels, and help the patient reach and maintain his ideal body weight. A dietitian estimates the total amount of energy the patient needs daily based on ideal body weight. Then she plans meals with the appropriate carbohydrate, fat, and protein content. For the diet to work, the patient must follow it consistently and eat at regular times. (See *Diabetes mellitus teaching topics.*)

In type 1 diabetes, the calorie allotment may be high, depending on the patient's growth stage and activity level. Weight reduction is a goal for an obese patient with type 2 diabetes.

OTHER TREATMENTS

Exercise is useful in managing type 2 diabetes because it increases insulin sensitivity, improves glucose tolerance, and promotes weight loss.

Treatment for long-term complications may include:
■ dialysis or kidney transplantation for renal failure
■ photocoagulation for retinopathy

- vascular surgery for large vessel disease
- pancreas transplantation.

GOITER

A goiter is an enlargement of the thyroid gland. It isn't caused by in-flammation or neoplasm and isn't initially tied to hyperthyroidism or hypothyroidism. This condition has two forms: nontoxic goiter and toxic goiter.

Nontoxic goiter is most common in females, especially during adolescence, pregnancy, and menopause. At these times, the de-mand for thyroid hormone increases. Nontoxic goiter is classified in two ways:

- endemic, caused by lack of iodine in the diet
- sporadic, related to ingestion of certain drugs or food and occur-ring randomly.

Toxic goiter arises from long-standing nontoxic goiter and oc-curs in elderly people. The enlarged thyroid gland develops small rounded masses and secretes excess thyroid hormone. Symptoms are the same as those of hyperthyroidism except that exophthalmos doesn't develop.

Pathophysiology

Nontoxic goiter occurs when the thyroid gland can't secrete enough thyroid hormone to meet metabolic needs. As a result, the thyroid mass increases to compensate. This response usually overcomes mild to moderate hormonal impairment.

TSH levels in nontoxic goiter typically are normal. Enlargement of the gland probably results from impaired hormone production in the thyroid and depleted iodine, which increases the thyroid gland's reaction to TSH.

Endemic nontoxic goiter usually results from inadequate di-etary intake of iodine, which leads to inadequate synthesis of thy-roid hormone. In Japan, goiter resulting from iodine excess from ex-cessive ingestion of seaweed has been found. Some areas, called goi-ter belts, have a high occurrence of endemic goiter. This is caused by iodine-deficient soil and water. Goiter belts include areas in the Midwest, Northwest, and Great Lakes region.

Sporadic nontoxic goiter commonly results from ingestion of large amounts of goitrogenic foods or use of goitrogenic drugs, each of which contains agents that decrease T_4 production. Goitrogenic foods include:

- rutabagas
- cabbage

- soybeans
- peanuts
- peaches
- peas
- strawberries
- spinach
- radishes.

Goitrogenic drugs include:
- propylthiouracil (PTU)
- iodides
- phenylbutazone (Cotylbutazone)
- aminosalicylic acid
- cobalt
- lithium (Eskalith).

Here's a more detailed account of what happens in goiter. Depletion of glandular organic iodine, along with impaired hormone synthesis, increases the thyroid gland's responsiveness to normal TSH levels. Resulting increases in thyroid mass and activity overcome mild impairment of hormone synthesis. Although the patient has a goiter, his metabolic function is normal. When the underlying disorder is severe, compensatory responses may cause both a goiter and hypothyroidism.

RED FLAG Complications from a large retrosternal goiter mainly result from compression and displacement of the trachea or esophagus. Thyroid cysts and hemorrhage into the cysts may increase the pressure on and compression of surrounding tissues and structures. Large goiters may obstruct venous return, prompt venous engorgement and, rarely, cause collateral circulation of the chest.

Signs and symptoms

A nontoxic goiter causes these signs and symptoms:
- single or multinodular, firm, irregular enlargement of the thyroid gland
- stridor
- respiratory distress and dysphagia from compression of the trachea and esophagus
- dizziness or syncope when arms are raised above the head due to obstructed venous return.

Enlargement of the thyroid gland undergoes frequent exacerbations and remissions and has areas of hypervolution and involution.

Fibrosis may alternate with hyperplasia, and nodules containing thyroid follicles may develop.

Production of excessive amounts of thyroid hormone may lead to thyrotoxicosis.

Test results
Several tests are used to diagnose nontoxic goiter and rule out other diseases with similar clinical effects.
■ Serum thyroid hormone levels are usually normal.
  – Abnormalities in T_3, T_4, and TSH levels rule out this diagnosis.
  – Transient increased levels of TSH, which occur infrequently, may be missed by diagnostic tests.
■ Thyroid antibody titers are usually normal. Increases indicate chronic thyroiditis.
■ Radioactive iodine (^{131}I) uptake is usually normal but may increase in the presence of iodine deficiency or a biosynthetic defect.
■ Urinalysis may show low urinary excretion of iodine.
■ Radioisotope scanning identifies thyroid neoplasms.

Treatment
With treatment, the prognosis is good for patients with either endemic or sporadic goiter. The goal of treatment for nontoxic goiter is to reduce thyroid hyperplasia. (See *Goiter teaching topics,* page 168.)

Hormone replacement
Thyroid hormone replacement is the treatment of choice because it inhibits thyroid-stimulating hormone secretion and allows the gland to rest. Replacements include:
■ levothyroxine (Synthroid)
■ desiccated thyroid
■ liothyronine (Cytomel).
　　Small doses of iodide (Lugol's solution or potassium iodide solution) may relieve goiter caused by iodine deficiency.

Diet
Patients with sporadic goiters must avoid goitrogenic drugs and foods.

Radiation
Radioiodine ablation therapy may be used to destroy the thyroid gland cells that concentrate iodine to make thyroxine.

TEACHING FOCUS

Goiter teaching topics

● To maintain steady hormone levels, instruct the patient to take prescribed thyroid hormone replacement at the same time each day on an empty stomach.
● Instruct the patient and his family to identify and immediately report signs and symptoms of thyrotoxicosis. They include increased pulse rate, palpitations, diarrhea, sweating, tremors, agitation, and shortness of breath.
● Instruct a patient with endemic goiter to use iodized salt to supply the daily 150 to 300 mcg of iodine needed to prevent goiter.

SURGERY

In rare cases of a large goiter unresponsive to treatment, partial removal of the thyroid gland may relieve pressure on surrounding structures.

HYPERTHYROIDISM

When thyroid hormone is overproduced, it creates a metabolic imbalance called hyperthyroidism or thyrotoxicosis. Excess thyroid hormone can cause various thyroid disorders; Graves' disease is the most common. (See *Types of hyperthyroidism*.)

Graves' disease is an autoimmune disorder that causes goiter and multiple systemic changes. It occurs mostly in people ages 30 to 60; usually, their family histories include thyroid abnormalities. Only 5% of patients are younger than age 15.

Thyrotoxic crisis, also known as thyroid storm, is an acute exacerbation of hyperthyroidism. It's a medical emergency that may lead to life-threatening cardiac, hepatic, or renal failure. Inadequately treated hyperthyroidism and stressful conditions, such as surgery, infection, toxemia of pregnancy, and DKA, can lead to thyrotoxic crisis. (See *Understanding thyroid storm,* page 170.)

Pathophysiology

In Graves' disease, thyroid-stimulating antibodies bind to and stimulate the TSH receptors of the thyroid gland. The trigger for this autoimmune response is unclear; it may have several causes. Genetic factors may play a part; the disease tends to occur in identical twins. Immunologic factors may also be the culprit; the disease occasionally coexists with other autoimmune endocrine abnormalities, such as type 1 diabetes mellitus, thyroiditis, and hyperparathyroidism. Graves' disease is also associated with production of several autoan-

Types of hyperthyroidism

In addition to Graves' disease, other forms of hyperthyroidism include toxic adenoma, thyrotoxicosis factitia, functioning metastatic thyroid carcinoma, thyroid-stimulating hormone (TSH)–secreting pituitary tumor, and subacute thyroiditis.

TOXIC ADENOMA
The second most common cause of hyperthyroidism, toxic adenoma is a small, benign nodule in the thyroid gland that secretes thyroid hormone. The cause of toxic adenoma is unknown; it's most common in elderly people. Clinical effects are similar to those of Graves' disease except that toxic adenoma doesn't cause ophthalmopathy, pretibial myxedema, or acropachy (clubbing of fingers or toes). A radioactive iodine (^{131}I) uptake test and a thyroid scan show a single hyperfunctioning nodule suppressing the rest of the gland. Treatment includes ^{131}I therapy or surgery to remove the adenoma after antithyroid drugs restore normal gland function.

THYROTOXICOSIS FACTITIA
Thyrotoxicosis factitia results from long-term ingestion of thyroid hormone for TSH suppression in patients with thyroid carcinoma. It also may result from thyroid hormone abuse by people trying to lose weight.

FUNCTIONING METASTATIC THYROID CARCINOMA
Functioning metastatic thyroid carcinoma is a rare disease that causes excess production of thyroid hormone.

TSH-SECRETING PITUITARY TUMOR
TSH-secreting pituitary tumor is a form of hyperthyroidism that causes excess production of thyroid hormone.

SUBACUTE THYROIDITIS
A virus-induced granulomatous inflammation of the thyroid, subacute thyroiditis produces transient hyperthyroidism with fever, pain, pharyngitis, and tenderness of the thyroid gland.

tibodies formed because of a defect in suppressor T-lymphocyte function.

In a person with latent hyperthyroidism, excessive iodine intake and, possibly, stress can cause active hyperthyroidism.

Signs and symptoms
Signs and symptoms typically arise after a period of acute physical or emotional stress. The classic features of Graves' disease are:
■ diarrhea
■ enlarged thyroid gland
■ excessive sweating

Understanding thyroid storm

Thyrotoxic crisis – also known as thyroid storm – usually occurs in patients with preexisting, though often unrecognized, thyrotoxicosis. Left untreated, it's usually fatal.

PATHOPHYSIOLOGY
The thyroid gland secretes the thyroid hormones triiodothyronine (T_3) and thyroxine (T_4). When T_3 and T_4 are overproduced, systemic adrenergic activity increases. The result is epinephrine overproduction and severe hypermetabolism, leading rapidly to cardiac, GI, and sympathetic nervous system decompensation.

ASSESSMENT FINDINGS
At first the patient may have marked tachycardia, vomiting, and stupor. If left untreated he may experience vascular collapse, hypotension, coma, and death. Other findings may include irritability, restlessness, visual disturbance (such as diplopia), tremor, weakness, angina, shortness of breath, cough, and swollen limbs. The patient may have warm, moist, flushed skin and a high fever that

starts insidiously and rises rapidly to a lethal level.

PRECIPITATING FACTORS
Onset is almost always abrupt and evoked by a stressful event, such as trauma, surgery, or infection. Other less common precipitating factors include:
● insulin-induced ketoacidosis
● hypoglycemia or diabetic ketoacidosis
● stroke
● myocardial infarction
● pulmonary embolism
● sudden stopping of antithyroid drug therapy
● start of radioactive iodine therapy
● preeclampsia
● subtotal thyroidectomy with excessive intake of synthetic thyroid hormone.

■ exophthalmos (abnormal protrusion of the eyes)
■ heat intolerance
■ nervousness and irritability
■ palpitations
■ tachycardia
■ tremors
■ weight loss despite increased appetite.

Many other signs and symptoms are common with hyperthyroidism because thyroid hormones have widespread effects on almost all body systems, including the CNS, cardiovascular system, integumentary system, respiratory system, GI system, musculoskeletal system, reproductive system, and eyes.

CNS signs and symptoms are most common in younger patients. They include:

■ anxiety
■ clumsiness
■ emotional instability
■ excitability or nervousness
■ fine tremor
■ mood swings ranging from occasional outbursts to overt psychosis
■ shaky handwriting
■ trouble concentrating.

Cardiovascular signs and symptoms are most common in elderly patients. They include:

■ arrhythmias, especially atrial fibrillation
■ cardiac decompensation
■ cardiac insufficiency
■ resistance to the usual therapeutic dose of digoxin.

Integumentary signs and symptoms include:

■ fine, soft hair
■ fragile nails
■ hair loss in both sexes
■ onycholysis (separation of distal nail from nail bed)
■ premature graying
■ pretibial myxedema producing raised, thickened skin and plaquelike or nodular lesions
■ vitiligo and skin hyperpigmentation
■ warm, moist, flushed skin with a velvety texture.

Respiratory signs and symptoms include:

■ breathlessness when climbing stairs
■ dyspnea on exertion and possibly at rest.

GI signs and symptoms include:

■ anorexia
■ nausea
■ vomiting.

Musculoskeletal signs and symptoms include:

■ acropachy (soft-tissue swelling with underlying bone changes where new bone formation occurs)
■ generalized or localized muscle atrophy
■ muscle weakness
■ osteoporosis.

Reproductive signs and symptoms include:

■ decreased libido

- gynecomastia (abnormal development of mammary glands in men)
- impaired fertility
- menstrual abnormalities.
   Signs and symptoms involving the eyes include:
- blurred vision
- convergence
- corneal ulcers
- exophthalmos, which causes the characteristic staring gaze
- impaired upward gaze
- infrequent blinking
- lid lag
- photophobia
- reddened conjunctiva and cornea
- strabismus (eye deviation).

On palpation, the thyroid gland may feel asymmetrical, lobular, and enlarged to three or four times its normal size. The liver also may be enlarged. You may notice a full, bounding, palpable pulse. Hyperreflexia is present.

Auscultation of the heart may reveal an accelerated heart rate. It may prove to be paroxysmal supraventricular tachycardia or atrial fibrillation when verified by electrocardiogram, especially in elderly patients. Occasionally, a systolic murmur occurs at the left sternal border.

Wide pulse pressures may be audible when blood pressure readings are taken. In Graves' disease, an audible bruit over the thyroid gland indicates thyrotoxicity but it may also be present in other hyperthyroid disorders.

With treatment, most patients can lead normal lives.

Test results

- These laboratory tests confirm Graves' disease:
   - Radioimmunoassay shows increased serum T_3 and T_4 concentrations.
   - TSH level is low in primary hyperthyroidism and elevated when excessive TSH secretion is the cause.
   - Thyroid scan reveals increased uptake of ^{131}I.
- Other tests show increased serum protein-bound iodine and decreased serum cholesterol and total lipid levels.

Treatment

In Graves' disease, the most common hyperthyroid disorder, treatment consists of drug therapy, including radioactive iodine (^{131}I) therapy, and surgery. (See *Hyperthyroidism teaching topics*.)

TEACHING FOCUS

Hyperthyroidism teaching topics

● Stress the importance of regular medical follow-up after discharge because hypothyroidism may develop 2 to 4 weeks postoperatively. Drug therapy and radioactive iodine therapy require careful monitoring and comprehensive patient teaching.

● If the patient has exophthalmos or another ophthalmopathy, suggest sunglasses or eye patches to protect the eyes from light. Moisten the conjunctivae often with artificial tears. If the patient has severe lid retraction, advise against sudden physical movements that might cause the lid to slip behind the eyeball. Elevate the head of the bed to reduce periorbital edema.

● If the patient is pregnant, tell her to watch closely during the first trimester for signs of spontaneous abortion (spotting, occasional mild cramps) and to report such signs to the physician immediately.

DRUG THERAPY
Antithyroid drugs are used for children, young adults, pregnant women, and patients who refuse other treatments. They include:
■ propylthiouracil (PTU)
■ methimazole (Tapazole).

RADIOACTIVE IODINE THERAPY
A single oral dose of ^{131}I is the treatment of choice. Radioactive iodine should be used cautiously in patients younger than age 20. It's contraindicated during pregnancy, which should be ruled out before treatment starts. Women should be cautioned to avoid pregnancy for 3 months after treatment.

During treatment, the thyroid gland picks up the radioactive element as it would regular iodine. The radioactivity destroys some of the cells that normally concentrate iodine and produce thyroxine (T_4), thus decreasing thyroid hormone production and normalizing thyroid size and function. In most patients, hypermetabolic symptoms diminish in 6 to 8 weeks. Some patients may need a second dose.

SURGERY
Partial thyroidectomy is indicated for certain patients:
■ those younger than age 40 who have a very large goiter and whose hyperthyroidism has repeatedly relapsed after drug therapy

■ pregnant patients
■ patients allergic to ^{131}I and other antithyroid drugs.

Before surgery, the patient may receive iodide (Lugol's or potassium iodide solution), antithyroid drugs, or high doses of propranolol (Inderal) to help prevent thyroid storm. If normal thyroid function isn't achieved, surgery should be delayed and propranolol given to decrease the risk of arrhythmias.

During surgery, part of the thyroid gland is removed, decreasing its size and capacity for hormone production.

OTHER TREATMENTS

Therapy for hyperthyroid ophthalmopathy includes local applications of topical drugs and may include high doses of corticosteroids. If severe exophthalmos presses on the optic nerve, the patient may need surgical decompression to reduce pressure on the orbital contents.

Treatment for thyrotoxic crisis includes:
■ an antithyroid drug
■ I.V. propranolol to block sympathetic effects
■ a corticosteroid to inhibit conversion of triiodothyronine to T_4 and replace depleted cortisol
■ an iodide to block release of thyroid hormones
■ supportive measures, including administration of nutrients, vitamins, fluids, and sedatives.

HYPOTHYROIDISM

In thyroid hormone deficiency (hypothyroidism) in adults, a deficit in T_3 or T_4 level causes metabolic processes to slow down. Hypothyroidism is most common in women and in people with Down syndrome. In the United States, it's becoming more common in people ages 40 to 50.

Hypothyroidism is classified as primary or secondary. The primary form stems from a disorder of the thyroid gland itself. The secondary form stems from a failure to stimulate normal thyroid function. Secondary hypothyroidism may progress to myxedema coma, a medical emergency. (See *Understanding myxedema coma.*)

Pathophysiology

Primary hypothyroidism has several possible causes:
■ thyroidectomy
■ inflammation from radiation therapy
■ other inflammatory conditions, such as amyloidosis and sarcoidosis

Understanding myxedema coma

A medical emergency, myxedema coma is commonly fatal. Progression is usually gradual, but coma may develop abruptly when stress — such as infection, exposure to cold, or trauma — aggravates severe or prolonged hypothyroidism. Other precipitating factors are withdrawal of thyroid drugs and the use of sedatives, opioids, or anesthetics.

WHAT HAPPENS
Patients in myxedema coma have significantly depressed respirations; their partial pressure of carbon dioxide in arterial blood may rise. Decreased cardiac output and worsening cerebral hypoxia may also occur. The patient becomes stuporous and hypothermic. Vital signs reflect bradycardia and hypotension. Lifesaving interventions are needed.

■ chronic autoimmune thyroiditis (Hashimoto's disease).

Secondary hypothyroidism is caused by a failure to stimulate normal thyroid function. The pituitary may fail to produce TSH (thyrotropin). The hypothalamus may fail to produce thyrotropin-releasing hormone. Secondary hypothyroidism also may be caused by an inability to synthesize thyroid hormones because of iodine deficiency (usually dietary) or the use of antithyroid drugs. (See *Thyroid disease and aging*, page 176.)

RED FLAG Possible complications of hypothyroidism include heart failure, myxedema coma, infection, megacolon, organic psychosis, and infertility.

Signs and symptoms

Because insufficient synthesis of thyroid hormones affects almost every organ system, signs and symptoms may be vague and may vary with the organs involved and the duration and severity of the condition. Early ones include:
■ constipation
■ energy loss
■ fatigue
■ forgetfulness
■ sensitivity to cold
■ unexplained weight gain.

As the disease progresses, the patient may experience:
■ anorexia
■ decreased libido

Thyroid disease and aging

As a person ages, structural changes occur in the thyroid gland that may contribute to the development of thyroid disease. The size of the gland may increase or decrease, depending on dietary intake of iodine. The gland also becomes more nodular.

Of those older than age 60, 0.5% to 2.3% have hyperthyroidism; 2.3% to 7% have hypothyroidism. By age 50, 10% of women have elevated thyroid-stimulating hormone (TSH) levels – a sign of thyroid failure; by age 60, 17% of women and 8% of men have elevated TSH levels.

Many of the signs and symptoms of thyroid disease may be overlooked and attributed to the normal aging process (signs of hypothyroidism include fatigue, constipation, hair loss, and forgetfulness; signs of hyperthyroidism include weight loss, hyperactivity, weakness, palpitations, tremors, nervousness, and insomnia).

While there's no accepted screening schedule for thyroid disease, hyperthyroidism and hypothyroidism should be considered if a mature patient has signs and symptoms, and appropriate blood tests should be drawn to evaluate thyroid function.

- impotence
- joint stiffness
- menorrhagia (painful menstruation)
- muscle cramps
- paresthesia (numbness, prickling, or tingling).

Other signs and symptoms affect various body systems, including the central nervous system, integumentary system, cardiovascular system, GI system, reproductive system, hematologic system, and eyes and ears.

Central nervous system signs and symptoms include:
- ataxia (loss of coordination)
- behavioral changes ranging from slight mental slowing to severe impairment
- benign intracranial hypertension
- carpal tunnel syndrome
- intention tremor (tremor during voluntary motion)
- psychiatric disturbances.

Integumentary signs and symptoms include:
- dry, flaky, inelastic skin
- dry, sparse hair with patchy hair loss and loss of the outer third of the eyebrow

- puffy face, hands, and feet
- thick, brittle nails with transverse and longitudinal grooves
- thick, dry tongue, causing hoarseness and slow, slurred speech.
    Cardiovascular signs and symptoms include:
- heart enlargement
- heart failure
- hypercholesterolemia (high cholesterol) with arteriosclerosis and ischemic heart disease
- pleural and pericardial effusions
- poor peripheral circulation.
    GI signs and symptoms include:
- achlorhydria (absence of free hydrochloric acid in the stomach)
- adynamic (weak) colon resulting in megacolon (extremely dilated colon) and intestinal obstruction
- pernicious anemia.
    Reproductive signs and symptoms include:
- impaired fertility.
    Hematologic signs and symptoms include:
- anemia, which may result in bleeding tendencies
- iron deficiency anemia.
    Signs and symptoms involving the eyes and ears include:
- conductive or sensorineural deafness
- nystagmus.
    Severe hypothyroidism, or myxedema, is characterized by
- bradycardia
- delayed reflex relaxation time (especially in the Achilles tendon)
- hyponatremia (low blood sodium), which may result from impaired water excretion and from poor regulation of ADH secretion
- induration of skin
- muscle weakness
- sacral or peripheral edema
- skin that feels rough, doughy, and cool
- thickening of facial features
- thyroid tissue that isn't easily palpable unless a goiter is present
- weak pulse.

Test results

- Primary hypothyroidism is confirmed by an elevated TSH level and low serum level of free T_4.
- Serum TSH levels determine whether the disorder is primary or secondary. An increased serum TSH level is from thyroid insufficiency. A decreased or normal level is from hypothalamic or pituitary insufficiency.

TEACHING FOCUS

Hypothyroidism teaching topics

- Teach the patient to watch for signs of hyperthyroidism – such as restlessness, sweating, and excessive weight loss – while taking thyroid replacement therapy.
- To prevent myxedema coma, tell the patient to continue the prescribed course of thyroid drug even if his symptoms subside.
- Tell the patient to report signs of aggravated cardiovascular disease, such as chest pain and tachycardia.
- Warn the patient to report infection immediately and to make sure any physician who prescribes drugs for him knows about the underlying hypothyroidism.

- Serum antithyroid antibodies are elevated in autoimmune thyroiditis.
- Perchlorate discharge tests identify enzyme deficiency in the thyroid gland. A deficiency affects iodine uptake.
- Radioisotope scanning identifies ectopic thyroid tissue.
- In secondary hypothyroidism, skull X-ray, CT scan, and MRI may locate pituitary or hypothalamic lesions.

Treatment
Treatment includes gradual thyroid hormone replacement with the synthetic hormone levothyroxine (Synthroid). To avoid adverse cardiovascular effects, treatment starts slowly, particularly in elderly patients. The dosage is increased every 2 to 3 weeks until the desired response is obtained. (See *Hypothyroidism teaching topics*.)

In underdeveloped areas, prophylactic iodine supplements have decreased the occurrence of iodine-deficient goiter.

Patients with myxedema coma and those having emergency surgery need rapid treatment that includes I.V. administration of levothyroxine and hydrocortisone (Solu-Cortef).

7

RESPIRATORY SYSTEM

Understanding the respiratory system

The respiratory system includes conducting airways, two lungs, and associated blood vessels. These structures work together to accomplish gas exchange, the major function of the respiratory system.

During inhalation (inspiration), air is taken into the body and travels through respiratory passages to the lungs. During perfusion, oxygen in the lungs changes places with carbon dioxide in the blood. During exhalation (expiration), carbon dioxide is expelled from the body.

Disease or injury may affect any of part of the respiratory system—conducting airways, lungs, breathing mechanics, and neurochemical control of ventilation—and, as a result, may interfere with the respiratory system's vital work.

CONDUCTING AIRWAYS

The conducting airways bring air into and out of gas-exchanging structures in the lungs. Conducting airways include the upper and lower airways.

Upper airways

The upper airways consist of the nose, mouth, pharynx, and larynx. These structures warm, humidify, and filter inspired air and protect the lower airways from foreign matter.

When the nose, mouth, pharynx, or larynx becomes partly or totally blocked, the oxygen supply to the lungs is reduced or cut off. Several conditions can cause upper airway obstruction, including:
- foreign objects
- trauma
- tumors.

A close look at a lobule

As illustrated here, each lobule contains terminal bronchioles and the acinus, consisting of respiratory bronchioles and alveolar sacs.

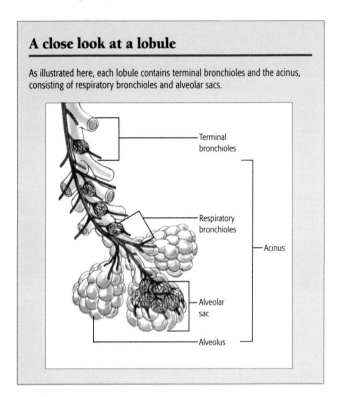

If not treated promptly, upper airway obstruction can lead to hypoxemia (insufficient oxygen in the blood) and then progress quickly to severe hypoxia (lack of oxygen available to body tissues), loss of consciousness, and death.

Lower airways
The lower airways include the trachea, the right and left mainstem bronchi, five secondary bronchi, and the bronchioles. Each bronchiole descends from a lobule and contains terminal bronchioles, alveolar ducts, and alveoli.

Terminal bronchioles are anatomic dead spaces because they don't participate in gas exchange. Alveoli are the chief units of gas exchange. (See *A close look at a lobule.*)

The lower airways facilitate gas exchange and continue the process of warming, humidifying, and filtering inspired air. Like the upper airways, the lower airways can become partly or totally blocked by inflammation, tumors, foreign bodies, bronchospasm, or trauma. This blockage can lead to respiratory distress and failure. Defense systems used by the lower airways to protect the lungs include the irritant reflex, the mucociliary system, and secretory immunity.

IRRITANT REFLEX
The irritant reflex is triggered when inhaled particles, cold air, or toxins stimulate irritant receptors. Reflex bronchospasm then occurs to limit the exposure, followed by coughing, which expels the irritant.

MUCOCILIARY SYSTEM
The mucociliary system produces mucus, which traps foreign particles. Foreign matter is then swept to the upper airway for expectoration. A breakdown in the epithelium of the lungs or the mucociliary system can cause the defense mechanisms to malfunction. This allows atmospheric pollutants and irritants to enter and inflame the lungs.

SECRETORY IMMUNITY
Secretory immunity protects the lungs by releasing an antibody in respiratory mucosal secretions. The antibody launches an immune response against antigens that contact the mucosa.

LUNGS
The lungs are air-filled, spongelike organs. They're divided into lobes: three lobes on the right, two lobes on the left. The lobes are further divided into lobules and segments.

The lungs contain about 300 million pulmonary alveoli, which are grapelike clusters of air-filled sacs at the ends of the respiratory passages. Here, gas exchange takes place by diffusion. In diffusion, gas molecules pass through respiratory membranes. Oxygen is passed to the blood for circulation through the body. At the same time, carbon dioxide — a cellular waste product that's gathered by the blood as it circulates — is collected from the blood for disposal out of the body through the lungs.

Alveoli consist of type I and type II epithelial cells. Type I cells form the alveolar walls, through which gas exchange occurs. Type II cells produce surfactant, a lipid-type substance that coats the alveoli. During inspiration, surfactant allows the alveoli to expand uniformly. During expiration, surfactant prevents alveolar collapse.

The amount of oxygen and carbon dioxide that trade places in the alveoli depends largely on the amount of air in the alveoli (ventilation) and the amount of blood in the pulmonary capillaries (perfusion). The ratio of ventilation to perfusion is called the $\dot{V}/\dot{Q}$ ratio. The $\dot{V}/\dot{Q}$ ratio expresses the effectiveness of gas exchange.

For effective gas exchange, ventilation and perfusion must match as closely as possible. In normal lung function, the alveoli receive air at a rate of about 4 L/minute, while the capillaries supply blood to the alveoli at a rate of about 5 L/minute, creating a $\dot{V}/\dot{Q}$ ratio of 4:5 or 0.8. (See *Understanding ventilation and perfusion*.) A $\dot{V}/\dot{Q}$ mismatch, resulting from ventilation-perfusion dysfunction or altered lung mechanics, accounts for most of the impaired gas exchange in respiratory disorders.

Ineffective gas exchange between the alveoli and the pulmonary capillaries can affect all body systems by altering the amount of oxygen delivered to the cells. It may have three outcomes:
■ shunting (reduced ventilation to a lung unit)
■ dead-space ventilation (reduced perfusion to a lung unit)
■ silent unit (combination of shunting and dead-space ventilation).

Respiratory disorders are commonly classified as shunt-producing if the $\dot{V}/\dot{Q}$ ratio falls below 0.8 and dead space-producing if the $\dot{V}/\dot{Q}$ ratio exceeds 0.8.

Shunting causes unoxygenated blood to move from the right side of the heart to the left side. A shunt may result from a physical defect that lets unoxygenated blood bypass fully functioning alveoli. It also may result when airway obstruction prevents oxygen from reaching an adequately perfused area of the lung.

Dead-space ventilation occurs when blood supply to the alveoli is inadequate for gas exchange to occur. This occurs in pulmonary emboli, pulmonary infarction, and cardiogenic shock.

A silent unit occurs when little or no ventilation and perfusion are present, such as in pneumothorax and acute respiratory distress syndrome (ARDS).

BREATHING MECHANICS

The amount of air that reaches the lungs carrying oxygen and then departs carrying carbon dioxide depends on three factors:
■ lung volume and capacity
■ compliance (the lungs' ability to expand)
■ resistance to airflow.

Lung volume and capacity is the amount of air that's moved in and out of the lungs. Conditions that reduce the lungs' capacity for air include polio and tuberculosis.

Understanding ventilation and perfusion

Effective gas exchange depends on the relationship between ventilation and perfusion, or the $\dot{V}/\dot{Q}$ ratio. The diagrams below show what happens when the $\dot{V}/\dot{Q}$ ratio is normal and abnormal.

NORMAL VENTILATION AND PERFUSION

When ventilation and perfusion are matched, unoxygenated blood from the venous system returns to the right side of the heart through the pulmonary artery to the lungs, carrying carbon dioxide (CO_2). The arteries branch into the alveolar capillaries. Gas exchange takes place in the alveolar capillaries.

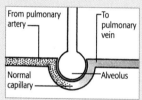

INADEQUATE PERFUSION (DEAD-SPACE VENTILATION)

When the $\dot{V}/\dot{Q}$ ratio is high, as shown here, ventilation is normal, but alveolar perfusion is reduced or absent. Note the narrowed capillary, indicating poor perfusion. This commonly results from a perfusion defect, such as a pulmonary embolism or a disorder that decreases cardiac output.

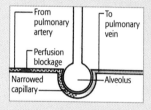

INADEQUATE VENTILATION (SHUNT)

When the $\dot{V}/\dot{Q}$ ratio is low, pulmonary circulation is adequate, but not enough oxygen (O_2) is available to the alveoli for normal diffusion. A portion of the blood flowing through the pulmonary vessels doesn't become oxygenated.

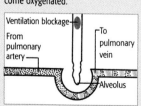

INADEQUATE VENTILATION AND PERFUSION (SILENT UNIT)

The silent unit indicates an absence of ventilation and perfusion to the lung area. The silent unit may help compensate for a $\dot{V}/\dot{Q}$ imbalance by delivering blood flow to better-ventilated lung areas.

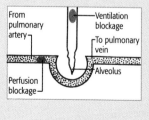

⬛ Blood with CO_2 ⬜ Blood with O_2 ▨ Blood with CO_2 and O_2

Compliance may change in either the lung or chest wall. Destruction of the lung's elastic fibers, which occurs in ARDS, decreases lung compliance. The lungs become stiff, making breathing difficult. The alveolocapillary membrane also may be affected, causing hypoxia. Chest-wall compliance is affected by thoracic deformity, muscle spasm, and abdominal distention.

Resistance refers to opposition to airflow. Changes in resistance may occur in the lung tissue, chest wall, or airways. Airway resistance accounts for about 80% of all respiratory system resistance. It's increased in such obstructive diseases as asthma, chronic bronchitis, and emphysema. With increased resistance, a person has to work harder to breathe, especially during expiration, to compensate for narrowed airways and diminished gas exchange.

NEUROCHEMICAL CONTROL

The respiratory center of the central nervous system is located in the lateral medulla oblongata of the brain stem. Impulses travel down the phrenic nerves to the diaphragm and then down the intercostal nerves to the intercostal muscles between the ribs. There, they change the rate and depth of respiration.

The respiratory center consists of different groups of neurons:
- The dorsal respiratory group of neurons determines the autonomic rhythm of respiration.
- The ventral respiratory group of neurons is inactive during normal respiration but becomes active when increased ventilatory effort is needed. It contains inspiratory and expiratory neurons.
- The pneumotaxic and apneustic centers don't generate a rhythm but modulate an established rhythm. The pneumotaxic center affects the inspiratory effort by limiting the volume of air inspired. The apneustic center prevents excessive inflation of the lungs.

Chemoreceptors respond to the pH of arterial blood, the partial pressure of arterial carbon dioxide ($PaCO_2$), and the partial pressure of arterial oxygen (PaO_2). Central chemoreceptors respond indirectly to arterial blood by sensing changes in the pH of cerebrospinal fluid (CSF). Peripheral chemoreceptors in the carotid and aortic bodies (small neurovascular structures in the carotid arteries and aorta) respond to decreased PaO_2 and decreased pH. Either change results in increased respiratory drive within minutes.

The $PaCO_2$ also helps regulate ventilation (by impacting the pH of CSF). If the $PaCO_2$ is high, the respiratory rate increases. If the $PaCO_2$ is low, the respiratory rate decreases.

Respiratory disorders

The respiratory disorders discussed in this section include:

■ acute respiratory distress syndrome (ARDS)
■ acute respiratory failure (ARF)
■ asbestosis
■ asthma
■ chronic bronchitis
■ cor pulmonale
■ emphysema
■ pneumonia
■ pneumothorax
■ pulmonary edema
■ pulmonary embolism
■ severe acute respiratory syndrome (SARS)
■ tuberculosis.

ACUTE RESPIRATORY DISTRESS SYNDROME

ARDS is a form of pulmonary edema that can quickly lead to ARF. ARDS is also known as *shock, stiff, white, wet,* or *Da Nang lung.* It may follow a direct or indirect lung injury. ARDS is difficult to diagnose and, if not promptly diagnosed and treated, can prove fatal within 48 hours. In about 50% to 70% of people who develop it, ARDS is fatal.

Pathophysiology

The most common causes of ARDS are shock, sepsis, and trauma-related factors, such as fat emboli, pulmonary contusions, and multiple transfusions, which may increase the risk of microemboli. Other causes of ARDS include:

■ acute miliary tuberculosis
■ anaphylaxis
■ aspiration of gastric contents
■ coronary artery bypass grafting
■ decreased surfactant production
■ diffuse pneumonia, especially viral pneumonia
■ drug overdose (for example, heroin, aspirin, or ethchlorvynol)
■ fluid overload
■ hemodialysis
■ idiosyncratic reaction to ampicillin (Principen) or hydrochlorothiazide (Microzide)

- inhalation of noxious gases, such as nitrous oxide, ammonia, or chlorine
- leukemia
- near-drowning
- neurologic injuries
- oxygen toxicity
- pancreatitis
- thrombotic thrombocytopenic purpura (embolism and thrombosis of small blood vessels in the brain)
- uremia
- venous air embolism.

In ARDS, fluid accumulates in the lungs' interstitium, alveolar spaces, and small airways, causing the lungs to stiffen. This impairs ventilation and reduces oxygenation of pulmonary capillary blood. Here's what happens.

Injury reduces normal blood flow to the lungs, allowing platelets to aggregate. These platelets release substances, such as serotonin, bradykinin, and histamine, that inflame and damage the alveolar membrane and later increase capillary permeability. Histamines and other inflammatory substances increase capillary permeability, and fluid shifts into the interstitial space.

As capillary permeability increases, proteins and more fluid leak out, causing pulmonary edema. Fluid in the alveoli and decreased blood flow damage surfactant in the alveoli. This reduces the alveolar cells' ability to produce more surfactant. Without surfactant, alveoli collapse, impairing gas exchange. The patient breathes faster, but sufficient oxygen can't cross the alveolocapillary membrane.

Carbon dioxide, however, crosses more easily and is lost with every exhalation. Oxygen and carbon dioxide levels in the blood decrease. Pulmonary edema worsens. Meanwhile, inflammation leads to fibrosis, which further impedes gas exchange, resulting in hypoxemia. Hypoxemia leads to respiratory acidosis, and carbon dioxide levels rise from resulting hypoventilation.

RED FLAG Severe ARDS causes overwhelming hypoxemia. If uncorrected, this results in hypotension, decreased urine output, and respiratory and metabolic acidosis. Eventually, ventricular fibrillation or standstill may occur.

Signs and symptoms

Within hours to days of the initial injury, ARDS produces rapid, shallow breathing and dyspnea. Hypoxemia develops, causing an increased drive for ventilation. Because of the effort required to expand the stiff lungs, intercostal and suprasternal retractions develop. Fluid accumulation produces crackles and rhonchi. Worsening hypoxemia causes restlessness, apprehension, mental sluggishness, motor dysfunction, and tachycardia.

Test results

■ Initially, arterial blood gas (ABG) analysis with the patient breathing room air shows a reduced partial pressure of arterial oxygen (PaO_2) (less than 60 mm Hg) and a decreased partial pressure of arterial carbon dioxide ($PaCO_2$) (less than 35 mm Hg).

■ Hypoxemia despite increased supplemental oxygen indicates the presence of a characteristic ARDS shunt. The resulting blood pH usually reflects respiratory alkalosis.

■ As ARDS worsens, ABG values show respiratory acidosis ($PaCO_2$ increasing to more than 45 mm Hg), metabolic acidosis (bicarbonate [HCO_3^-] levels decreasing to less than 22 mEq/L), declining PaO_2 despite oxygen therapy, and declining oxygen saturation (SaO_2).

■ Pulmonary artery catheterization identifies the cause of edema by measuring pulmonary artery wedge pressure (PAWP) (12 mm Hg or less in ARDS). Pulmonary artery mixed venous blood shows hypoxia.

■ Serial chest X-rays in early stages show bilateral infiltrates. In later stages, the lung fields have a ground-glass appearance. With irreversible hypoxemia, X-rays show "whiteouts" of both lung fields.

■ Pulse oximetry shows a decreasing SaO_2.

■ Differential diagnosis rules out cardiogenic pulmonary edema, pulmonary vasculitis, and diffuse pulmonary hemorrhage.

■ Tests that aid in the diagnosis include:
  – sputum analysis, including Gram stain and culture and sensitivity tests, to identify organisms and help determine the disease process
  – blood cultures to identify infectious organisms
  – toxicology tests to screen for drug ingestion
  – serum amylase tests to rule out pancreatitis.

Treatment

Therapy focuses on correcting the cause of ARDS and preventing the progression of hypoxemia and respiratory acidosis. Supportive care includes administering continuous positive airway pressure. This therapy alone seldom fulfills the patient's ventilatory requirements, so several other treatments are used. (See *Acute respiratory distress syndrome teaching topics.*)

VENTILATION

The primary treatment for ARDS is intubation and mechanical ventilation to increase lung volume, open airways, and improve oxygenation. Positive end-expiratory pressure (PEEP) is also added to increase lung volume and open alveoli. Two other techniques can maximize the benefits and minimize the risks of mechanical ventilation:

■ Pressure-controlled inverse ratio ventilation reverses the conventional inspiration to expiration ratio and minimizes the risk of barotrauma. The mechanical breaths are pressure-limited.
■ Permissive hypercapnia limits peak inspiratory pressure. Although carbon dioxide removal is compromised, no treatment is given for subsequent changes in blood hydrogen and oxygen concentration.

DRUGS

During mechanical ventilation, drugs may be ordered to facilitate ventilation and minimize restlessness, oxygen consumption, and carbon dioxide production. They include sedatives such as propofol (Diprivan) or midazolam (Versed), opioids, and neuromuscular blocking agents such as vecuronium.

When ARDS results from fat emboli or a chemical injury, a short course of high-dose corticosteroids may be given. Sodium bicarbonate may reverse severe metabolic acidosis. Fluids and vasopressors help maintain blood pressure. Nonviral infections require treatment with antimicrobial drugs.

ADDITIONAL SUPPORT

Supportive measures include diuretic therapy, correction of electrolyte and acid-base imbalances, prone positioning, and fluid restriction (because even small increases in capillary pressure from I.V. fluids can greatly increase interstitial and alveolar edema).

ACUTE RESPIRATORY FAILURE

When the lungs can't adequately maintain oxygenation or eliminate carbon dioxide, ARF results, which can lead to tissue hypoxia. About 150,000 people develop ARF annually in the United States. In about 50% to 70% of people who develop it, ARF is fatal.

Pathophysiology

In patients with normal lung tissue, ARF usually means a $PaCO_2$ above 50 mm Hg and a PaO_2 below 50 mm Hg. These limits don't apply to patients with chronic obstructive pulmonary disease (COPD), who usually have a consistently high $PaCO_2$. In patients with COPD, only acute deterioration in ABG values with corresponding clinical deterioration indicates ARF.

ARF results from impaired gas exchange. Conditions that can lead to ARF include:

■ ARDS
■ atelectasis
■ bronchitis
■ bronchospasm
■ central nervous system (CNS) depression — head trauma or the use of sedatives, opioids, tranquilizers, or oxygen
■ CNS disease
■ COPD
■ cor pulmonale
■ pneumonia
■ pneumothorax
■ pulmonary edema
■ pulmonary emboli
■ ventilatory failure.

If left untreated, conditions associated with alveolar hypoventilation (deficient movement of air into and out of the alveoli), V̇/Q̇ (ventilation-perfusion) mismatch, and intrapulmonary (right-to-left) shunting can cause ARF.

Decreased SaO_2 may result from alveolar hypoventilation, in which chronic airway obstruction reduces alveolar minute ventilation (the volume of air inhaled and exhaled in 60 seconds). PaO_2 levels fall and $PaCO_2$ levels rise, resulting in hypoxemia.

Hypoventilation can result from a decrease in the respiratory rate or duration or from the inspiratory signal from the respiratory center, as with CNS conditions, trauma, or CNS depressant drugs. The most common cause of alveolar hypoventilation is airway obstruction, commonly seen with COPD (emphysema or bronchitis).

Hypoxemia — $\dot{V}/\dot{Q}$ imbalance — most commonly occurs when such conditions as pulmonary embolism or ARDS interrupt normal gas exchange in a specific lung region. Too little ventilation with normal blood flow or too little blood flow with normal ventilation may cause the imbalance, resulting in decreased PaO_2 levels and, thus, hypoxemia.

RED FLAG The hypoxemia and hypercapnia characteristic of ARF stimulate strong compensatory responses by all body systems, including the respiratory system, cardiovascular system, and CNS. In response to hypoxemia, for example, the sympathetic nervous system triggers vasoconstriction and increases peripheral resistance and heart rate.

■ *Untreated $\dot{V}/\dot{Q}$ imbalances can lead to right-to-left shunting, in which blood passes from the heart's right side to its left without being oxygenated. Tissue hypoxemia also occurs in ARF, resulting in anaerobic metabolism and lactic acidosis.*

■ *Respiratory acidosis is caused by hypercapnia. The heart rate increases, the stroke volume increases, and heart failure may occur. Cyanosis occurs because of increased amounts of unoxygenated blood. Hypoxia of the kidneys results in the release of erythropoietin from renal cells, which in turn causes the bone marrow to increase red blood cell (RBC) production — an attempt by the body to increase the blood's oxygen-carrying capacity.*

■ *The body responds to hypercapnia with cerebral depression, hypotension, circulatory failure, and increased heart rate and cardiac output. Hypoxemia, hypercapnia, or both cause the brain's respiratory control center first to increase respiratory depth (tidal volume) and then to increase the respiratory rate. As ARF worsens, retractions may also occur.*

Signs and symptoms

Specific symptoms vary with the underlying cause of ARF, and the following body systems may be affected.

RESPIRATORY SYSTEM

The respiratory rate may be increased, decreased, or normal depending on the cause; respirations may be shallow or deep or alternate between the two. The patient may experience air hunger. Cyanosis may occur depending on hemoglobin level and arterial oxygenation. Auscultation of the chest may reveal crackles, rhonchi, wheezing, or diminished breath sounds.

CENTRAL NERVOUS SYSTEM
The patient may be restless and confused. He may have a loss of concentration, irritability, and tremulousness. He may develop diminished tendon reflexes, papilledema, and coma.

CARDIOVASCULAR SYSTEM
Tachycardia, increased cardiac output, and mildly elevated blood pressure occur early in response to a low PaO_2. With myocardial hypoxia, arrhythmias may develop. Pulmonary hypertension may cause increased pressure on the right side of the heart, jugular vein distention, an enlarged liver, and peripheral edema.

Test results
■ ABG analysis shows deteriorating values and a pH below 7.35. Patients with COPD may have a lower than normal pH compared with previous levels.
■ Chest X-rays identify pulmonary diseases or conditions, such as emphysema, atelectasis, lesions, pneumothorax, infiltrates, and effusions.
■ Electrocardiography (ECG) can show ventricular arrhythmias (indicating myocardial hypoxia) or right ventricular hypertrophy (indicating cor pulmonale).
■ Pulse oximetry reveals decreasing SaO_2.
■ The white blood cell (WBC) count detects the underlying infection.
■ Abnormally low hemoglobin level and hematocrit signal blood loss, which indicates a decreased oxygen-carrying capacity.
■ Pulmonary artery catheterization helps to distinguish pulmonary and cardiovascular causes of ARF and monitors hemodynamic pressures.

Treatment
Therapy for ARF focuses on correcting hypoxemia and preventing respiratory acidosis. (See *Acute respiratory failure teaching topics,* page 192.) These measures can be used to improve oxygenation in patients with ARF:
■ deep breathing with pursed lips, if the patient isn't intubated and mechanically ventilated, to help keep the airway patent
■ incentive spirometry and chest physiotherapy with postural drainage to increase lung volume
■ oxygen therapy to promote oxygenation and raise the PaO_2 level

TEACHING FOCUS

Acute respiratory failure teaching topics

● Most patients with acute respiratory failure are treated in the intensive care unit; orient the patient to the environment, procedures, and routines to minimize anxiety.
● If the patient is intubated or has a tracheostomy, explain why he can't speak. Suggest alternative means of communication.
● Teach the patient how to perform deep breathing and incentive spirometry. Encourage him to perform these techniques as often as tolerated to help lower carbon dioxide levels.
● Help the patient learn to recognize reportable signs of respiratory infection.

■ mechanical ventilation with an endotracheal or tracheostomy tube, if needed, to provide adequate oxygenation and reverse acidosis
■ high-frequency ventilation, if the patient doesn't respond to treatment, to force the airways open, promoting oxygenation and preventing alveolar collapse.

ASBESTOSIS

Asbestosis is characterized by diffuse interstitial pulmonary fibrosis. Prolonged exposure to airborne asbestos particles causes pleural plaques and tumors of the pleura and peritoneum. (See *A close look at asbestosis*.)

Asbestos is a potent cocarcinogen, increasing a cigarette smoker's risk of lung cancer. An asbestos worker who smokes is 90 times more likely to develop lung cancer than a smoker who has never worked with asbestos. Asbestosis may develop 15 to 20 years after regular exposure to asbestos has ended.

Pathophysiology

Asbestosis is caused by prolonged inhalation of asbestos fibers. People at high risk include workers in the mining, milling, construction, fireproofing, and textile industries. Asbestos is also used in paints, plastics, and brake and clutch linings. Family members of asbestos workers may develop asbestosis from exposure to stray fibers shaken off the workers' clothing. The general public may be exposed to fibrous asbestos dust in deteriorating buildings or in waste piles from asbestos plants.

In asbestosis, inhaled asbestos fibers travel down the airways and penetrate respiratory bronchioles and alveolar walls. Fibers be-

A close look at asbestosis

After years of exposure to asbestos, healthy lung tissue progresses to massive pulmonary fibrosis, as shown here.

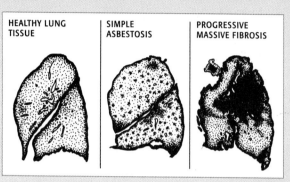

| HEALTHY LUNG TISSUE | SIMPLE ASBESTOSIS | PROGRESSIVE MASSIVE FIBROSIS |

come encased in a brown, iron-rich, proteinlike sheath in sputum or lung tissue. Interstitial fibrosis may develop in lower lung zones, affecting lung parenchyma and the pleurae. Raised hyaline plaques may form in the parietal pleura, the diaphragm, and the pleura adjacent to the pericardium.

RED FLAG Asbestosis may progress to pulmonary fibrosis with respiratory failure and cardiovascular complications, including pulmonary hypertension and cor pulmonale.

Signs and symptoms
Signs and symptoms of asbestosis include:
■ chest pain (typically pleuritic)
■ decreased forced expiratory volume and vital capacity
■ decreased lung inflation
■ dyspnea at rest with extensive fibrosis
■ dyspnea on exertion
■ finger clubbing
■ pleural friction rub and crackles on auscultation
■ productive cough in smokers
■ recurrent pleural effusions
■ recurrent respiratory tract infections
■ severe, nonproductive cough in nonsmokers.

TEACHING FOCUS

Asbestosis teaching topics

- Explain the disease process and its treatments.
- Teach the patient to prevent infections by avoiding crowds and people with infections and by receiving flu and pneumonia vaccines.
- Explain the importance of increasing fluid intake.
- Discuss prescribed drugs and how to take them correctly.
- Demonstrate how to perform bronchial drainage and chest percussion and vibration.
- Explain the safe use of oxygen in the home.
- Urge the patient to avoid exposure to bronchial irritants.

Test results

■ Chest X-rays may show fine, irregular, linear, diffuse infiltrates. With extensive fibrosis, the lungs have a honeycomb or ground-glass appearance. Other findings include pleural thickening and calcification, bilateral obliteration of costophrenic angles and, in later disease stages, an enlarged heart with a classic "shaggy" border.

■ Pulmonary function tests (PFTs) may identify decreased vital capacity, decreased forced vital capacity (FVC), decreased total lung capacity, decreased or normal forced expiratory volume in 1 second (FEV_1), a normal ratio of FEV_1 to FVC, and a reduced diffusing capacity for carbon monoxide when fibrosis destroys alveolar walls and thickens the alveolocapillary membrane.

■ ABG analysis may reveal decreased PaO_2 and $PaCO_2$ from hyperventilation.

Treatment

Asbestosis can't be cured. The goal of treatment is to relieve symptoms and control complications. (See *Asbestosis teaching topics*.)

Chest physiotherapy, such as controlled coughing and postural drainage with chest percussion and vibration, helps relieve respiratory signs and symptoms. In advanced disease, it's used to manage hypoxia and cor pulmonale.

Aerosol therapy, inhaled mucolytics, and fluid intake of at least 3 L daily help relieve respiratory symptoms.

Antibiotics should be given promptly for respiratory tract infections.

Oxygen administration relieves hypoxia. It's given by cannula, mask, or mechanical ventilation.

Patients with cor pulmonale may need diuretics, digoxin (Lanoxin), and salt restriction.

ASTHMA

Asthma is a chronic reactive airway disorder that may cause acute attacks — episodic airway obstruction — resulting from broncho-spasms, increased mucus secretion, and mucosal edema. Asthma is one type of COPD, a long-term pulmonary disease characterized by airflow resistance. Chronic bronchitis and emphysema are other types of COPD. (See *Understanding chronic obstructive pulmonary disease,* page 196.)

Asthma is becoming more common. It currently affects an esti-mated 17 million Americans. Children account for 4.8 million asth-ma sufferers in the United States. Twice as many boys as girls are af-fected. About one-third of patients develop asthma between ages 10 and 30. In this group, it's about equally common in both sexes. About one-third of all patients have at least one immediate family member who also has asthma.

Pathophysiology

In asthma, bronchial linings overreact to various stimuli, causing episodic smooth-muscle spasms that severely constrict the airways. Mucosal edema and thickened secretions further block the airways. (See *Understanding asthma,* page 197.) Asthma can be described in two ways: extrinsic (or atopic) asthma and intrinsic (or nonatopic) asthma. Many people with asthma, especially children, have both intrinsic and extrinsic asthma. (See *Asthma: A complex disease,* page 198.)

EXTRINSIC ASTHMA

Extrinsic asthma begins in childhood and is commonly accompa-nied by other hereditary allergies, such as eczema and allergic rhini-tis. This form of asthma is sensitive to specific external allergens, which include animal dander, cockroach allergen (major allergen for inner-city children), food additives containing sulfites, house dust or mold, kapok or feather pillows, pollen, and any other sensitizing substance.

INTRINSIC ASTHMA

This form of asthma is a reaction to internal, nonallergenic factors. No external substance can be implicated. Most episodes occur after a severe respiratory tract infection, especially in adults. Other pre-disposing conditions include emotional stress; endocrine changes;

Understanding chronic obstructive pulmonary disease

Chronic obstructive pulmonary disease (COPD) refers to long-term pulmonary disorders characterized by airflow resistance. Such disorders include asthma, chronic bronchitis, and emphysema. Chronic bronchitis and emphysema are more closely related in cause, pathogenesis, and treatment and are more likely to occur together. Asthma is more acute and intermittent than chronic bronchitis or emphysema.

PREDISPOSING FACTORS

Factors that predispose a patient to COPD include:

● smoking
● recurrent or chronic respiratory infections
● allergies
● hereditary factors such as an inherited deficiency in alpha$_1$-protease inhibitor, an inhibitor to the enzyme protease.

Smoking is the most important predisposing factor. It impairs ciliary action and macrophage function, causing inflammation in the airway, increased mucus production, alveolar destruction, and peribronchiolar fibrosis.

exposure to noxious fumes, such as nitrogen dioxide, which is produced by tobacco smoking among family members and inadequately vented stoves and heating appliances; fatigue; irritants; and temperature and humidity variations.

 RED FLAG *Complications of asthma may include pneumonia, respiratory failure, and status asthmaticus.*

Signs and symptoms

Signs and symptoms vary depending on the severity of a patient's asthma.

MILD INTERMITTENT ASTHMA

The patient has adequate air exchange and is asymptomatic between attacks. Coughing, wheezing, chest tightness, or trouble breathing occurs less than twice weekly. Flare-ups are brief but may vary in intensity. Nighttime symptoms occur less than twice monthly.

MILD PERSISTENT ASTHMA

The patient has adequate air exchange and is asymptomatic between attacks. Coughing, wheezing, chest tightness, or trouble breathing occurs three to six times weekly. Flare-ups may affect the patient's

Understanding asthma

Asthma is an inflammatory disease characterized by bronchospasm and hyper-responsiveness of the airway. These illustrations show the progression of an asthma attack.

1. Histamine (H) attaches to receptor sites in the larger bronchi, where it causes swelling in smooth muscles.

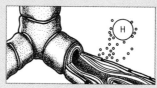

2. Leukotrienes attach to receptor sites in the smaller bronchi and cause swelling of smooth muscle there. Leukotrienes also cause fatty acids called prostaglandins to travel by way of the bloodstream to the lungs, where they enhance histamine's effects.

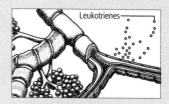

3. Histamine stimulates the mucous membranes to secrete excessive mucus, further narrowing the bronchial lumen, as shown.

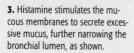

4. On inhalation (shown at left), the narrowed bronchial lumen can still expand slightly, allowing air to reach the alveoli. On exhalation (shown at right), increased intrathoracic pressure closes the bronchial lumen completely.

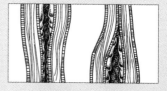

5. Mucus fills the lung bases, inhibiting alveolar ventilation, as shown. Blood, shunted to alveoli in other lung parts, still can't compensate for diminished ventilation.

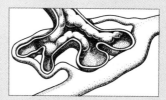

activity level. Nighttime symptoms occur three or four times per month.

MODERATE PERSISTENT ASTHMA
The patient has normal or below-normal air exchange. Coughing, wheezing, chest tightness, or trouble breathing occurs daily. Flare-ups may affect the patient's level of activity. Nighttime symptoms occur five or more times monthly.

SEVERE PERSISTENT ASTHMA
The patient has below-normal air exchange. Coughing, wheezing, chest tightness, and trouble breathing are continually present. The patient's activity level is greatly affected. Nighttime symptoms occur often.

STATUS ASTHMATICUS
Patients with any type of asthma may develop status asthmaticus, a severe acute attack that doesn't respond to conventional treatment. Signs and symptoms include marked respiratory distress, marked wheezing or absent breath sounds, pulsus paradoxus greater than 10 mm Hg, and chest wall contractions.

Test results
■ PFTs reveal signs of obstructive airway disease. These include low-normal or decreased vital capacity, and increased total lung and residual capacities. Pulmonary function may be normal between attacks. The PaO_2 and $PaCO_2$ usually are decreased, except in severe asthma, when the $PaCO_2$ may be normal or increased, indicating severe bronchial obstruction.
■ Serum immunoglobulin (Ig) E levels may increase from an allergic reaction.

Asthma teaching topics

- Teach the patient to avoid known allergens and irritants.
- Describe prescribed drugs, including their names, dosages, actions, adverse effects, and special instructions.
- Teach the patient how to use a metered-dose inhaler.
- If the patient has moderate to severe asthma, explain how to use a peak flowmeter to measure the degree of airway obstruction. Urge him to keep a record of peak flow readings and to bring the record to medical appointments.
- Explain the importance of seeking immediate medical attention if the peak flow drops suddenly (which may forecast severe respiratory problems).
- Tell the patient to seek immediate medical attention if he develops a fever above 100° F (37.8° C), chest pain, shortness of breath without coughing or exercising, or uncontrollable coughing.
- Teach diaphragmatic and pursed-lip breathing and effective coughing techniques.
- Urge the patient to drink at least 3 qt (3 L) of fluids daily to help loosen secretions and maintain hydration.

- Complete blood count (CBC) with differential reveals an increased eosinophil count.
- Chest X-rays can diagnose or monitor asthma's progress and may show hyperinflation with areas of atelectasis.
- ABG analysis detects hypoxemia and guides treatment.
- Skin testing may identify specific allergens. Test results are read in 1 to 2 days to detect an early reaction and again after 4 to 5 days to reveal a late reaction.
- Bronchial challenge testing evaluates the clinical significance of allergens identified by skin testing.
- Pulse oximetry may show a reduced SaO_2 level.

Treatment

The best treatment for asthma is prevention, which includes identifying and avoiding precipitating factors, such as environmental allergens and irritants. (See *Asthma teaching topics.*) Usually, such stimuli can't be removed entirely, so desensitization to specific antigens may be helpful, especially in children. Other common treatments include drug therapy and oxygen.

DRUG THERAPY

Bronchodilators decrease bronchoconstriction, reduce bronchial airway edema, and increase pulmonary ventilation. These include quick-relief drugs, such as inhaled short-acting beta$_2$ agonists (albuterol [Ventolin]) and long-term control drugs, such as long-acting beta$_2$ agonists (salmeterol [Serevent Diskus]).

Corticosteroids decrease airway inflammation and edema. Systemic corticosteroids, such as hydrocortisone sodium succinate (Solu-Cortef), are used for acute exacerbations. Inhaled corticosteroids, such as fluticasone propionate (Flovent), are considered the gold standard of long-term asthma control.

Mast cell stabilizers are effective in patients with atopic asthma who have seasonal disease. These drugs include cromolyn (Intal) and nedocromil (Tilade). Given prophylactically, they block the acute obstructive effects of antigen exposure by inhibiting the degranulation of mast cells, thereby preventing the release of the chemical mediators responsible for anaphylaxis.

Leukotriene modifiers (zileuton [Zyflo]) and leukotriene receptor antagonists (montelukast [Singulair] and zafirlukast [Accolate]) inhibit potent bronchoconstriction and inflammatory effects of cysteinyl leukotrienes and also can act as adjunctive therapy to avoid high-dose inhaled corticosteroids.

Anticholinergic bronchodilators, such as ipratropium bromide (Atrovent), block acetylcholine, another chemical mediator.

OXYGEN THERAPY
Low-flow humidified oxygen may be needed to treat dyspnea, cyanosis, and hypoxemia. The amount delivered is designed to maintain the PaO$_2$ between 65 and 85 mm Hg, as determined by ABG analysis. If the patient doesn't respond to initial ventilatory and drug therapy or develops respiratory failure, mechanical ventilation will be needed.

ALTERNATIVE THERAPY
Relaxation exercises, such as yoga, may help increase circulation and help a patient recover from an asthma attack.

CHRONIC BRONCHITIS
Chronic bronchitis, a form of COPD, is inflammation of the bronchi caused by irritants or infection. Hypersecretion of mucus and a chronic productive cough last for 3 months of the year and occur for at least 2 consecutive years. The distinguishing characteristic of bronchitis is the obstruction of airflow by mucus.

Pathophysiology
Chronic bronchitis occurs when irritants are inhaled for a prolonged period. The result is resistance in the small airways and severe V̇/Q̇

imbalance that decreases arterial oxygenation. Patients have a diminished respiratory drive, so they usually hypoventilate. Chronic hypoxia causes the kidneys to produce erythropoietin. This stimulates excessive RBC production, leading to polycythemia. The hemoglobin level is high, but the amount of reduced hemoglobin that comes in contact with oxygen is low; therefore, cyanosis develops.

RED FLAG *Complications of chronic bronchitis include pulmonary hypertension, ARF, cor pulmonale, and heart failure.*

Signs and symptoms
Signs and symptoms of advanced chronic bronchitis include:
■ cyanosis
■ dyspnea
■ finger clubbing
■ productive cough
■ prolonged expiration
■ pulmonary hypertension
■ rhonchi and wheezes
■ use of accessory muscles for breathing
■ weight gain and edema.

As pulmonary hypertension continues, right ventricular end-diastolic pressure increases. This leads to cor pulmonale (right ventricular hypertrophy with right-sided heart failure). Heart failure results in increased venous pressure, liver engorgement, epigastric distress, an S_3 gallop, and dependent edema.

Test results
■ Chest X-rays may show hyperinflation and increased bronchovascular markings.
■ PFTs indicate increased residual volume, decreased vital capacity and forced expiratory flow, and normal static compliance and diffusing capacity.
■ ABG analysis displays decreased PaO_2 and normal or increased $PaCO_2$.
■ Sputum culture may reveal many microorganisms and neutrophils.
■ ECG may show atrial arrhythmias; peaked P waves in leads II, III, and aV_F; and, occasionally, right ventricular hypertrophy.
■ Pulse oximetry shows decreased SaO_2.

Treatment
The most effective treatment for chronic bronchitis is to avoid air pollutants and, if the patient is a smoker, to stop smoking. (See

TEACHING FOCUS

Chronic bronchitis teaching topics

● Explain the disease process and its treatments.
● Discuss the importance of not smoking and of avoiding other bronchial irritants, such as second-hand smoke, allergens, pollution, aerosol sprays, and adverse weather conditions.
● Advise the patient to avoid crowds and people with infections and to obtain influenza and pneumococcal immunizations.
● Warn the patient that exposure to blasts of cold air may trigger bronchospasm; suggest that he avoid

cold, windy weather and that he cover his mouth and nose with a scarf or mask if he must go outside.
● Explain all drugs, including their indications, dosages, adverse effects, and special considerations.
● Demonstrate how to use a metered-dose inhaler.
● Show the proper use of safe home oxygen therapy.
● Teach the patient and his family how to perform postural drainage and chest physiotherapy.
● Discuss the importance of drinking plenty of fluids to liquefy secretions.

Chronic bronchitis teaching topics.) Other common treatments include:
■ adequate hydration
■ antibiotics to treat recurring infections
■ bronchodilators to relieve bronchospasm and facilitate mucus clearance
■ chest physiotherapy to mobilize secretions
■ corticosteroids to combat inflammation
■ diuretics for edema
■ nebulizer treatments to loosen and mobilize secretions
■ oxygen for hypoxia.

COR PULMONALE

In cor pulmonale, hypertrophy and dilation of the right ventricle develop secondary to a disease that affects the structure or function of the lungs or related structures. This condition occurs at the end stage of various chronic disorders of the lungs, pulmonary vessels, chest wall, and respiratory control center. It doesn't occur with disorders stemming from congenital heart disease or those affecting the left side of the heart.

Cor pulmonale causes about 25% of all types of heart failure. About 85% of patients with cor pulmonale also have COPD, and about 25% of patients with bronchial COPD eventually develop cor pulmonale. Cor pulmonale is most common in smokers and in middle-aged and elderly men; however, it's becoming more common in women.

Pathophysiology

Cor pulmonale may result from:

■ disorders that affect the pulmonary parenchyma
■ pulmonary diseases that affect the airways, such as COPD
■ vascular diseases, such as vasculitis, pulmonary emboli, and external vascular obstruction resulting from a tumor or aneurysm
■ chest wall abnormalities, including such thoracic deformities as kyphoscoliosis and pectus excavatum (funnel chest)
■ neuromuscular disorders, such as muscular dystrophy and poliomyelitis
■ external factors, such as obesity and living at a high altitude.

In cor pulmonale, pulmonary hypertension increases the heart's workload. To compensate, the right ventricle hypertrophies to force blood through the lungs. As long as the heart can compensate for the increased pulmonary vascular resistance, signs and symptoms reflect only the underlying disorder.

Red Flag Eventually, cor pulmonale may lead to biventricular failure, edema, ascites, and pleural effusions. Polycythemia — which develops when the bone marrow produces more RBCs in response to hypoxia — aggravates pulmonary hypertension and increases the risk of right-sided heart failure and thromboembolism. Because cor pulmonale occurs late in the course of COPD and other irreversible diseases, the prognosis is poor. (See Understanding cor pulmonale, *page 204.)*

Signs and symptoms

In early stages of cor pulmonale, patients are most likely to report chronic productive cough, exertional dyspnea, fatigue, weakness, and wheezing respirations.

As compensatory mechanisms begin to fail, larger amounts of blood remain in the right ventricle at the end of diastole, causing ventricular dilation. As cor pulmonale progresses, these additional symptoms occur:

■ decreased cardiac output
■ dependent edema
■ dyspnea at rest
■ hepatojugular reflux (jugular vein distention produced by pressure over the liver)

Understanding cor pulmonale

Three types of disorders are responsible for cor pulmonale:
● restrictive pulmonary disorders, such as fibrosis or obesity
● obstructive pulmonary disorders, such as chronic obstructive pulmonary disease
● primary vascular disorders, such as recurrent pulmonary emboli.

These disorders share a common pathway to the formation of cor pulmonale. Hypoxic constriction of pulmonary blood vessels and obstruction of pulmonary blood flow lead to increased pulmonary resistance, which progresses to cor pulmonale.

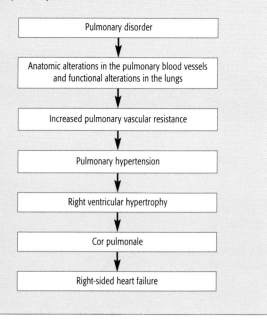

Pulmonary disorder
↓
Anatomic alterations in the pulmonary blood vessels and functional alterations in the lungs
↓
Increased pulmonary vascular resistance
↓
Pulmonary hypertension
↓
Right ventricular hypertrophy
↓
Cor pulmonale
↓
Right-sided heart failure

■ hepatomegaly (enlarged, tender liver)
■ orthopnea
■ jugular vein distention
■ right upper quadrant discomfort
■ tachycardia
■ tachypnea
■ weight gain.

Chest examination reveals characteristics of the underlying lung disease.

Test results

- Pulmonary artery catheterization shows increased right ventricular and pulmonary artery pressures, resulting from increased pulmonary vascular resistance. Right ventricular systolic and pulmonary artery systolic pressures are greater than 30 mm Hg. Pulmonary artery diastolic pressure is greater than 15 mm Hg.
- Echocardiography or angiography demonstrates right ventricular enlargement.
- Chest X-rays reveal large central pulmonary arteries and right ventricular enlargement.
- ABG analysis detects decreased PaO_2 (usually less than 70 mm Hg and never more than 90 mm Hg).
- Pulse oximetry shows reduced SaO_2.
- ECG may disclose arrhythmias, such as premature atrial and ventricular contractions and atrial fibrillation during severe hypoxia; right bundle-branch block; right axis deviation; prominent P waves; and an inverted T wave in right precordial leads.
- PFTs reflect underlying pulmonary disease.
- Magnetic resonance imaging (MRI) measures right ventricular mass, wall thickness, and ejection fraction.
- Cardiac catheterization measures pulmonary vascular pressures.
- Hematocrit is typically over 50%.
- Hepatic enzyme tests show an increased aspartate aminotransferase level with hepatic congestion and decreased liver function.
- Serum bilirubin levels may be elevated if liver dysfunction and hepatomegaly are present.

Treatment

Therapy for a patient with cor pulmonale aims to reduce hypoxemia and pulmonary vasoconstriction, increase exercise tolerance, and correct the underlying condition if possible. Treatment includes:
- bed rest
- antibiotics for an underlying respiratory tract infection
- oral calcium channel blockers, such as nifedipine (Procardia), nicardipine (Cardene), amlodipine (Norvasc), and diltiazem (Cardizem) for vasodilation
- potent pulmonary artery vasodilators, such as diazoxide (Hyperstat IV), nitroprusside (Nitropress), or hydralazine (Apresoline), to treat primary pulmonary hypertension

Cor pulmonale teaching topics

● Make sure that the patient understands the importance of maintaining a low-salt diet, weighing himself daily, and watching for increased edema. Teach him to look for edema by pressing the skin over a shin with one finger, holding it for a second or two, and then checking for a finger impression. Increased weight, increased edema, or respiratory difficulty should be reported to the physician.

● Instruct the patient to plan for frequent rest periods and to do breathing exercises regularly.

● If the patient has been placed on anticoagulant therapy, emphasize the need to watch for bleeding (epistaxis, hematuria, bruising) and to report signs to the physician. Also encourage him to return for periodic laboratory tests to monitor partial thrombo-

plastin time, fibrinogen level, platelet count, hematocrit, hemoglobin level, and prothrombin time.

● Because pulmonary infection commonly worsens chronic obstructive pulmonary disease and cor pulmonale, tell the patient to watch for and immediately report early signs of infection, such as increased sputum production, change in sputum color, increased coughing or wheezing, chest pain, fever, and tightness in the chest. Tell the patient to avoid crowds and people with pulmonary infections, especially during the flu season. Patients should receive pneumonia and annual flu vaccines.

● Warn the patient to avoid substances that may depress the ventilatory drive, such as sedatives and alcohol.

■ I.V. prostacyclin (Flolan) therapy to dilate blood vessels and reduce clotting by stopping platelet aggregation
■ endolithin receptor antagonists, such as bosentan (Tracleer), to reduce vasoconstriction
■ continuous administration of low concentrations of oxygen to decrease polycythemia and tachypnea
■ mechanical ventilation in acute disease
■ low-sodium diet with restricted fluids
■ phlebotomy to decrease RBC mass and anticoagulation with small doses of heparin to decrease the risk of thromboembolism. (See *Cor pulmonale teaching topics*.)

ADDITIONAL THERAPIES

Additional treatment may vary, depending on the underlying cause. For example, the patient may need a tracheotomy if he has an upper airway obstruction. The patient may need corticosteroids if he has vasculitis or an autoimmune disorder.

LIFE STAGES

Age-related changes and emphysema

Age-related changes in the respiratory system can worsen the symptoms of emphysema. Decreased peak airflow, gas exchange, and vital capacity can increase the shortness of breath experienced by the patient as he ages. These changes can be complicated by smoking, which actually speeds up the process of aging in the lungs and further worsens symptoms. What's more, defense mechanisms in the lungs and immune system decrease, increasing the aging person's risk of developing pneumonia after a bacterial or viral infection.

EMPHYSEMA

A form of COPD, emphysema is the abnormal, permanent enlargement of the acini accompanied by destruction of the alveolar walls. Obstruction results from tissue changes, rather than mucus production, which is the case in asthma and chronic bronchitis. The distinguishing characteristic of emphysema is airflow limitation caused by the lack of elastic recoil in the lungs.

Pathophysiology

Emphysema may be caused by a deficiency of alpha$_1$-protease inhibitor or by cigarette smoking. (See *Age-related changes and emphysema.*) Recurrent inflammation is associated with the release of proteolytic enzymes (enzymes that promote splitting of proteins by hydrolysis of peptide bonds) from lung cells. This causes irreversible enlargement of the air spaces distal to the terminal bronchioles. Enlargement of air spaces destroys the alveolar walls, which results in a breakdown of elasticity and loss of fibrous and muscle tissues, making the lungs less compliant. (See *Understanding emphysema,* page 208.)

RED FLAG In emphysema, complications may include recurrent respiratory tract infections, cor pulmonale, and respiratory failure. Also, alveolar blebs and bullae may rupture, leading to spontaneous pneumothorax or pneumomediastinum.

Signs and symptoms

Signs and symptoms of emphysema include:
■ anorexia and weight loss
■ barrel-shaped chest from lung overdistention
■ decreased breath sounds
■ dyspnea on exertion (initial symptom)
■ finger clubbing

Understanding emphysema

In normal, healthy breathing, air moves in and out of the lungs to meet metabolic needs. Any change in airway size compromises the lungs' ability to circulate sufficient air.

In a patient with emphysema, recurrent pulmonary inflammation damages and eventually destroys the alveolar walls, creating large air spaces. This breakdown leaves the alveoli unable to recoil normally after expanding and results in bronchiolar collapse on expiration. This traps air in the lungs, leading to overdistention.

Pulmonary capillary destruction usually allows a patient with severe emphysema to match ventilation to perfusion and thereby avoid cyanosis. The lungs are usually enlarged; therefore, total lung capacity and residual volume increase.

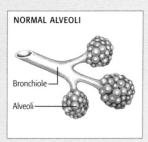

NORMAL ALVEOLI

Bronchiole

Alveoli

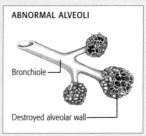

ABNORMAL ALVEOLI

Bronchiole

Destroyed alveolar wall

■ prolonged expiration because accessory muscles are used for inspiration and abdominal muscles are used to force air out of the lungs.

Because minimal V̇/Q̇ imbalance occurs, hyperventilation keeps blood gases within the normal range until late in the disease.

Test results

■ Chest X-rays in advanced disease may show a flattened diaphragm, reduced vascular markings at the lung periphery, overaeration of the lungs, a vertical heart, an enlarged anteroposterior chest diameter, and a large retrosternal air space.
■ PFTs indicate increased residual volume and total lung capacity, reduced diffusing capacity, and increased inspiratory flow.
■ ABG analysis usually shows reduced PaO_2 and normal $PaCO_2$ until late in the disease, when $PaCO_2$ is elevated. As the body compensates to maintain a normal pH, HCO_3^- levels rise.

TEACHING FOCUS

Emphysema teaching topics

- Explain the disease process and treatments.
- Urge the patient to avoid inhaled irritants, such as automobile exhaust fumes, aerosol sprays, and industrial pollutants.
- Advise the patient to avoid crowds and people with infections and to obtain pneumonia and annual flu vaccines.
- Warn the patient that exposure to blasts of cold air may trigger bronchospasm; suggest that he avoid cold, windy weather and that he cover his mouth and nose with a scarf or mask if he must go outside in such conditions.
- Explain all drugs, including their indications, dosages, adverse effects, and special considerations.

- Inform the patient about signs and symptoms that suggest ruptured alveolar blebs and bullae, and urge him to seek immediate medical attention if they occur.
- Demonstrate how to use a metered-dose inhaler.
- Teach the safe use of home oxygen therapy.
- Teach the patient and his family how to perform postural drainage and chest physiotherapy.
- Discuss the importance of drinking plenty of fluids to liquefy secretions.
- For family members of a patient with familial emphysema, recommend a blood test for alpha$_1$-antitrypsin. If a deficiency is found, stress the importance of not smoking and avoiding areas (if possible) where smoking is permitted.

- ECG may reveal tall, symmetrical P waves in leads II, III, and aV$_F$; vertical QRS axis; and signs of right ventricular hypertrophy late in the disease.
- CBC usually shows an increased hemoglobin level late in the disease, when the patient has persistent severe hypoxia.
- Pulse oximetry may show reduced SaO$_2$.

Treatment

Counsel patients with emphysema to avoid smoking and air pollution. (See *Emphysema teaching topics*.) Additional treatment includes:

- bronchodilators, such as beta blockers, albuterol (Ventolin), and ipratropium bromide (Atrovent) to reverse bronchospasm and promote mucociliary clearance
- mucolytics to thin secretions and aid mucus expectoration
- antibiotics to treat respiratory tract infections
- immunizations to prevent influenza and pneumococcal pneumonia
- adequate hydration

- chest physiotherapy to mobilize secretions
- oxygen therapy at low concentrations to increase the patient's PaO_2 to 55 to 65 mm Hg
- lung volume reduction surgery to allow functional lung tissue to expand and the diaphragm to return to its normally elevated position
- corticosteroids to reduce inflammation.

PNEUMONIA

Pneumonia is an acute infection of the lung parenchyma that commonly impairs gas exchange. It's the leading cause of death from infectious disease, and it occurs in both sexes and all ages. More than 4 million cases of pneumonia occur annually in the United States. In patients with normal lungs and adequate immune systems, the prognosis is good. In debilitated patients, bacterial pneumonia is the leading cause of death.

Pathophysiology

Pneumonia may be classified in three ways: by origin, location, and type.

ORIGIN

Pneumonia may be viral, bacterial, fungal, or protozoal in origin.

LOCATION

Bronchopneumonia involves distal airways and alveoli. Lobular pneumonia involves part of a lobe. Lobar pneumonia involves an entire lobe.

TYPE

Primary pneumonia results from inhalation or aspiration of a pathogen, such as bacteria or a virus, and includes pneumococcal and viral pneumonia. Secondary pneumonia may follow lung damage from a noxious chemical or other insult or may result from hematogenous spread of bacteria. Aspiration pneumonia results from inhalation of foreign matter, such as vomitus or food particles, into the bronchi.

In general, the lower respiratory tract can be exposed to pathogens by inhalation, aspiration, vascular dissemination, or direct contact with contaminated equipment such as suction catheters. After pathogens get inside, they begin to colonize and infection develops.

A close look at atelectatic alveoli

Normally, air-filled alveoli exchange oxygen and carbon dioxide with capillary blood. However, in atelectasis, airless, shrunken alveoli can't accomplish gas exchange.

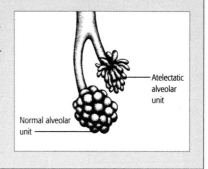

Atelectatic alveolar unit

Normal alveolar unit

In bacterial pneumonia, which can occur in any part of the lungs, an infection initially triggers alveolar inflammation and edema. This produces an area of low ventilation with normal perfusion. Capillaries become engorged with blood, causing stasis. As the alveolocapillary membrane breaks down, alveoli fill with blood and exudate, resulting in atelectasis (lung collapse). (See *A close look at atelectatic alveoli*.) In severe bacterial infections, the lungs look heavy and liverlike — reminiscent of ARDS.

In viral pneumonia, the virus first attacks bronchiolar epithelial cells. This causes interstitial inflammation and desquamation. The virus also invades bronchial mucous glands and goblet cells. It then spreads to the alveoli, which fill with blood and fluid. In advanced infection, a hyaline membrane may form. Like bacterial infections, viral pneumonia clinically resembles ARDS.

In aspiration pneumonia, inhalation of gastric juices or hydrocarbons triggers inflammatory changes and also inactivates surfactant over a large area. Decreased surfactant leads to alveolar collapse. Also, acidic gastric juices may damage the airways and alveoli. And particles containing aspirated gastric juices may obstruct the airways and reduce airflow, leading to secondary bacterial pneumonia.

RISK FACTORS
Certain predisposing factors increase the risk of pneumonia. For bacterial and viral pneumonia, these include:
■ abdominal and thoracic surgery

- alcoholism
- aspiration
- atelectasis
- cancer (particularly lung cancer)
- chronic illness and debilitation
- chronic respiratory disease, such as COPD, bronchiectasis, or cystic fibrosis
- colds or other viral respiratory infections
- exposure to noxious gases
- immunosuppressive therapy
- influenza
- malnutrition
- premature birth
- sickle cell disease
- smoking
- tracheostomy.
  For aspiration pneumonia, these include:
- a debilitated state
- a decreased level of consciousness
- an impaired gag reflex
- old age
- poor oral hygiene
- presence of nasogastric tube feedings.

RED FLAG Complications include hypoxemia, respiratory failure, pleural effusion, empyema, lung abscess, and bacteremia, with spread of infection to other parts of the body, resulting in meningitis, endocarditis, and pericarditis.

Signs and symptoms
The signs and symptoms of different types of pneumonia vary. (See *Distinguishing types of pneumonia*.)

Test results
- Chest X-rays confirm the diagnosis by disclosing infiltrates.
- Sputum specimen, Gram stain, and culture and sensitivity tests help differentiate the type of infection and the drugs that are effective in treatment.
- WBC count indicates leukocytosis in bacterial pneumonia and a normal or low count in viral or mycoplasmal pneumonia.
- Blood cultures reflect bacteremia and are used to determine the causative organism.
- ABG levels vary, depending on the severity of pneumonia and the underlying lung state.

Distinguishing types of pneumonia

The characteristics and prognosis of different types of pneumonia vary.

TYPE	CHARACTERISTICS
VIRAL	
Influenza	• Prognosis poor even with treatment • 50% mortality from cardiopulmonary collapse • Cough (initially nonproductive; later, purulent sputum), marked cyanosis, dyspnea, high fever, chills, substernal pain and discomfort, moist crackles, frontal headache, and myalgia
Adenovirus	• Insidious onset • Typically affects young adults • Good prognosis; usually clears with no residual effects • Sore throat, fever, cough, chills, malaise, small amounts of mucoid sputum, retrosternal chest pain, anorexia, rhinitis, adenopathy, scattered crackles, and rhonchi
Respiratory syncytial virus	• Most common in infants and children • Complete recovery in 1 to 3 weeks; may cause death in premature infants younger than age 6 months • Listlessness, irritability, tachypnea with retraction of intercostal muscles, slight sputum production, fever, severe malaise, possible cough or croup, and fine, moist crackles
Measles (rubeola)	• Typically more severe in adults than in children • Fever, dyspnea, cough, small amounts of sputum, rash, cervical adenopathy, and profusely runny nose
Chickenpox (varicella pneumonia)	• Uncommon in children but present in 30% of adults with varicella • Characteristic rash, cough, dyspnea, cyanosis, tachypnea, pleuritic chest pain, and hemoptysis and rhonchi 1 to 6 days after onset of rash
Cytomegalovirus	• Difficult to distinguish from other nonbacterial pneumonias • In adults with healthy lung tissue, resembles mononucleosis and typically is benign; in neonates, occurs as devastating multisystemic infection; in immunocompromised hosts, varies from clinically inapparent to fatal infection • Fever, cough, shaking chills, dyspnea, cyanosis, weakness, and diffuse crackles

(continued)

Distinguishing types of pneumonia (*continued*)

TYPE	CHARACTERISTICS
BACTERIAL	
Streptococcus	• Sudden onset of a single, shaking chill, and sustained temperature of 102° to 104° F (38.9° to 40° C); commonly preceded by upper respiratory tract infection
Klebsiella	• More likely in patients with chronic alcoholism, pulmonary disease, and diabetes • Fever and recurrent chills; cough producing rusty, bloody, viscous sputum (currant jelly); cyanosis of lips and nail beds from hypoxemia; and shallow, grunting respirations
Staphylococcus	• Commonly occurs in patients with viral illness, such as influenza or measles, and in those with cystic fibrosis • Temperature of 102° to 104° F, recurrent shaking chills, bloody sputum, dyspnea, tachypnea, and hypoxemia
ASPIRATION	
Aspiration of gastric or oropharyngeal contents into trachea and lungs	• Noncardiogenic pulmonary edema possible with damage to respiratory epithelium from contact with gastric acid • Subacute pneumonia possible with cavity formation • Lung abscess possible if foreign body present • Crackles, dyspnea, cyanosis, hypotension, and tachycardia

■ Bronchoscopy or transtracheal aspiration allows the collection of material for culture.
■ Pulse oximetry may show reduced SaO_2.

Treatment

A patient with pneumonia needs antimicrobial therapy based on the causative agent. Reevaluation should be done early in treatment. (See *Pneumonia teaching topics*.)

Supportive measures include analgesics to relieve pleuritic chest pain, antitussives, bed rest, bronchodilator therapy, chest physiotherapy and postural drainage, a high-calorie diet and adequate fluid intake, humidified oxygen therapy for hypoxia, mechanical ventilation for respiratory failure, and PEEP ventilation to main-

TEACHING FOCUS

Pneumonia teaching topics

● Explain the disease process and the treatment plan.

● Teach the patient how to cough and perform deep-breathing exercises to clear secretions; encourage him to do so often.

● Give emotional support by explaining all procedures (especially intubation and suctioning) to the patient and his family. Encourage family visits.

● To control the spread of infection, dispose of secretions properly. Tell the patient to sneeze and cough into a disposable tissue; tape a lined bag to the side of the bed for used tissues.

● Teach the patient strategies to prevent pneumonia:

  – Advise against using antibiotics indiscriminately during minor viral infections because doing so may encourage upper airway colonization by antibiotic-resistant bacteria.

  – Encourage pneumonia and annual flu vaccination for high-risk patients, such as those with chronic obstructive pulmonary disease, chronic heart disease, or sickle cell disease.

  – Urge all bedridden and postoperative patients to perform deep-breathing and coughing exercises often. Reposition such patients frequently to promote full aeration and drainage of secretions. Encourage early ambulation in postoperative patients.

tain adequate oxygenation for patients with severe pneumonia on mechanical ventilation.

PNEUMOTHORAX

Pneumothorax is an accumulation of air in the pleural cavity that leads to partial or complete lung collapse. When the amount of air between the visceral and parietal pleurae increases, increasing tension in the pleural cavity can cause the lung to progressively collapse. In some cases, venous return to the heart is impeded, causing a life-threatening condition called tension pneumothorax.

Pneumothorax is classified as either traumatic or spontaneous. Traumatic pneumothorax may be further classified as open (sucking chest wound) or closed (blunt or penetrating trauma). An open (penetrating) wound may cause closed pneumothorax if communication between the atmosphere and the pleural space seals itself off. Spontaneous pneumothorax, which is also considered closed, can be further classified as primary (idiopathic) or secondary (related to a specific disease).

Understanding tension pneumothorax

In tension pneumothorax, air accumulates in the intrapleural space and can't escape. Intrapleural pressure rises, collapsing the ipsilateral lung.

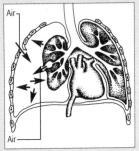

On inspiration, the mediastinum shifts toward the unaffected lung, impairing ventilation.

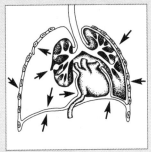

On expiration, the mediastinal shift distorts the vena cava and reduces venous return.

Pathophysiology

The causes of pneumothorax vary according to the classification.

Traumatic open pneumothorax, traumatic closed pneumothorax, or hemothorax (accumulation of blood in the pleural cavity) may result from a penetrating injury, such as a stab wound, a gunshot wound, or impalement. Traumatic closed pneumothorax or hemothorax also may result from blunt trauma, as from a car accident, a fall, or a crushing chest injury.

Traumatic pneumothorax also may result from insertion of a central line, thoracic surgery, thoracentesis, pleural or transbronchial biopsy, or tracheotomy. Tension pneumothorax can develop from either spontaneous or traumatic pneumothorax. (See *Understanding tension pneumothorax*.)

Open pneumothorax results when atmospheric air (positive pressure) flows directly into the pleural cavity (negative pressure). As the air pressure in the pleural cavity becomes positive, the lung collapses on the affected side. Lung collapse leads to decreased total lung capacity. The patient then develops $\dot{V}/\dot{Q}$ imbalance leading to hypoxia.

Closed pneumothorax occurs when air enters the pleural space from inside the lung. This increases pleural pressure and prevents lung expansion during inspiration. It may be called *traumatic pneu-*

mothorax when blunt chest trauma causes lung tissue to rupture, resulting in air leakage.

Spontaneous pneumothorax is a type of closed pneumothorax. It's more common in men and in older patients with chronic pulmonary disease. It also occurs in healthy young adults. The usual cause is rupture of a subpleural bleb (a small cystic space) at the surface of the lung. This causes air leakage into the pleural spaces; then the lung collapses, causing decreased total lung capacity, vital capacity, and lung compliance — leading, in turn, to hypoxia. The total amount of lung collapse can range from 5% to 95%.

 RED FLAG *Extensive pneumothorax and tension pneumothorax can lead to fatal pulmonary and circulatory impairment.*

Signs and symptoms

Although the causes of traumatic and spontaneous pneumothorax vary greatly, the effects are similar. The cardinal signs and symptoms of pneumothorax include:

- asymmetric chest wall movement
- cyanosis
- hyperresonance or tympany heard with percussion
- respiratory distress
- shortness of breath
- sudden, sharp, pleuritic pain worsened by chest movement, breathing, and coughing.

  Signs and symptoms of open pneumothorax also include:

- absent breath sounds on the affected side
- chest rigidity on the affected side
- crackling beneath the skin on palpation, indicating subcutaneous emphysema (air in the tissues)
- tachycardia.

  Tension pneumothorax produces the most severe respiratory symptoms, including:

- cardiac arrest
- compensatory tachycardia
- decreased cardiac output
- hypotension
- lung collapse from air or blood in the intrapleural space
- mediastinal shift and tracheal deviation to the opposite side
- tachypnea.

Test results

- Chest X-rays confirm the diagnosis by revealing air in the pleural space and, possibly, a mediastinal shift. Sequential chest X-rays

TEACHING FOCUS

Pneumothorax teaching topics

● To reassure the patient, explain what pneumothorax is, what causes it, and all planned diagnostic tests and procedures. Make him as comfortable as possible. (A patient with pneumothorax is usually most comfortable sitting upright.)
● Urge the patient to control coughing and gasping during chest tube insertion. However, after the chest tube is in place, encourage him to cough and perform deep-breathing exercises (at least once per hour) to facilitate lung expansion.
● Discuss the risk of recurrent spontaneous pneumothorax, and review its signs and symptoms. Emphasize the need for immediate medical intervention if they occur.

show whether thoracostomy was effective in resolving pneumothorax.
■ ABG analysis may show hypoxemia, possibly with respiratory acidosis and hypercapnia. SaO_2 levels may decrease at first but typically return to normal within 24 hours.
■ Pulse oximetry reveals hypoxemia.

Treatment
Treatment of pneumothorax depends on its type. (See *Pneumothorax teaching topics*.)

SPONTANEOUS PNEUMOTHORAX
Treatment is usually conservative for spontaneous pneumothorax when there's no sign of increased pleural pressure, less than 30% lung collapse, and no dyspnea or indication of physiologic compromise. Such treatment includes bed rest; careful monitoring of blood pressure, pulse, and respiratory rate; pulse oximetry; oxygen administration; and possible aspiration of air with a large-bore needle attached to a syringe.

If more than 30% of the lung collapses, a thoracostomy tube is typically placed in the second intercostal space in the midclavicular line to try to reexpand the lung. The tube then connects to an underwater seal or to low-pressure suction. If blood is present in the pleural space, a second thoracostomy tube is placed in the fourth, fifth, or sixth intercostal space to drain the blood.

Treatment for recurring spontaneous pneumothorax is thoracotomy and pleurectomy, which causes the lung to adhere to the parietal pleura.

TRAUMATIC PNEUMOTHORAX
Traumatic pneumothorax requires thoracostomy tube insertion and chest drainage and may also require surgical repair.

TENSION PNEUMOTHORAX
Tension pneumothorax is a medical emergency. If the tension in the pleural space isn't relieved, the patient will die from inadequate cardiac output or hypoxemia. A large-bore needle is inserted into the pleural space through the second intercostal space. If large amounts of air escape through the needle after insertion, the needle is left in place until a thoracostomy tube can be inserted.

PULMONARY EDEMA
Pulmonary edema is a common complication of cardiac disorders. It may occur as a chronic condition or develop quickly and rapidly become fatal. It's marked by accumulated fluid in the extravascular spaces of the lung.

Pathophysiology
Pulmonary edema may result from left-sided heart failure caused by arteriosclerotic, cardiomyopathic, hypertensive, or valvular heart disease. Normally, pulmonary capillary hydrostatic pressure, capillary oncotic pressure, capillary permeability, and lymphatic drainage are in balance, which prevents fluid infiltration to the lungs.

When this balance changes, or the lymphatic drainage system is obstructed, pulmonary edema results. If colloid osmotic pressure decreases, the hydrostatic force that regulates intravascular fluids is lost because nothing opposes it. Fluid flows freely into the interstitium and alveoli, impairing gas exchange and leading to pulmonary edema. (See *Understanding pulmonary edema,* page 220.)

RED FLAG Acute pulmonary edema may progress to respiratory and metabolic acidosis with subsequent cardiac and respiratory arrest.

Signs and symptoms
Signs and symptoms vary with the stage of pulmonary edema. In the early stages, look for:
- cough
- dependent crackles
- diastolic S_3 gallop
- dyspnea on exertion
- increased blood pressure
- jugular vein distention

Understanding pulmonary edema

In pulmonary edema, diminished function of the left ventricle causes blood to pool there and in the left atrium. Eventually, blood backs up into the pulmonary veins and capillaries.

Increasing capillary hydrostatic pressure pushes fluid into the interstitial spaces and alveoli. These illustrations show a normal alveolus and the effects of pulmonary edema.

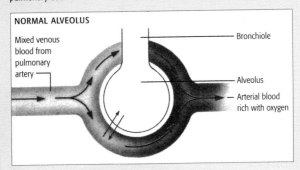

NORMAL ALVEOLUS

Mixed venous blood from pulmonary artery

Bronchiole

Alveolus

Arterial blood rich with oxygen

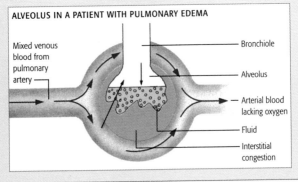

ALVEOLUS IN A PATIENT WITH PULMONARY EDEMA

Mixed venous blood from pulmonary artery

Bronchiole

Alveolus

Arterial blood lacking oxygen

Fluid

Interstitial congestion

■ mild tachypnea
■ orthopnea
■ paroxysmal nocturnal dyspnea
■ tachycardia.

As tissue hypoxia and decreased cardiac output occur, you'll see:

■ arrhythmias
■ cold, clammy skin

- cough producing frothy, bloody sputum
- cyanosis
- diaphoresis
- falling blood pressure
- increased tachycardia
- labored, rapid respiration
- more diffuse crackles
- thready pulse.

Test results

- Clinical features of pulmonary edema permit a working diagnosis. Diagnostic tests are used to confirm the disease.
- ABG analysis usually shows hypoxia with variable $PaCO_2$, depending on the patient's degree of fatigue. Metabolic acidosis may be revealed.
- Chest X-rays show diffuse haziness of the lung fields and, usually, cardiomegaly and pleural effusion.
- Pulse oximetry may reveal decreasing SaO_2.
- Pulmonary artery catheterization identifies left-sided heart failure and helps rule out ARDS.
- ECG may show previous or current myocardial infarction (MI).

Treatment

Treatment for pulmonary edema aims to reduce extravascular fluid, improve gas exchange and myocardial function, and correct the underlying disease, if possible. (See *Pulmonary edema teaching topics*, page 222.) Treatments include:

- antiarrhythmics for arrhythmias related to decreased cardiac output
- arterial vasodilators, such as nitroprusside (Nitropress), to decrease peripheral vascular resistance, preload, and afterload
- assisted ventilation to improve oxygen delivery to the tissues and acid-base balance for persistently low arterial oxygen levels
- diuretics, such as furosemide (Lasix), ethacrynic acid (Edecrin), and bumetanide (Bumex), to increase urination, which helps mobilize extravascular fluid
- high concentrations of oxygen given by nasal cannula (the patient probbaly can't tolerate a mask)
- human B-type natriuretic peptide, such as nesiritide (Natrecor), to reduce PAWP and systemic arterial pressure
- morphine to reduce anxiety and dyspnea and dilate the systemic venous bed, promoting blood flow from pulmonary circulation to the periphery

TEACHING FOCUS

Pulmonary edema teaching topics

- Explain all procedures to the patient and his family.
- Review all prescribed drugs with the patient. If he takes digoxin (Lanoxin), show him how to monitor his own pulse rate and warn him to report signs of toxicity.
- Encourage the patient to eat potassium-rich foods to lower the risk of toxicity and cardiac arrhythmias.
- If the patient takes a vasodilator, teach him the signs of hypotension and emphasize the need to avoid alcohol.
- Urge the patient to comply with the prescribed drug regimen to avoid future episodes of pulmonary edema.
- Emphasize the need to report early signs of fluid overload.
- Discuss ways to conserve physical energy.

■ positive inotropic agents, such as digoxin (Lanoxin), milrinone (Primacor), and inamrinone, to enhance contractility in myocardial dysfunction
■ pressor agents to enhance contractility and promote vasoconstriction in peripheral vessels.

PULMONARY EMBOLISM

Pulmonary embolism is an obstruction of the pulmonary arterial bed by a dislodged thrombus, heart valve growth, or foreign substance. It strikes an estimated 6 million adults each year in the United States, resulting in 100,000 deaths. Although pulmonary infarction that results from embolism may be so mild as to produce no symptoms, massive embolism (more than a 50% obstruction of pulmonary arterial circulation) and the accompanying infarction can be rapidly fatal.

Pathophysiology

Pulmonary embolism typically results from thrombi dislodged from the leg veins or pelvis. More than half of such thrombi arise in the deep veins of the legs. Predisposing factors include advanced age, atrial fibrillation, autoimmune hemolytic anemia, burns, cancer, central venous catheter insertion, chronic pulmonary disease, heart failure, hormonal contraceptives, I.V. drug abuse, leg fractures or surgery, long-term immobility or prolonged bed rest, obesity, polycythemia vera, pregnancy, recent surgery, sickle cell disease, thrombocytosis, thrombophlebitis, varicose veins, and vascular injury.

Thrombus formation results directly from vascular wall damage, venostasis, or hypercoagulability of the blood. Trauma, clot dissolution, sudden muscle spasm, intravascular pressure changes, or a change in peripheral blood flow can cause the thrombus to loosen or fragment. Then the thrombus — now called an *embolus* — floats to the heart's right side and enters the lung through the pulmonary artery. There, the embolus may dissolve, continue to fragment, or grow.

🚩 **RED FLAG** *By occluding the pulmonary artery, the embolus prevents alveoli from producing enough surfactant to maintain alveolar integrity. As a result, alveoli collapse and atelectasis develops. If the embolus enlarges, it may clog most or all of the pulmonary vessels and be fatal.*

Signs and symptoms
Total occlusion of the main pulmonary artery is rapidly fatal; smaller or fragmented emboli produce symptoms that vary with the size, number, and location of the emboli. Usually, the first symptom of pulmonary embolism is dyspnea, which may be accompanied by anginal or pleuritic chest pain. Other clinical features include:
■ low-grade fever
■ pleural effusion
■ productive cough (sputum may be blood-tinged)
■ tachycardia.
    Less common signs include:
■ cyanosis, syncope, and jugular vein distention (with a large embolus)
■ hypoxia (restlessness and anxiety)
■ leg edema
■ massive hemoptysis
■ pleural friction rub
■ signs of circulatory collapse (weak, rapid pulse and hypotension)
■ splinting of the chest.

Test results
■ The patient's history probably will reveal predisposing conditions as well as risk factors, including long car or plane trips, cancer, pregnancy, hypercoagulability, and previous deep vein thromboses or pulmonary emboli.
■ Chest X-rays help to rule out other pulmonary diseases.
■ Lung scan shows perfusion defects in areas beyond occluded vessels; however, it doesn't rule out microemboli.
■ Pulmonary angiography is the most definitive test, but it poses some risk to the patient. Its use depends on the uncertainty of

TEACHING FOCUS

Pulmonary embolism teaching topics

- Explain all procedures and treatments to the patient and his family.
- Teach the patient and his family the signs and symptoms of thrombophlebitis and pulmonary embolism.
- Teach the patient receiving anticoagulant therapy the signs of bleeding to watch for (bloody stools, blood in urine, large bruises).
- Tell the patient he can help prevent bleeding by shaving with an electric razor and by brushing his teeth with a soft toothbrush.
- Make sure that the patient understands the importance of taking drugs exactly as prescribed. Tell him not to take other drugs, especially aspirin, without asking the physician.
- Stress the importance of follow-up laboratory tests, such as prothrombin time, to monitor anticoagulant therapy.
- Tell the patient that he must inform all his health care providers – including dentists – that he's receiving anticoagulant therapy.
- To prevent pulmonary emboli in a high-risk patient, encourage him to walk and exercise his legs and to wear support or antiembolism stockings. Tell him not to cross or massage his legs.

the diagnosis and the need to avoid unnecessary anticoagulant therapy in a high-risk patient.

- ECG is inconclusive but helps distinguish a pulmonary embolism from an MI.
- Auscultation occasionally reveals a right ventricular S_3 gallop and increased intensity of a pulmonic component of S_2. Also, crackles and a pleural rub may be heard at the embolism site.
- ABG analysis showing decreased PaO_2 and $PaCO_2$ is characteristic but doesn't always occur.
- If pleural effusion is present, thoracentesis may rule out empyema, which indicates pneumonia.

Treatment

Treatment of pulmonary embolism is designed to maintain adequate cardiovascular and pulmonary function during resolution of the obstruction and to prevent embolus recurrence. (See *Pulmonary embolism teaching topics*.)

HEPARIN AND NONDRUG THERAPIES

Because most emboli resolve within 10 to 14 days, treatment consists of oxygen therapy, as needed; anticoagulation with heparin to inhibit new thrombus formation; and pneumatic compression devices. Heparin therapy is monitored with daily coagulation studies (partial thromboplastin time).

FIBRINOLYTIC THERAPY
Patients with massive pulmonary embolism and shock may need fibrinolytic therapy with streptokinase (Streptase) or alteplase (Activase) to enhance fibrinolysis of the pulmonary emboli and remaining thrombi. Emboli that cause hypotension may require the use of vasopressors.

SURGERY
Surgery is performed on patients who can't take anticoagulants (because of recent surgery or blood dyscrasias) and patients who have recurrent emboli during anticoagulant therapy. Surgery consists of vena caval ligation or insertion of a device (umbrella filter) to filter blood returning to the heart and lungs.

SEVERE ACUTE RESPIRATORY SYNDROME
SARS, a viral respiratory illness caused by a coronavirus, was first reported in Asia in February 2003. According to the World Health Organization (WHO), a total of 8,422 people worldwide became sick with SARS during the 2003 outbreak. Of these, 916 died. In the United States, 192 cases were reported; all of these patients recovered.

Pathophysiology
The coronavirus that causes SARS seems to spread by close person-to-person contact, probably by respiratory droplets produced when an infected person coughs or sneezes. Droplets are propelled a short distance (typically up to 3′ [1 m]) through the air and deposited on the mucous membranes of the mouth, nose, or eyes of a person who's nearby. The virus can also spread when a person touches a surface or object contaminated with infectious droplets and then touches his mouth, nose, or eyes. The virus incubates for 2 to 10 days.

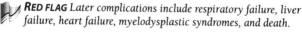 *RED FLAG Later complications include respiratory failure, liver failure, heart failure, myelodysplastic syndromes, and death.*

Signs and symptoms
SARS mimics many other respiratory diseases. It begins with a high fever (usually a temperature greater than 100.4° F [38° C]), chills, and achiness. Respiratory symptoms develop 4 to 7 days after the onset of fever. Respiratory symptoms can be mild to severe and include:

- diarrhea (in up to 20% of patients)
- dry cough
- hypoxemia
- pneumonia
- shortness of breath.

Test results

- The patient history is one of the most valuable sources of information when diagnosing suspected SARS. The diagnosis is fairly certain if the patient traveled to an area with documented SARS cases or has had close contact during the past 10 days with a person suspected of having SARS.
- Chest X-ray reveals hazy opacities and ground-glass appearance that progresses to bilateral consolidation in 24 to 48 hours.
- Suspect SARS in patients with severe atypical pneumonia.
- The SARS virus may be detected in nasopharyngeal or oropharyngeal secretions, blood, or stool.
- The WHO developed three types of diagnostic tests for SARS, including:
  - reverse transcription polymerase chain reaction test to detect ribonucleic acid of the SARS virus. To confirm SARS, two tests on two different specimens must be positive.
  - serum tests to detect IgM and IgG antibodies. The test result is considered negative if no SARS virus antibodies are found in serum obtained more than 28 days after the onset of symptoms.
  - cell culture test.
- A positive result for any of these tests confirms the diagnosis of SARS, but negative results don't necessarily rule out the diagnosis.

Treatment

The Centers for Disease Control and Prevention recommends using the same treatment for patients with SARS as for patients with serious community-acquired pneumonia, including oxygen support, as needed. Some experts advocate the use of antiviral drugs, such as oseltamivir (Tamiflu) or ribavirin (Virazole). Corticosteroid use is controversial. (See *Severe acute respiratory syndrome teaching topics.*) Other treatments being studied include:

- interferon beta (Betaseron) to block the virus from entering the cell; however, stopping the virus may require 10 times the normal dose

TEACHING FOCUS

Severe acute respiratory syndrome teaching topics

● Teach the patient about the need for isolation. Provide emotional support to help him deal with anxiety and fear related to the diagnosis of severe acute respiratory syndrome and as a result of isolation.
● Emphasize the importance of frequent hand washing, covering the mouth and nose when coughing or sneezing, and avoiding close personal contact while infected or potentially infected.
● Instruct the patient and his family that such items as eating utensils, towels, and bedding shouldn't be shared until they've been washed with soap and hot water, and that disposable gloves and household disinfectant should be used to clean any surface that may have been exposed to the patient's body fluids.
● Emphasize to the patient the importance of not going to work, school, or other public places, as recommended by the health care provider.

■ cysteine protease inhibitors to inhibit SARS virus replication; however, this has been effective in only 30% of cases
■ Surfaxin, a liquid surfactant.

TUBERCULOSIS

Tuberculosis is an infectious disease that affects mainly the lungs but can invade other body systems as well. Pulmonary infiltrates accumulate, cavities develop, and masses of granulated tissue form in the lungs.

Tuberculosis may occur as an acute or a chronic infection. The American Lung Association estimates that active tuberculosis afflicts 5.2 of every 100,000 people in the United States, which is a 43.5% decrease over the past 10 years. Tuberculosis is 63% more common in men and four times as common in nonwhites.

The disease is most common among people who live in crowded, poorly ventilated, unsanitary conditions, such as prisons, tenement houses, and homeless shelters. Others at high risk for tuberculosis include alcoholics, I.V. drug abusers, elderly people, and those who are immunocompromised.

Pathophysiology

Tuberculosis results from exposure to *Mycobacterium tuberculosis* and, sometimes, other strains of mycobacteria. Here's what happens.

TRANSMISSION

An infected person coughs or sneezes, spreading infected droplets. When someone without immunity inhales these droplets, the bacilli are deposited in the lungs.

IMMUNE RESPONSE

The immune system responds by sending leukocytes, and inflammation results. After a few days, leukocytes are replaced by macrophages. Bacilli are then ingested by the macrophages and carried off by the lymphatics to the lymph nodes.

TUBERCLE FORMATION

Macrophages that ingest the bacilli fuse to form epithelioid cell tubercles, tiny nodules surrounded by lymphocytes. In the lesion, caseous necrosis develops and scar tissue encapsulates the tubercle. The organism may be killed in the process.

DISSEMINATION

If the tubercles and inflamed nodes rupture, the infection contaminates the surrounding tissue and may spread through the blood and lymphatic circulation to distant sites. This process is called hematogenous dissemination. (See *Understanding tuberculosis invasion.*)

🚩 **RED FLAG** *Tuberculosis can cause massive pulmonary tissue damage, with inflammation and tissue necrosis eventually leading to respiratory failure. Bronchopleural fistulas can develop from lung tissue damage, resulting in pneumothorax. The disease also can lead to hemorrhage, pleural effusion, and pneumonia. Small mycobacterial foci can infect other organs and structures, including the kidneys, skeleton, and CNS. With proper treatment, the prognosis for a patient with tuberculosis is usually excellent.*

Signs and symptoms

After exposure to *M. tuberculosis*, roughly 5% of infected people develop active tuberculosis within 1 year. They may complain of a low-grade fever at night, a productive cough that lasts longer than 3 weeks, and symptoms of airway obstruction from lymph node involvement.

In other infected people, microorganisms cause a latent infection. The host's immunologic defense system may destroy the bacillus. Alternatively, the encapsulated bacillus may live in the tubercle. It may lie dormant for years, reactivating later to cause active infection.

Understanding tuberculosis invasion

After infected droplets are inhaled, they enter the lungs and are deposited either in the lower part of the upper lobe or in the upper part of the lower lobe. Leukocytes surround the droplets, which leads to inflammation. As part of the inflammatory response, some mycobacteria are carried off in the lymphatic circulation by the lymph nodes.

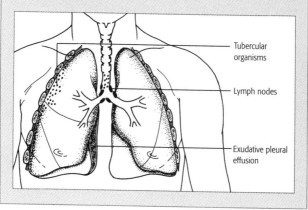

Tubercular organisms

Lymph nodes

Exudative pleural effusion

Test results
- Chest X-rays show nodular lesions, patchy infiltrates (mainly in upper lobes), cavity formation, scar tissue, and calcium deposits.
- A tuberculin skin test reveals infection at some point but doesn't indicate active disease.
- Stains and cultures of sputum, cerebrospinal fluid, urine, drainage from abscesses, or pleural fluid show heat-sensitive, nonmotile, aerobic, acid-fast bacilli.
- Computed tomography or MRI scans allow the evaluation of lung damage and may confirm a difficult diagnosis.
- Bronchoscopy shows inflammation and altered lung tissue. It also may be performed to obtain sputum if the patient can't produce an adequate sputum specimen.
- Several of these tests may be needed to distinguish tuberculosis from other diseases that mimic it, such as lung cancer, lung abscess, pneumoconiosis, and bronchiectasis.

Tuberculosis teaching topics

- Teach the infectious patient to cough and sneeze into tissues and to dispose of all secretions properly. Place a covered trash can nearby or tape a lined bag to the side of the bed to dispose of used tissues.
- Instruct the patient to wear a mask when out of his room.
- Advise visitors and staff members to wear particulate respirators that fit closely around the face when they're in the patient's room.
- Remind the patient to get plenty of rest. Stress the importance of eating balanced meals to promote recovery. If the patient is anorectic, urge him to eat small, frequent meals.
- Before discharge, advise the patient to watch for adverse drug effects and to report them immediately. Emphasize the importance of regular follow-up examinations. Teach the patient and his family about signs and symptoms of recurring tuberculosis. Stress the need to follow long-term treatment faithfully.
- Advise staff members and others who have been exposed to infected patients to receive tuberculin tests; chest X-rays and prophylactic isoniazid (Nydrazid) may also be ordered.
- Emphasize to the patient the importance of taking the drugs daily as prescribed. To avoid the development of drug-resistant organisms, he may participate in a supervised administration program.

Treatment

The usual treatment is at least 9 months of daily oral doses of isoniazid (Nydrazid) or rifampin (Rifadin). In some cases, ethambutol (Myambutol) is added. After 2 to 4 weeks, the disease is no longer infectious, and the patient can resume normal activities while continuing the drug regimen.

A patient with atypical mycobacterial disease or drug-resistant tuberculosis may require second-line drugs, such as capreomycin (Capastat), streptomycin, para-aminosalicylic acid, pyrazinamide, or cycloserine (Seromycin). (See *Tuberculosis teaching topics.*)

THE RISE OF RESISTANT STRAINS

Many patients find it difficult to follow this lengthy treatment regimen, and noncompliance is common. This has led to the development of resistant strains of tuberculosis in recent years.

8

CARDIOVASCULAR SYSTEM

The cardiovascular system is made up of the heart, arteries, veins, and lymphatics. These structures transport life-supporting oxygen and nutrients to cells, remove metabolic waste products, and carry hormones from one part of the body to another. The cardiovascular system starts working when a fetus is barely 1 month old, and it's the last system to stop working at the end of life.

Circulation requires normal heart function, which propels blood through the system by continuous rhythmic contractions. Despite advances in disease detection and treatment, cardiovascular disease remains the leading cause of death in the United States. Myocardial infarction, or heart attack, is the primary cause of cardiovascular-related deaths. It typically occurs with little or no warning.

OXYGEN BALANCING ACT

A critical balance exists between myocardial oxygen supply and demand. A decrease in oxygen supply or an increase in oxygen demand can disturb this balance and threaten myocardial function.

The four major determinants of myocardial oxygen demand are heart rate, contractile force, muscle mass, and ventricular wall tension. Cardiac workload and oxygen demand increase if the heart rate speeds up or if the force of contractions becomes stronger. This can occur in hypertension, ventricular dilation, or heart muscle hypertrophy.

If myocardial oxygen demand increases, so must oxygen supply. To effectively increase oxygen supply, coronary perfusion must

231

also increase. Tissue hypoxia — the most potent stimulus — causes coronary arteries to dilate and increases coronary blood flow. Normal coronary vessels can dilate and increase blood flow five to six times above resting levels. However, stenotic, diseased vessels can't dilate, so an oxygen deficit may result.

Normally, blood flows unimpeded across the valves in one direction. The valves open and close in response to a pressure gradient. When the pressure in the chamber proximal to the valve exceeds the pressure in the chamber beyond the valve, the valves open. When the pressure beyond the valve exceeds the pressure in the proximal chamber, the valves close. The valve leaflets, or cusps, are so responsive that a pressure difference of less than 1 mm Hg between chambers will open and close them.

Valvular disease is the major cause of low blood flow. A diseased valve allows blood to flow backward across leaflets that haven't closed securely. This phenomenon is called *regurgitation*. The backflow of blood through the valves forces the heart to pump more blood, increasing cardiac workload. The valve opening also may become restricted and impede the forward flow of blood. The heart may fail to meet the tissues' metabolic requirements for blood and fail to function as a pump. Eventually, the circulatory system may fail to perfuse body tissues, and blood volume and vascular tone may be altered.

The body closely monitors blood volume and vascular tone. Blood flow to each tissue is monitored by microvessels, which measure how much blood each tissue needs and control the local blood flow. The nerves that control circulation also help direct blood flow to tissues. The heart pays attention to the tissues' demands. It responds to the return of blood through the veins and to nerve signals that make it pump the required amounts of blood.

Arterial pressure is carefully regulated by the body: If it falls below or rises above its normal mean level, immediate circulatory changes occur. If arterial pressure falls below normal, heart rate, force of contraction, and arteriolar constriction increase. If arterial pressure rises above normal, the person will have reflex slowing of the heart rate, decreased force of contraction, and vasodilation.

RISK FACTORS

Risk factors for cardiovascular disease fall into two categories: those that are modifiable and those that are nonmodifiable.

Modifiable risk factors

Some risk factors can be avoided or altered, possibly slowing the disease process or even reversing it. They include:

- cigarette smoking
- diabetes mellitus
- elevated serum lipid levels
- excessive intake of saturated fats, carbohydrates, and salt
- hypertension
- obesity
- sedentary lifestyle
- stress.

Nonmodifiable risk factors

Four nonmodifiable factors increase a person's risk of cardiovascular disease:

- age
- male gender
- family history
- race.

Susceptibility to cardiovascular disease increases with age; disease before age 40 is unusual. However, the age-disease correlation may simply reflect the longer duration of exposure to other risk factors.

Women are less susceptible than men to heart disease until after menopause; then they become as susceptible as men. One theory proposes that estrogen has a protective effect.

A family history also increases a person's chance of developing premature cardiovascular disease. For example, genetic factors can cause some pronounced, accelerated forms of atherosclerosis such as lipid disease. However, a family history of cardiovascular disease may reflect a strong environmental component. Risk factors — such as obesity or a lifestyle that causes tension — may recur in families.

Although cardiovascular disease affects all races, Blacks are most susceptible.

Cardiovascular disorders

The disorders discussed in this section include:

- abdominal aortic aneurysm
- cardiac tamponade
- cardiogenic shock
- coronary artery disease (CAD)
- dilated cardiomyopathy
- heart failure
- hypertension
- hypertrophic cardiomyopathy

- myocardial infarction (MI)
- pericarditis
- rheumatic fever and rheumatic heart disease.

ABDOMINAL AORTIC ANEURYSM

In abdominal aortic aneurysm, the wall of the aorta dilates abnormally between the renal arteries and the iliac branches. Such aneurysms are four times more common in men than in women and are most prevalent in Whites ages 50 to 80. An aneurysm that measures $2\frac{3}{8}''$ (6 cm) has a 20% chance of rupturing within 1 year.

Pathophysiology

About 95% of abdominal aortic aneurysms result from arteriosclerosis; the rest, from cystic medial necrosis, trauma, syphilis, and other infections. These aneurysms develop slowly over time. First, a local weakness in the muscular layer of the aorta (tunica media), because of degenerative changes, allows the inner layer (tunica intima) and outer layer (tunica adventitia) to stretch outward. Blood pressure in the aorta progressively weakens the vessel walls and enlarges the aneurysm.

RED FLAG Rupture of an abdominal aortic aneurysm may occur spontaneously in those left untreated. Patients with such rupture may remain stable for hours before shock and death occur, although 20% die immediately.

Signs and symptoms

Although abdominal aortic aneurysms usually don't produce symptoms, most are evident (unless the patient is obese) as a pulsating mass in the periumbilical area, accompanied by a systolic bruit over the aorta. A large aneurysm may continue to enlarge and eventually rupture. Lumbar pain that radiates to the flank and groin from pressure on lumbar nerves may signify enlargement and imminent rupture. If the aneurysm ruptures into the peritoneal cavity, it causes severe, persistent abdominal and back pain.

Other signs and symptoms of enlargement and rupture include weakness, sweating, tachycardia, and hypotension, which may be subtle if rupture into the retroperitoneal space produces a tamponade effect that prevents continued hemorrhage.

Test results

Because an abdominal aortic aneurysm rarely produces symptoms, in many cases it's detected accidentally as the result of an X-ray or a routine physical examination. Several tests can confirm suspected abdominal aortic aneurysm.

TEACHING FOCUS

Abdominal aortic aneurysm teaching topics

● Provide psychological support for the patient and his family. Help ease their fears about the intensive care unit (ICU), the threat of impending rupture, and surgery by providing appropriate explanations and answering all questions.
● Explain the surgical procedure and the expected postoperative care in the ICU for patients undergoing complex abdominal surgery (I.V. lines, endotracheal and nasogastric intubation, and mechanical ventilation).
● Tell the patient not to push, pull, or lift heavy objects until cleared by the physician.

▨ Serial ultrasonography allows accurate determination of aneurysm size, shape, and location.
▨ Anteroposterior and lateral X-rays of the abdomen can detect aortic calcification, which outlines the mass at least 75% of the time.
▨ Computed tomography can visualize the aneurysm's effect on nearby organs, particularly the position of the renal arteries in relation to the aneurysm.
▨ Aortography shows the condition of vessels proximal and distal to the aneurysm and the extent of the aneurysm, but may underestimate the aneurysm's diameter because it visualizes only the flow channel and not the surrounding clot.

Treatment

Treatments for abdominal aortic aneurysm are few. They include invasive interventions and drug therapy. (See *Abdominal aortic aneurysm teaching topics.*)

INVASIVE INTERVENTIONS

Usually, an abdominal aortic aneurysm requires resection of the aneurysm and replacement of the damaged aortic section with a Dacron or polytetrafluoroethylene graft. Surgery is advised when the aneurysm is $1\frac{7}{8}''$ to $2\frac{3}{8}''$ (5 to 6 cm) in diameter.

Another invasive treatment option is a procedure known as endoluminal stent grafting. In this procedure, the physician inserts a catheter through the femoral artery. Guided by angiography, he advances the catheter to the aneurysm. A balloon in the catheter is then inflated, pushing the stent open. The stent attaches with tiny hooks above and below the aneurysm. This creates a path for blood flow that bypasses the aneurysm.

DRUG OPTIONS
If the patient's aneurysm is small and produces no symptoms, surgery may be delayed. Beta blockers may be given to decrease the rate of the aneurysm's growth.

CARDIAC TAMPONADE

In cardiac tamponade, a rapid rise in intrapericardial pressure impairs diastolic filling of the heart. The rise in pressure usually results from blood or fluid accumulation in the pericardial sac. As little as 200 ml of fluid can create an emergency if it accumulates rapidly. If the condition is left untreated, cardiogenic shock and death can occur.

If fluid accumulates slowly and pressure rises — as in pericardial effusion caused by cancer — signs and symptoms may not be immediate. This is because the fibrous wall of the pericardial sac can stretch to accommodate up to 2 L of fluid.

Pathophysiology

Cardiac tamponade may result from:

■ effusion, as in cancer, bacterial infections, tuberculosis and, rarely, acute rheumatic fever
■ hemorrhage caused by trauma, such as from a gunshot or stab wound in the chest; cardiac surgery; or perforation by a catheter during cardiac or central venous catheterization and pacemaker insertion
■ hemorrhage from nontraumatic causes, such as from rupture of the heart or great vessels and anticoagulant therapy in a patient with pericarditis
■ viral, postirradiation, or idiopathic pericarditis
■ acute MI
■ chronic renal failure during dialysis
■ drug reaction from procainamide, hydralazine (Apresoline), minoxidil (Loniten), isoniazid (Nydrazid), penicillin, or daunorubicin (Cerubidine)
■ connective tissue disorders, such as rheumatoid arthritis, systemic lupus erythematosus, rheumatic fever, vasculitis, and scleroderma.

In cardiac tamponade, progressive accumulation of fluid in the pericardium compresses the heart chambers, obstructing blood flow into the ventricles and reducing the amount of blood that can be pumped out of the heart with each contraction. Every time the ventricles contract, more fluid accumulates in the pericardial sac. This further limits the amount of blood that can fill the chamber during the next cardiac cycle and reduces cardiac output.

RED FLAG *Decreased ventricular filling and cardiac output may result in cardiogenic shock and death if untreated.*

The amount of fluid needed to cause cardiac tamponade varies greatly. It may be as small as 200 ml if the fluid accumulates rapidly. It may be more than 2 L if the fluid accumulates slowly and the pericardium stretches to adapt. (See *Understanding cardiac tamponade,* page 238.)

Signs and symptoms

Cardiac tamponade has three classic features known as *Beck's triad:*
- elevated central venous pressure (CVP) with jugular vein distention
- muffled heart sounds
- pulsus paradoxus (inspiratory drop in systemic blood pressure greater than 15 mm Hg).

Other signs and symptoms include orthopnea, diaphoresis, anxiety, restlessness, cyanosis, and a weak, rapid peripheral pulse.

Test results

- Chest X-ray shows a slightly widened mediastinum and enlargement of the cardiac silhouette.
- Electrocardiography (ECG) rules out other cardiac disorders. The QRS amplitude may be reduced. Electrical alternans of the P wave, QRS complex, and T wave may be present. Generalized ST-segment elevation appears in all leads.
- Pulmonary artery pressure (PAP) monitoring reveals increased right atrial pressure or CVP and right ventricular diastolic pressure.
- Echocardiography records pericardial effusion with signs of right ventricular and atrial compression.

Treatment

The goal of treatment for cardiac tamponade is to relieve intrapericardial pressure and cardiac compression by removing the accumulated blood or fluid. This can be done by pericardiocentesis (needle aspiration of the pericardial cavity), by surgical creation of an opening, commonly called a *pericardial window,* or by insertion of a drain into the pericardial sac to drain the effusion.

In hypotensive patients, cardiac output is maintained through trial volume loading with I.V. normal saline solution, albumin, and perhaps an inotropic drug, such as dopamine (Intropin), or a vasopressor such as phenylephrine (Neo-Synephrine).

Depending on the cause of tamponade, additional treatment may be needed. For example, in traumatic injury, the patient may

Understanding cardiac tamponade

A healthy heart (top illustration) can deliver oxygen, nutrients, and other substances to all the body's cells.

In cardiac tamponade (bottom illustration), blood or fluid fills the pericardial space, compressing the heart chambers, increasing intracardial pressure, and obstructing venous return.

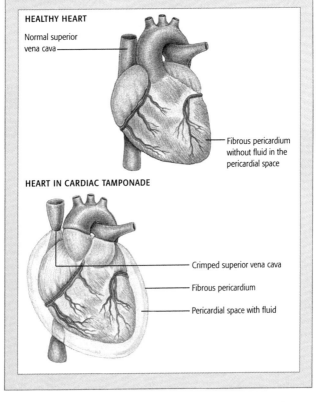

HEALTHY HEART

Normal superior vena cava

Fibrous pericardium without fluid in the pericardial space

HEART IN CARDIAC TAMPONADE

Crimped superior vena cava

Fibrous pericardium

Pericardial space with fluid

need a blood transfusion or a thoracotomy to drain reaccumulating fluid or to repair bleeding sites. In heparin-induced tamponade, the patient may need the heparin antagonist protamine. In warfarin-induced tamponade, the patient may need vitamin K and infusion of fresh frozen plasma. (See *Cardiac tamponade teaching topics*.)

TEACHING FOCUS

Cardiac tamponade teaching topics

● Reassure the patient to help reduce his anxiety.
● If the patient needs pericardiocentesis or thoracotomy, explain the procedure to him. Tell him what to expect postoperatively (chest tubes, drainage bottles, and oxygen administration). Teach him how to turn, deep breathe, and cough.

CARDIOGENIC SHOCK

Sometimes called *pump failure,* cardiogenic shock is a condition of diminished cardiac output that severely impairs tissue perfusion and oxygen delivery to the tissues. It reflects severe left-sided heart failure and occurs as a serious complication in some patients hospitalized with an acute MI.

Cardiogenic shock typically affects patients whose area of infarction exceeds 40% of the heart's muscle mass. In these patients, mortality may exceed 85%. Most patients with cardiogenic shock die within 24 hours of onset. The prognosis for those who survive is extremely poor.

Pathophysiology

Regardless of the underlying cause, left ventricular dysfunction triggers a series of compensatory mechanisms that attempt to increase cardiac output and, in turn, maintain vital organ function. As cardiac output falls, baroreceptors in the aorta and carotid arteries launch responses in the sympathetic nervous system. These responses, in turn, increase the heart rate, left ventricular filling pressure, and peripheral resistance to flow to enhance venous return to the heart.

These compensatory responses initially stabilize the patient, but later cause his condition to deteriorate as the oxygen demands of the already compromised heart rise. These events create a vicious cycle of low cardiac output, sympathetic compensation, myocardial ischemia, and even lower cardiac output.

 RED FLAG Death usually ensues because the vital organs can't overcome the deleterious effects of extended hypoperfusion.

Signs and symptoms

Cardiogenic shock produces signs of poor tissue perfusion, such as:
■ cold, pale, clammy skin

- confusion
- cyanosis
- drop in systolic blood pressure to 30 mm Hg below baseline or a sustained reading below 80 mm Hg that isn't caused by drug therapy
- narrowing pulse pressure
- oliguria (urine output less than 20 ml/hour)
- rapid, shallow respirations
- restlessness
- S_3 and S_4 heart sounds
- tachycardia
- weak peripheral pulses.

Test results

- PAP monitoring shows increased PAP and pulmonary artery wedge pressure (PAWP), which reflects a rise in left ventricular end-diastolic pressure (preload) and increased resistance to left ventricular emptying (afterload).
- Cardiac output measured by thermodilution reveals diminished cardiac output.
- Invasive arterial pressure monitoring shows hypotension.
- Arterial blood gas analysis reveals metabolic acidosis and hypoxia.
- ECG may reveal evidence of an acute MI, myocardial ischemia, or ventricular aneurysm.
- Cardiac enzymes and troponin levels are elevated.
- Echocardiography shows left ventricular dysfunction, valvular disease, dilation caused by an aneurysm, and ventricular septal defects.

Treatment

The aim of treatment is to enhance cardiovascular status by increasing cardiac output, improving myocardial perfusion, and decreasing cardiac workload. (See *Cardiogenic shock teaching topics*.) Treatment combines various cardiovascular drugs and mechanical assist techniques.

CARDIOVASCULAR DRUGS

Drug therapy may include I.V. dopamine (Intropin), a vasopressor that increases blood pressure and blood flow to the kidneys, and I.V. inamrinone, milrinone (Primacor), or dobutamine (Dobutrex), which are inotropic agents that increase myocardial contractility and cardiac output.

TEACHING FOCUS

Cardiogenic shock teaching topics

● Provide psychological support and reassurance because the patient and his family may be anxious about the intensive care unit, an intra-aortic balloon pump, and other tubes and devices.
● If needed, prepare the patient and his family for a possible fatal outcome, and help them find effective coping strategies.

Norepinephrine (Levophed) or phenylephrine (Neo-Synephrine) may be used when a potent vasoconstrictor is needed. I.V. nitroprusside (Nitropress), a vasodilator, may be used with a vasopressor to further improve cardiac output by decreasing afterload and reducing preload. However the patient's blood pressure must be adequate to support nitroprusside therapy and must be monitored closely.

MECHANICAL ASSIST TECHNIQUES
The intra-aortic balloon pump (IABP) is a mechanical assist device that attempts to improve coronary artery perfusion and decrease cardiac workload. An inflatable balloon pump is surgically inserted through the femoral artery into the descending thoracic aorta. After it's in place, the balloon inflates during diastole to increase coronary artery perfusion pressure and deflates before systole (before the aortic valve opens) to reduce resistance to ejection (afterload) and therefore lessen cardiac workload. Improved cardiac output and vasodilation in the peripheral blood vessels lead to a lower preload.

When drug therapy and IABP insertion fail, treatment may require a ventricular assist device until transplantation is possible.

CORONARY ARTERY DISEASE
CAD causes the loss of oxygen and nutrients to myocardial tissue because of poor coronary blood flow. CAD is nearly epidemic in the Western world. About 250,000 people per year die in the United States of CAD without being hospitalized — about half of all the deaths caused by CAD. It's most common in white, middle-aged men and in elderly people, with more than half of men age 60 or older showing signs of CAD on autopsy.

Pathophysiology
Atherosclerosis is the most common cause of CAD. In this condition, fatty, fibrous plaques, possibly including calcium deposits, pro-

gressively narrow the coronary artery lumens, which reduces the volume of blood that can flow through them. This can lead to myocardial ischemia (a temporary deficiency of blood flow to the heart) and eventually necrosis (heart tissue death).

RISK FACTORS
Many risk factors are associated with atherosclerosis and CAD. Some are modifiable and some are nonmodifiable. Nonmodifiable risk factors include:
■ being older than age 40
■ being male
■ being white
■ having a family history of CAD. (See *Genes implicated in coronary artery disease*.)

Modifiable risk factors include:
■ diabetes mellitus, especially in women
■ inactivity
■ increased homocysteine level
■ increased low-density and decreased high-density lipoprotein levels
■ obesity, which increases the risk of diabetes mellitus, hypertension, and high cholesterol level
■ smoking (risk dramatically drops within 1 year of quitting)
■ stress
■ systolic blood pressure greater than 140 mm Hg or diastolic blood pressure greater than 95 mm Hg.

Other risk factors that can be modified include:
■ high resting heart rate
■ increased hematocrit
■ increased levels of serum fibrinogen and uric acid
■ reduced vital capacity
■ thyrotoxicosis
■ use of hormonal contraceptives.

Other factors that can reduce blood flow include:
■ congenital defects in the coronary vascular system
■ dissecting aneurysm
■ infectious vasculitis
■ syphilis.

Coronary artery spasms can also impede blood flow. These spontaneous, sustained contractions of one or more coronary arteries occlude the vessel, reduce blood flow to the myocardium, and cause angina pectoris (chest pain). Without treatment, ischemia and, eventually, MI result.

Genes implicated in coronary artery disease

Overwhelming evidence confirms a genetic link to coronary artery disease (CAD). Indeed, researchers have identified more than 250 genes that may play a role in the disease. CAD commonly results from combined effects of multiple genes. These effects complicate the genetics of CAD because many genes can influence a person's risk.

Some of the best understood genes linked to CAD include:
- low-density lipoprotein (LDL) receptor – This protein removes LDL from the bloodstream. A mutation in this gene is responsible for familial hypercholesterolemia.
- apolipoprotein E – Mutations in this gene, commonly called *apo E*, also affect blood levels of LDL.
- apolipoprotein B-100 – Commonly called *apo B-100*, it's a component of

LDL. Mutations of this gene cause LDL to stay in the blood longer than normal, leading to very high LDL levels
- apolipoprotein A – This glycoprotein combines with LDL to form a particle called *Lp(a)*. Lp(a) appears as part of plaque on blood vessels.
- MTHFR – This is one of the enzymes that clears homocysteine from the blood. Mutations in MTHFR genes may increase homocysteine levels.
- cystathionine B-synthase – Also known as *CBS,* this is another enzyme involved in homocysteine metabolism. CBS mutations cause a condition known as *homocystinuria.* Homocysteine levels are so high that homocysteine can be detected in urine.

DISEASE PROCESS

As atherosclerosis progresses, luminal narrowing is accompanied by vascular changes that impair the diseased vessel's ability to dilate. This causes an imbalance between myocardial oxygen supply and demand, threatening the myocardium beyond the lesion. When oxygen demand exceeds what the diseased vessels can supply, localized myocardial ischemia results.

Transient ischemia causes reversible changes at the cellular and tissue levels, depressing myocardial function. Untreated, it can lead to tissue injury or necrosis. Oxygen deprivation forces the myocardium to shift from aerobic to anaerobic metabolism. As a result, lactic acid (the end product of anaerobic metabolism) accumulates. This reduces cellular pH.

The combination of hypoxia, reduced energy availability, and acidosis rapidly impairs left ventricular function. The strength of contractions in the affected myocardial region declines as the fibers shorten inadequately with less force and velocity. In addition, the ischemic section's wall motion is abnormal. This typically results in less blood being ejected from the heart with each contraction. Because of reduced contractility and impaired wall motion, the hemodynamic response becomes variable. It depends on the ischemic segment's size and the degree of reflex compensatory response by the autonomic nervous system.

Depression of left ventricular function may reduce stroke volume and thereby lower cardiac output. Reduction in systolic emptying increases ventricular volumes. As a result, left-sided heart pressures and PAWP increase. These increases in left-sided heart pressures and PAWP are magnified by changes in wall compliance induced by ischemia. Compliance is reduced, magnifying the elevation in pressure.

During ischemia, sympathetic nervous system response leads to slight elevations in blood pressure and heart rate before the onset of pain. With the onset of pain, further sympathetic activation occurs.

RED FLAG Complications of CAD may include arrhythmias, heart failure, ischemic cardiomyopathy, and MI.

Signs and symptoms

Angina is the classic sign of CAD. If the pain is predictable and relieved by rest or nitrates, it's called *stable angina*. If it increases in frequency and duration and is more easily induced, it's called *unstable* or *unpredictable angina*. Left untreated, either type of angina may progress to MI.

Angina commonly occurs after physical exertion but may also follow emotional excitement, exposure to cold, or the consumption of a large meal. Sometimes, it develops during sleep and wakes the patient. The patient may describe a burning, squeezing, or crushing tightness in the substernal or precordial area that radiates to the left arm, neck, jaw, or shoulder blade. He may clench his fist over his chest or rub his left arm when describing it. Pain is commonly accompanied by nausea, vomiting, fainting, sweating, and cool extremities.

Test results

- ECG during an episode of angina shows ischemia, as demonstrated by T-wave inversion, ST-segment depression and, possibly, arrhythmias such as premature ventricular contractions. Results may be normal during pain-free periods. Arrhythmias may occur without infarction, secondary to ischemia.
- Treadmill or bicycle exercise stress testing may provoke chest pain and ECG signs of myocardial ischemia. Monitoring of elec-

TEACHING FOCUS

Coronary artery disease teaching topics

● Explain the disease process and its treatments.
● Review the complications of coronary artery disease, such as myocardial infarction, and when to seek medical attention.
● Help the patient recognize cardiac risk factors and devise a plan of lifestyle modifications, such as exercise, dietary restrictions, stress reduction, weight control, and smoking cessation.

● Discuss the signs and symptoms of angina as well as how to prevent and treat it.
● If the patient is scheduled for surgery, explain the procedure to him and his family; give them a tour of the intensive care unit and introduce them to the staff.
● Explain drugs the patient is taking, including their names, dosages, frequencies, adverse effects, and special considerations.

trical rhythm may demonstrate T-wave inversion or ST-segment depression in the ischemic areas.

■ Coronary angiography reveals the location and extent of coronary artery stenosis or obstruction, collateral circulation, and the arteries' condition beyond the narrowing.

■ Myocardial perfusion imaging with thallium-201 during treadmill exercise detects ischemic areas of the myocardium, visualized as "cold spots."

Treatment

Because CAD is so widespread, controlling risk factors is important. Other treatment may focus on reducing myocardial oxygen demand or increasing the oxygen supply and alleviating pain. Interventions may be noninvasive, such as drug therapy, or invasive, such as coronary artery bypass graft (CABG) surgery, percutaneous transluminal coronary angioplasty (PTCA), and laser angioplasty. (See *Coronary artery disease teaching topics*.)

CONTROLLING RISK

Patients should limit calories and their intake of salt, fats, and cholesterol as well as stop smoking. Regular exercise is important, although it may need to be done more slowly to prevent pain. If stress is a known pain trigger, patients should learn stress reduction techniques. Other preventive actions include:

- controlling hypertension with diuretics, beta blockers, or angiotensin-converting enzyme (ACE) inhibitors
- controlling elevated serum cholesterol or triglyceride levels with antilipemics
- minimizing platelet aggregation and blood clot formation with aspirin.

DRUG THERAPY

Drug therapy may include nitrates, such as nitroglycerin or isosorbide dinitrate (Sorbitrate), and beta blockers that dilate vessels.

CABG SURGERY

Critically narrowed or blocked arteries may need CABG surgery to alleviate uncontrollable angina and prevent an MI. In this procedure, a part of the saphenous vein in the leg or the internal mammary artery in the chest is grafted between the aorta and the affected artery beyond the obstruction.

Minimally invasive CABG surgery requires a shorter recovery period and has fewer postoperative complications. Instead of sawing open the patient's sternum and spreading the ribs apart, several small cuts are made in the torso through which small surgical instruments and fiber-optic cameras are inserted. This procedure was designed to correct blockages in one or two easily reached arteries and may not be appropriate for more complicated cases.

PTCA

PTCA may be performed during cardiac catheterization to compress fatty deposits and relieve occlusion. In patients with calcification, this procedure may reduce the obstruction by fracturing the plaque. PTCA causes fewer complications than surgery, but it does have risks, which include:

- circulatory insufficiency
- MI
- restenosis of the vessels
- retroperitoneal bleeding
- sudden coronary reocclusions
- vasovagal response and arrhythmias
- death (rarely).

PTCA is a good alternative to bypass grafting in elderly patients and others who can't tolerate cardiac surgery. However, patients with left main coronary artery occlusions or lesions in extremely tortuous vessels aren't candidates for PTCA.

Stenting may also be done in conjunction with PTCA. A stent is introduced into the artery and placed in the area where the vessel has narrowed to keep the artery open.

LASER ANGIOPLASTY

Laser angioplasty corrects occlusion by vaporizing fatty deposits with a hot-tip laser device. Rotational ablation, or rotational atherectomy, removes plaque with a high-speed, rotating burr covered with diamond crystals.

DILATED CARDIOMYOPATHY

Also called *congestive cardiomyopathy,* dilated cardiomyopathy results from extensively damaged myocardial muscle fibers. It interferes with myocardial metabolism and grossly dilates every heart chamber, giving the heart a globular shape.

This disorder usually affects middle-aged men but can occur in any age-group. Because it usually isn't diagnosed until an advanced stage, the prognosis typically is poor. Most patients, especially those older than age 55, die within 2 years of symptom onset.

Pathophysiology

The exact cause of dilated cardiomyopathy is unknown. It may be linked to myocardial destruction caused by:

- infectious agents, such as viral myocarditis (especially after infection with coxsackievirus B, poliovirus, or influenza virus) and acquired immunodeficiency syndrome
- metabolic agents that cause endocrine and electrolyte disorders and nutritional deficiencies, such as hyperthyroidism, pheochromocytoma, beriberi, and kwashiorkor
- muscle disorders, such as myasthenia gravis, muscular dystrophy, and myotonic dystrophy
- infiltrative disorders, such as hemochromatosis and amyloidosis
- sarcoidosis
- rheumatic fever, especially in children with myocarditis
- alcoholism
- use of doxorubicin (Adriamycin), cyclophosphamide (Cytoxan), cocaine, or fluorouracil (Adrucil)
- X-linked inheritance patterns.

Dilated cardiomyopathy also may develop during the last trimester of pregnancy or a few months after delivery. Its cause is unknown, but it's most common in multiparous women older than age 30, particularly those with malnutrition or preeclampsia. In some pregnant patients, cardiomegaly and heart failure reverse with treatment, allowing a subsequent normal pregnancy. If cardiomegaly persists despite treatment, prognosis is poor.

Cardiomyopathy involves the ventricular myocardium as opposed to other heart structures, such as the valves or coronary arteries. Dilated cardiomyopathy is characterized by a grossly dilated, hypodynamic ventricle that contracts poorly and, to a lesser degree, myocardial hypertrophy. All four chambers become dilated as a result of increased volumes and pressures. Thrombi commonly develop in these chambers from blood pooling and stasis, which may lead to embolization. If hypertrophy coexists, the heart ejects blood less efficiently. A large volume remains in the left ventricle after systole, causing heart failure.

The onset of the disease is usually insidious. It may progress to end-stage refractory heart failure. If so, the patient's prognosis is poor. He may need heart transplantation.

RED FLAG *Dilated cardiomyopathy can lead to intractable heart failure, arrhythmias, and emboli. Ventricular arrhythmias may lead to syncope and sudden death.*

Signs and symptoms
Signs and symptoms of dilated cardiomyopathy include:
■ dry cough at night
■ dyspnea on exertion
■ fatigue
■ irregular rhythms
■ narrow pulse pressure
■ nausea
■ orthopnea
■ palpitations
■ pansystolic murmur
■ paroxysmal nocturnal dyspnea
■ peripheral edema
■ S_3 and S_4 gallop rhythms
■ shortness of breath
■ vague chest pain.

Test results
■ No single test confirms dilated cardiomyopathy. Diagnosis requires elimination of other possible causes of heart failure and arrhythmias.
■ ECG and angiography rule out ischemic heart disease. ECG also may show biventricular hypertrophy, sinus tachycardia, atrial enlargement, ST-segment and T-wave abnormalities and, in 20% of

patients, atrial fibrillation or left bundle-branch block. QRS complexes are decreased in amplitude.

■ Chest X-ray shows moderate to marked cardiomegaly, usually affecting all heart chambers, along with pulmonary congestion, pulmonary venous hypertension, and pleural effusion. Pericardial effusion may give the heart a globular shape.

■ Echocardiography may reveal ventricular thrombi, global hypokinesis, and degrees of left ventricular dilation and dysfunction.

■ Cardiac catheterization can show left ventricular dilation and dysfunction, elevated left ventricular and right ventricular filling pressures, and diminished cardiac output.

■ Gallium scans may identify patients with dilated cardiomyopathy and myocarditis.

■ Transvenous endomyocardial biopsy may be useful in some patients to determine the underlying disorder, such as amyloidosis or myocarditis.

Treatment

The goals of treatment for dilated cardiomyopathy are to correct the underlying causes and to improve the heart's pumping ability. The second goal is achieved with:

■ anticoagulants
■ cardiac glycosides
■ diuretics
■ low-sodium diet with vitamin suplementation
■ oxygen
■ vasodilators.

Antiarrhythmics may be used to treat arrhythmias.

Therapy also may include prolonged bed rest and selective use of corticosteroids, particularly if the patient has myocardial inflammation. Vasodilators reduce preload and afterload, decreasing congestion and increasing cardiac output. (See *Dilated cardiomyopathy teaching topics,* page 250.)

ACUTE AND LONG-TERM THERAPY

Acute heart failure requires vasodilation with I.V. nitroprusside (Nitropress) or nitroglycerin. Dopamine (Intropin), dobutamine (Dobutrex), milrinone (Primacor), and inamrinone may be useful during the acute stage. Long-term treatment may include prazosin (Minipress), hydralazine (Apresoline), isosorbide dinitrate (Sorbitrate), and anticoagulants if the patient is on bed rest. When these treatments fail, heart transplantation may be the only option for carefully selected patients.

TEACHING FOCUS

Dilated cardiomyopathy teaching topics

- Explain to the patient how dilated cardiomyopathy affects the heart muscle and circulation.
- Review signs and symptoms of the disease with the patient.
- Discuss signs and symptoms of complications, such as a weight gain of 3 lb (1.4 kg) or more over 1 to 2 days, which indicates heart failure and requires immediate medical attention.

- Teach the patient about sodium and fluid restrictions.
- Discuss the patient's drugs, dosages, how to take them, and their adverse effects.
- Emphasize the need to avoid alcohol and smoking.
- Explain preoperative and postoperative care to the patient undergoing heart surgery.
- Urge the family to learn cardiopulmonary resuscitation.

HEART FAILURE

When the myocardium can't pump effectively enough to meet the body's metabolic needs, heart failure occurs. Heart failure is classified as high-output or low-output, acute or chronic, left-sided or right-sided, and forward or backward (See *Classifying heart failure* and *Understanding left-sided and right-sided heart failure,* pages 252 and 253.) Pump failure usually occurs in a damaged left ventricle, but it also may happen in the right ventricle. Usually, left-sided heart failure develops first.

Heart failure affects about 5 million people in the United States. Its symptoms may restrict a person's ability to perform activities of daily living and severely affect quality of life. Advances in diagnostic and therapeutic techniques have greatly improved the outlook for these patients. However, the prognosis still depends on the underlying cause and its response to treatment.

Pathophysiology

Heart failure is commonly associated with systolic or diastolic overloading and myocardial weakness. It may result from a primary abnormality of the heart muscle — for example, an infarction — that impairs ventricular function and prevents the heart from pumping enough blood. It also may be caused by problems unrelated to MI, including the following:

Classifying heart failure

Heart failure may be classified different ways according to its pathophysiology.

RIGHT-SIDED OR LEFT-SIDED

Right-sided heart failure is a result of ineffective right ventricular contractile function. It may be caused by an acute right ventricular infarction or pulmonary embolus. However, the most common cause is profound backward flow from left-sided heart failure.

Left-sided heart failure is the result of ineffective left ventricular contractile function. It may lead to pulmonary congestion or pulmonary edema and decreased cardiac output. Left ventricular myocardial infarction, hypertension, and aortic and mitral valve stenosis or insufficiency are common causes.

As the decreased pumping ability of the left ventricle persists, fluid accumulates, backing up into the left atrium and then into the lungs. If this worsens, pulmonary edema and right-sided heart failure may result.

SYSTOLIC OR DIASTOLIC

In systolic heart failure, the left ventricle can't pump enough blood out to the systemic circulation during systole, and the ejection fraction falls. Consequently, blood backs up into the pulmonary circulation, pressure rises in the pulmonary venous system, and cardiac output falls.

In diastolic heart failure, the left ventricle can't relax and fill properly during diastole and the stroke volume falls. Therefore, larger ventricular volumes are needed to maintain cardiac output.

ACUTE OR CHRONIC

Acute refers to the timing of the onset of symptoms and whether compensatory mechanisms kick in. Typically, fluid status is normal or low, and sodium and water retention don't occur.

In chronic heart failure, signs and symptoms have been present for some time, compensatory mechanisms have taken effect, and fluid volume overload persists. Drugs, diet changes, and activity restrictions usually control symptoms.

- ▪ Mechanical disturbances in ventricular filling during diastole, from a blood volume that's too low for the ventricle to pump, occur in mitral stenosis secondary to rheumatic heart disease or constrictive pericarditis and in atrial fibrillation.
- ▪ Systolic hemodynamic disturbances — such as excessive cardiac workload caused by volume or pressure overload — limit the heart's pumping ability. This problem can result from mitral or aortic insufficiency, which leads to volume overload. It can also result from aortic stenosis or systemic hypertension, which causes increased resistance to ventricular emptying and decreased cardiac output.

(Text continues on page 254.)

Understanding left-sided and right-sided heart failure

These illustrations show how myocardial damage leads to heart failure.

LEFT-SIDED HEART FAILURE
1. Increased workload and end-diastolic volume enlarge the left ventricle (see illustration below). Because of lack of oxygen, the ventricle enlarges with stretched tissue rather than functional tissue. The patient may experience increased heart rate, pale and cool skin, tingling in the extremities, decreased cardiac output, and arrhythmias.

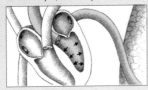

2. Diminished left ventricular function allows blood to pool in the ventricle and atrium and eventually back up into the pulmonary veins and capillaries, as shown below. At this stage, the patient may experience dyspnea on exertion, confusion, dizziness, orthostatic hypotension, decreased peripheral pulses and pulse pressure, cyanosis, and an S_3 gallop.

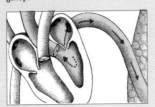

3. As the pulmonary circulation becomes engorged, rising capillary pressure pushes sodium and water into the interstitial space (as shown below), causing pulmonary edema. You'll note coughing, subclavian retractions, crackles, tachypnea, elevated pulmonary artery pressure, diminished pulmonary compliance, and increased partial pressure of carbon dioxide.

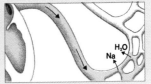

4. When the patient lies down, fluid in the extremities moves into the systemic circulation (see illustration below). Because the left ventricle can't handle the increased venous return, fluid pools in the pulmonary circulation, worsening pulmonary edema. You may note decreased breath sounds, dullness on percussion, crackles, and orthopnea.

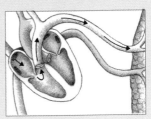

5. The right ventricle may now become stressed because it's pumping against greater pulmonary vascular resistance and left ventricular pressure (see illustration below). When this occurs, the patient's symptoms worsen.

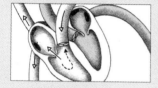

RIGHT-SIDED HEART FAILURE
6. The stressed right ventricle enlarges with the formation of stretched tissue (see illustration below). Increasing conduction time and deviation of the heart from its normal axis can cause arrhythmias. If the patient doesn't already have left-sided heart failure, he may experience increased heart rate, cool skin, cyanosis, decreased cardiac output, palpitations, and dyspnea.

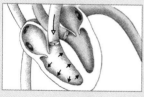

7. Blood pools in the right ventricle and right atrium. The backed-up blood causes pressure and congestion in the vena cava and systemic circulation (see illustration at top of next column). The patient will have elevated central venous pressure, jugular vein distention, and hepatojugular reflux.

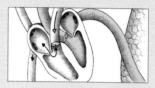

8. Backed-up blood also distends the visceral veins, especially the hepatic vein. As the liver and spleen become engorged (see illustration below), their function is impaired. The patient may develop anorexia, nausea, abdominal pain, a palpable liver and spleen, weakness, and dyspnea secondary to abdominal distention.

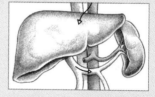

9. Rising capillary pressure forces excess fluid from the capillaries into the interstitial space (see illustration below). This causes tissue edema, especially in the lower extremities and abdomen. The patient may experience weight gain, pitting edema, and nocturia.

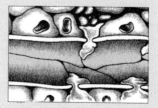

LIFE STAGES

Effects of aging and exercise on heart failure

Stiffening of the heart muscle has been thought to occur as an inevitable part of aging. A stiffened heart muscle impairs the heart's ability to circulate blood throughout the body and can result in heart failure, one of the most common age-related cardiovascular problems. Heart failure is the leading cause of hospitalization in people age 65 and older.

However, new research has shown that it's a sedentary lifestyle in addition to aging that results in stiffening of the heart muscle and impaired pumping action. Older adults who pursued lifelong endurance training programs have the same heart muscle pumping ability as that of their younger counterparts, while older, sedentary persons had 50% more stiffening than those who pursued lifelong exercise.

Certain conditions can predispose a patient to heart failure, especially if he has underlying heart disease. (See *Effects of aging and exercise on heart failure*.) These include:

■ arrhythmias, such as tachyarrhythmias, that reduce ventricular filling time
■ arrhythmias that disrupt the normal atrial and ventricular filling synchrony
■ bradycardia, which can reduce cardiac output
■ pregnancy and thyrotoxicosis, which increase cardiac output
■ pulmonary embolism, which elevates PAP, causing right-sided heart failure
■ infections, which increase metabolic demands and further burden the heart
■ anemia, which leads to increased cardiac output to meet the oxygen needs of the tissues
■ increased physical activity, increased salt or water intake, emotional stress, or failure to comply with the prescribed treatment regimen for the underlying heart disease.

The patient's underlying condition determines whether heart failure is acute or insidious.

The body's responses to decreased cardiac output include a reflex increase in sympathetic activity, release of renin from the juxtaglomerular cells of the kidney, anaerobic metabolism by affected cells, and increased extraction of oxygen by the peripheral cells. When blood in the ventricles increases, the heart compensates, or adapts. Adaptations may be short term or long term. In the former, as the end-diastolic fiber length increases, the ventricular muscle responds by dilating and increasing the force of contraction. (This is called the Starling curve.) In long-term adaptations, ventricular hypertrophy increases the heart muscle's ability to contract and push its volume of blood into the circulation.

Compensation may occur for long periods before signs and symptoms develop. As stress on the heart muscle reaches a critical level, the muscle's contractility is reduced and cardiac output declines despite the same venous input to the ventricle.

RED FLAG Eventually, sodium and water may enter the lungs, causing pulmonary edema, a life-threatening condition. Decreased perfusion to the brain, kidneys, and other major organs can cause them to fail. MI can occur because the oxygen demands of the overworked heart can't be met.

Signs and symptoms

Early signs and symptoms of heart failure include fatigue; exertional, paroxysmal, and nocturnal dyspnea; jugular vein engorgement; and hepatomegaly.

Later signs and symptoms include:

- anorexia
- chest tightness
- cyanosis
- dependent edema
- diaphoresis
- dullness over the lung bases
- gallop rhythm
- hemoptysis
- hypotension
- inspiratory crackles on auscultation
- marked hepatomegaly
- narrow pulse pressure
- nausea
- oliguria
- pallor
- palpitations
- pitting ankle enema
- sacral edema in bedridden patients
- slowed mental response
- tachypnea
- unexplained, steady weight gain.

Test results

- ECG reveals ischemia, tachycardia, and extrasystole.

TEACHING FOCUS

Heart failure teaching topics

- Teach the patient about the disease process, including its symptoms, complications, and treatments.
- Teach about prescribed drugs, their names, indications, dosages, adverse effects, and special considerations.
- Explain to the patient that the potassium lost through diuretic therapy may need to be replaced by taking a prescribed potassium supplement and eating high-potassium foods.
- Stress the importance of taking digoxin (Lanoxin) exactly as prescribed. Tell the patient to watch for and immediately report signs of toxicity, such as anorexia, vomiting, and yellow vision.
- Advise the patient to avoid foods high in sodium to curb fluid overload.

- Explain any fluid restrictions.
- Encourage the patient to participate in an outpatient cardiac rehabilitation program.
- Stress the need for regular checkups.
- Tell the patient to notify a physician promptly if his pulse is unusually irregular or measures less than 60 beats/minute; if he has dizziness, blurred vision, shortness of breath, a persistent dry cough, palpitations, increased fatigue, paroxysmal nocturnal dyspnea, swollen ankles, or decreased urine output; or if he notices rapid weight gain (3 to 5 lb [1.5 to 2.5 kg] in 1 week).
- Discuss the importance of smoking cessation.

- Echocardiogram identifies the underlying cause as well as the type and severity of the heart failure.
- Laboratory studies, such as B-type natriuretic peptide, confirm the presence of heart failure.
- Chest X-ray shows increased pulmonary vascular markings, interstitial edema, or pleural effusion and cardiomegaly.
- In left-sided heart failure, PAP monitoring shows elevated PAP and PAWP and elevated left ventricular end-diastolic pressure; in right-sided heart failure, it shows elevated right atrial pressure or elevated CVP.

Treatment

The goal of treatment for heart failure is to improve pump function, thereby reversing the compensatory mechanisms that produce or intensify the clinical effects. (See *Heart failure teaching topics.*) Heart failure can usually be controlled quickly with treatment, including:

- diuretics (such as furosemide [Lasix], hydrochlorothiazide [Microzide], ethacrynic acid [Edecrin], bumetanide [Bumex],

spironolactone [Aldactone], or triamterene [Dyrenium]) to reduce total blood volume and circulatory congestion
■ bed rest
■ oxygen administration to increase oxygen delivery to the myocardium and other vital organs
■ inotropic drugs (such as digoxin [Lanoxin]) to strengthen myocardial contractility; sympathomimetics (such as dopamine [Intropin] and dobutamine [Dobutrex]) in acute situations; or inamrinone or milrinone (Primacor) to increase contractility and cause arterial vasodilation
■ vasodilators to increase cardiac output or ACE inhibitors to decrease afterload
■ antiembolism stockings to prevent venostasis and thromboembolism formation.

ACUTE PULMONARY EDEMA
As a result of decreased contractility and elevated fluid volume and pressure, fluid may be driven from the pulmonary capillary beds into the alveoli, causing pulmonary edema. Treatment for acute pulmonary edema includes morphine; nitroglycerin or nitroprusside (Nitropress) to diminish blood return to the heart; dobutamine, dopamine, inamrinone, or milrinone to increase myocardial contractility and cardiac output; diuretics to reduce fluid volume; supplemental oxygen; and high Fowler's position.

CONTINUED CARE
After recovery, the patient must continue medical care and usually must continue taking digoxin, diuretics, and potassium supplements. A patient with valve dysfunction who has recurrent, acute heart failure may need surgical valve replacement.

Left ventricular remodeling surgery also may be performed. This procedure involves cutting a wedge about the size of a small slice of pie out of the left ventricle of an enlarged heart. The left ventricle is repaired. The result is a smaller ventricle that can pump blood more efficiently.

The only option for some patients is heart transplantation. A left ventricular assist device may be needed until a heart is available for transplantation.

HYPERTENSION
Hypertension is an intermittent or sustained elevation of diastolic or systolic blood pressure. A sustained systolic blood pressure of 140 mm Hg or higher or a diastolic blood pressure of 90 mm Hg or higher indicates hypertension.

Hypertension affects about 50 million adults in the United States. Blacks are more likely than Whites to be affected. The two major types of hypertension are essential (also called *primary* or *idiopathic*) and secondary. The cause of essential hypertension, the most common type, is complex. It involves several interacting homeostatic mechanisms. Hypertension is classified as secondary if it's related to a systemic disease that raises peripheral vascular resistance or cardiac output. Malignant hypertension is a severe, fulminant form of the disorder that may arise from either type.

Pathophysiology

Hypertension may be caused by increases in cardiac output, total peripheral resistance, or both. Cardiac output is increased by conditions that increase heart rate or stroke volume. Peripheral resistance is increased by factors that increase blood viscosity or reduce the lumen size of vessels, especially the arterioles. Family history, race, stress, obesity, a diet high in fat or sodium, use of tobacco or hormonal contraceptives, a sedentary lifestyle, and aging may all play a role. Their effects continue to be studied.

Essential hypertension usually begins insidiously as a benign disease, slowly progressing to a malignant state. If left untreated, even mild cases can cause major complications and death. Carefully managed treatment, which may include lifestyle modifications and drug therapy, improves the prognosis.

Several theories help to explain the development of hypertension. For example, it may arise from:
■ changes in the arteriolar bed that cause increased resistance
■ abnormally increased tone in the sensory nervous system that originates in the vasomotor system centers, causing increased peripheral vascular resistance
■ increased blood volume resulting from renal or hormonal dysfunction
■ an increase in arteriolar thickening caused by genetic factors, leading to increased peripheral vascular resistance
■ abnormal renin release resulting in the formation of angiotensin II, which constricts the arterioles and increases blood volume. (See *Understanding blood pressure regulation*.)

Secondary hypertension may be caused by renovascular disease; renal parenchymal disease; pheochromocytoma; primary hyperaldosteronism; Cushing's syndrome; diabetes mellitus; dysfunction of the thyroid, pituitary, or parathyroid gland; coarctation of the aorta; pregnancy; or neurologic disorders. The pathophysiology of secondary hypertension is related to the underlying disease. For example, consider these points.

Understanding blood pressure regulation

Hypertension may result from a disturbance in one of the body's intrinsic regulatory mechanisms.

RENIN-ANGIOTENSIN SYSTEM
Here's how the renin-angiotensin system acts to increase blood pressure:
● Sodium depletion, reduced blood pressure, and dehydration stimulate renin release.
● Renin reacts with angiotensinogen, a liver enzyme, and converts it to angiotensin I, which increases preload and afterload.
● Angiotensin I converts to angiotensin II in the lungs. Angiotensin II is a potent vasoconstrictor that targets the arterioles.
● Circulating angiotensin II works to increase preload and afterload by stimulating the adrenal cortex to secrete aldosterone. This increases blood volume by conserving sodium and water.

AUTOREGULATION
Several intrinsic mechanisms work to change an artery's diameter to maintain tissue and organ perfusion despite fluctuations in systemic blood pressure. These mechanisms include stress relaxation and capillary fluid shift:
● In stress relaxation, blood vessels gradually dilate when blood pressure rises to reduce peripheral resistance.
● In capillary fluid shift, plasma moves between vessels and extravascular spaces to maintain intravascular volume.

SYMPATHETIC STIMULATION
When blood pressure drops, baroreceptors in the aortic arch and carotid sinuses decrease their inhibition of the medulla's vasomotor center. This action increases sympathetic stimulation of the heart by norepinephrine. This increases cardiac output by strengthening the contractile force, raising the heart rate, and augmenting peripheral resistance by vasoconstriction. Stress can also stimulate the sympathetic nervous system to increase cardiac output and peripheral vascular resistance.

ANTIDIURETIC HORMONE
The release of antidiuretic hormone can regulate hypotension by causing reabsorption of water by the kidney. With reabsorption, blood plasma volume increases, raising blood pressure.

The most common cause of secondary hypertension is chronic renal disease. Insult to the kidney from chronic glomerulonephritis or renal artery stenosis interferes with sodium excretion, the renin-angiotensin-aldosterone system, or renal perfusion. This causes blood pressure to rise.

In Cushing's syndrome, increased cortisol levels raise blood pressure by increasing renal sodium retention, angiotensin II level, and vascular response to norepinephrine.

In primary aldosteronism, increased intravascular volume, altered sodium concentrations in vessel walls, or a very high aldosterone level cause vasoconstriction (increased resistance).

Pheochromocytoma is a secreting tumor of chromaffin cells, usually of the adrenal medulla. It causes hypertension because of increased secretion of epinephrine and norepinephrine. Epinephrine functions mainly to increase cardiac contractility and rate. Norepinephrine functions mainly to increase peripheral vascular resistance.

RED FLAG Complications occur late in the disease and can attack any organ system. Cardiac complications include CAD, angina, MI, heart failure, arrhythmias, and sudden death. Neurologic complications include stroke and hypertensive encephalopathy. Hypertensive retinopathy can cause blindness. Renovascular hypertension can lead to renal failure. (See A close look at blood vessel damage.)

Signs and symptoms

According to the Seventh Report of the Joint National Committee on Prevention, Detection, Evaluation, and Treatment of High Blood Pressure from the National Institutes of Health (NIH), serial blood pressure measurements are used to classify hypertension:

- Systolic blood pressure less than 120 mm Hg *and* diastolic blood pressure less than 80 mm Hg are considered normal.
- Prehypertension is characterized by systolic blood pressure of 120 to 139 mm Hg or diastolic blood pressure of 80 to 89 mm Hg.
- Stage 1 hypertension is characterized by systolic blood pressure of 140 to 159 mm Hg or diastolic blood pressure of 90 to 99 mm Hg.
- Stage 2 hypertension is characterized by systolic blood pressure of 160 mm Hg or higher or diastolic blood pressure of 100 mm Hg or higher.

Hypertension usually doesn't produce signs and symptoms until vascular changes occur in the heart, brain, or kidneys. Severely elevated blood pressure damages the intima of small vessels, resulting in fibrin accumulation in the vessels, local edema and, possibly, intravascular clotting. Symptoms depend on the location of the damaged vessels. For example, damage to vessels in the brain may cause stroke or transient ischemic attacks, damage to vessels in the retina may cause blindness, damage to vessels in the heart may cause MI, and damage to vessels in the kidneys may cause proteinuria, edema and, eventually, renal failure. Hypertension increases the heart's workload. This causes left ventricular hypertrophy and,

A close look at blood vessel damage

Sustained hypertension damages blood vessels. Vascular injury begins with alternating areas of dilation and constriction in the arterioles. Increased intra-arterial pressure damages the endothelium (as shown at right). Angiotensin induces endothelial wall contraction, allowing plasma to leak through interendothelial spaces (below left). Plasma constituents deposited in the vessel wall cause medial necrosis (below right).

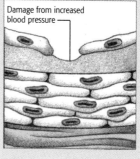

Damage from increased blood pressure

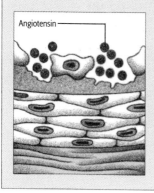

Angiotensin

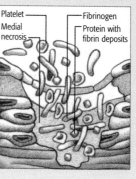

Platelet
Medial necrosis
Fibrinogen
Protein with fibrin deposits

later, left-sided heart failure, pulmonary edema, and right-sided heart failure.

Test results
Certain tests may reveal predisposing factors and help identify the cause of hypertension.

■ Urinalysis may show protein, red blood cells, or white blood cells (WBCs), suggesting renal disease; or glucose, suggesting diabetes mellitus.
■ Excretory urography may reveal renal atrophy, indicating chronic renal disease. One kidney that's more than ⅝″ (1.6 cm) shorter than the other suggests unilateral renal disease.

TEACHING FOCUS

Hypertension teaching topics

- Teach the patient about the disease process, including its complications and treatments.
- Explain the importance of complying with antihypertensive therapy and establishing a daily routine for taking prescribed drugs.
- Teach about prescribed drugs, including their names, indications, dosages, adverse effects, and special considerations.
- Show the patient how to use a blood pressure cuff; instruct him to record readings in a journal for review by the physician.

- Warn that uncontrolled hypertension may cause stroke and heart attack.
- Advise the patient to avoid high-sodium antacids and over-the-counter cold and sinus medicines, which contain harmful vasoconstrictors.
- Encourage the patient to avoid high-sodium foods and to achieve and maintain a healthy weight.
- Help the patient examine and modify his lifestyle (for example, by reducing stress and exercising regularly).
- Stress the importance of follow-up care.

■ Serum potassium level less than 3.5 mEq/L may indicate adrenal dysfunction (primary hyperaldosteronism).
■ Blood urea nitrogen (BUN) level elevated to more than 20 mg/dl and serum creatinine level elevated to more than 1.5 mg/dl suggest renal disease.
■ ECG may show left ventricular hypertrophy or ischemia.
■ Chest X-ray may demonstrate cardiomegaly.

Treatment

The NIH recommends a routine approach for treating primary hypertension. Lifestyle modifications should be made first, including weight reduction, moderation of alcohol intake, regular physical exercise, reduction of sodium intake, and smoking cessation. (See *Hypertension teaching topics*.)

Continue lifestyle modifications and begin drug therapy if the patient doesn't have the desired blood pressure or significant progress toward it. Thiazide-type diuretics are recommended for most patients with stage 1 hypertension who have no compelling indications, such as heart failure, post-MI, high CAD risk, diabetes, chronic kidney disease, or recurrent stroke prevention. An ACE inhibitor, a beta blocker, a calcium channel blocker, an angiotensin receptor blocker, or a combination also may be considered.

A two-drug combination (usually a thiazide-type diuretic and an ACE inhibitor, an angiotensin receptor blocker, a calcium channel blocker, or a beta blocker) may be ordered for a patient with stage 2 hypertension in the absence of compelling indications. If the patient has one or more compelling indications, drug treatment is based on benefits from outcome studies or existing clinical guidelines, such as these:

■ chronic kidney disease — ACE inhibitor or angiotensin receptor blocker
■ diabetes — diuretic, beta blocker, ACE inhibitor, angiotensin receptor blocker, or calcium channel blocker
■ heart failure — diuretic, beta blocker, ACE inhibitor, angiotensin receptor blocker, or aldosterone antagonist
■ high CAD risk — diuretic, beta blocker, ACE inhibitor, or calcium channel blocker
■ postmyocardial failure — beta blocker, ACE inhibitor, or aldosterone antagonist
■ recurrent stroke prevention — diuretic or ACE inhibitor.

If blood pressure remains outside the desired range, continue lifestyle modifications and optimize drug dosages until the goal blood pressure is achieved. Also, consider consultation with a hypertension specialist. Treatment of secondary hypertension includes correcting the underlying cause and controlling hypertensive effects. Hypertensive crisis, or severely elevated blood pressure, may not respond to drugs and may be fatal.

HYPERTROPHIC CARDIOMYOPATHY

Hypertrophic cardiomyopathy is a primary disease of the cardiac muscle. You may hear it called several other names, including *idiopathic hypertrophic subaortic stenosis, hypertrophic obstructive cardiomyopathy,* or *muscular aortic stenosis.* The course of this disorder varies. Some patients have progressive deterioration; others remain stable for years.

Pathophysiology

About half the time, hypertrophic cardiomyopathy is transmitted genetically as an autosomal dominant trait. Other causes aren't known.

Hypertrophic cardiomyopathy is characterized by left ventricular hypertrophy and an unusual cellular hypertrophy of the upper ventricular septum. These changes may result in an outflow tract pressure gradient, a pressure difference that results in an obstruction of blood outflow. The obstruction may change between examinations and even from beat to beat.

Hypertrophy of the intraventricular septum can pull the papillary muscle out of its usual alignment. This causes altered function of the anterior leaflet of the mitral valve and mitral insufficiency. The myocardial wall may stiffen over time, causing increased resistance to blood entering the right ventricle and an increase in diastolic filling pressures. Cardiac output may be low, normal, or high, depending on whether the stenosis is obstructive or nonobstructive. Eventually, left ventricular dysfunction—a result of rigidity and decreased compliance—causes pump failure.

RED FLAG Pulmonary hypertension and heart failure may occur secondary to left ventricular stiffness. Sudden death is also possible and usually results from ventricular arrhythmias, such as ventricular tachycardia and ventricular fibrillation.

Signs and symptoms

Signs and symptoms of hypertrophic cardiomyopathy include abdominal pain, angina, atrial fibrillation, dyspnea on exertion, edema, fatigue, migratory joint pain, orthopnea, syncope, and tachypnea.

Test results

- In obstructive disease, echocardiography shows left ventricular hypertrophy and a thick, asymmetrical intraventricular septum. Poor septal contraction, abnormal motion of the anterior mitral leaflet during systole, and narrowing or occlusion of the left ventricular outflow tract also may be seen. The left ventricular cavity looks small, with vigorous posterior wall motion but reduced septal excursion.
- In nonobstructive disease, echocardiography shows that ventricular areas are hypertrophied, and the septum may have a ground-glass appearance.
- Cardiac catheterization reveals elevated left ventricular end-diastolic pressure and, possibly, mitral insufficiency.
- ECG usually shows left ventricular hypertrophy; ST-segment and T-wave abnormalities; Q waves in leads II, III, aV_F, and in V_4 to V_6 (from hypertrophy, not infarction); left anterior hemiblock; left axis deviation; and ventricular and atrial arrhythmias.
- Chest X-ray may show a mild to moderate increase in heart size.
- Thallium scan usually reveals myocardial perfusion defects.

TEACHING FOCUS

Hypertrophic cardiomyopathy teaching topics

- Explain to the patient the way hypertrophic cardiomyopathy affects the heart muscle and circulation.
- Discuss signs and symptoms of the disease.
- Explain signs and symptoms of complications that require immediate medical attention, such as heart failure.
- Because syncope or sudden death may follow well-tolerated exercise, warn against strenuous physical activity, such as running.
- Warn the patient not to stop taking propranolol (Inderal) abruptly;

doing so may increase myocardial demand.
- Discuss dietary restrictions, including calorie and sodium reduction.
- Tell the patient to discuss antibiotic prophylaxis for subacute infective endocarditis with his health care provider before dental work or surgery.
- Prepare the patient for heart surgery if indicated.
- Because sudden cardiac arrest is possible, urge the patient's family to learn cardiopulmonary resuscitation.

Treatment

The goals of treatment for hypertrophic cardiomyopathy are to relax the ventricle and relieve outflow tract obstruction. Drugs are the first line of treatment. Surgery is performed rarely and only when all else fails. (See *Hypertrophic cardiomyopathy teaching topics*.)

DRUG THERAPY

Propranolol (Inderal) or metoprolol (Lopressor), each a beta blocker, is used to slow the heart rate and increase ventricular filling by relaxing the obstructing muscle, thereby reducing angina, syncope, dyspnea, and arrhythmias.

Calcium channel blockers may reduce elevated diastolic pressures, decrease the severity of outflow tract gradients, and increase exercise tolerance.

Disopyramide (Norpace) can be used to reduce left ventricular hypercontractility and the outflow gradient.

Heparin is given during episodes of atrial fibrillation. When accompanying hypertrophic cardiomyopathy, atrial fibrillation is a medical emergency that calls for cardioversion. Because of the high risk of systemic embolism, heparin must be given until fibrillation subsides.

Amiodarone (Cordarone) is given if heart failure occurs, unless the patient has an atrioventricular block. This drug also is effective in reducing ventricular and supraventricular arrhythmias and improving left ventricular pressure gradients.

The following drugs are contraindicated in the treatment of this disorder:

■ Vasodilators, such as nitroglycerin and diuretics, reduce venous return by permitting blood to pool in the periphery. This decreases ventricular volume and chamber size and may cause further obstruction.
■ Sympathetic stimulators and inotropic drugs increase cardiac contractility. If the septum is asymmetrically enlarged, it may obstruct left ventricular outflow, resulting in decreased cardiac output. Under these circumstances, any condition or drug that increases contractility also increases the degree of obstruction.

MYOCARDIAL INFARCTION

MI, an acute coronary syndrome, results from reduced blood flow through one of the coronary arteries. This causes myocardial ischemia, injury, and necrosis. In Q-wave (transmural) MI, tissue damage extends through all myocardial layers. In non–Q-wave (subendocardial) MI, usually only the innermost layer is damaged. (See *Understanding myocardial infarction,* pages 268 and 269.)

In North America and Western Europe, MI is one of the leading causes of death, usually from cardiac damage or complications. Mortality is about 25% in men and 38% in women within 1 year of an MI. However, more than half of sudden deaths occur within 1 hour after the onset of symptoms, before the patient reaches the hospital.

Men are more susceptible to MI than premenopausal women, although the risk is increasing in women who smoke and take hormonal contraceptives. The risk in postmenopausal women is similar to that in men.

Pathophysiology

MI results from occlusion of one or more of the coronary arteries. Occlusion can stem from atherosclerosis, thrombosis, platelet aggregation, and coronary artery stenosis or spasm.

Prolonged ischemia to the myocardium may cause irreversible cell damage and muscle death. Functionally, MI causes reduced contractility with abnormal wall motion, altered left ventricular compliance, reduced stroke volume, reduced ejection fraction, and elevated left ventricular end-diastolic pressure.

All MIs have a central area of necrosis or infarction surrounded by an area of injury. The area of injury is surrounded by a ring of ischemia. Tissue doesn't regenerate in the area of necrosis because the affected myocardial muscle is dead.

Scar tissue that forms on the necrotic area may inhibit contractility. When this occurs, compensatory mechanisms (vascular constriction, increased heart rate, and renal retention of sodium and water) act to try to maintain cardiac output. Ventricular dilation also may occur. If a lot of scar tissue forms, contractility may be greatly reduced, and heart failure or cardiogenic shock may develop.

The infarction site depends on the vessels involved. Occlusion of the circumflex coronary artery causes lateral wall infarctions. Occlusion of the left anterior coronary artery causes anterior wall infarctions. Occlusion of the right coronary artery or one of its branches causes posterior and inferior wall infarctions and right ventricular infarctions. Right ventricular infarctions can also accompany inferior infarctions and may cause right-sided heart failure.

Predisposing factors for MI include:
■ aging
■ diabetes mellitus
■ elevated serum triglyceride, low-density lipoprotein, cholesterol, and homocysteine levels and decreased serum high-density lipoprotein level
■ excessive intake of saturated fats, carbohydrates, or salt
■ family history of CAD
■ hypertension
■ obesity
■ sedentary lifestyle
■ smoking
■ stress
■ use of amphetamines or cocaine.

RED FLAG Elderly patients are more prone to complications and death. The most common complications after an acute MI include arrhythmias, cardiogenic shock, heart failure causing pulmonary edema, and pericarditis. Other complications include:
■ *rupture of the atrial or ventricular septum, ventricular wall, or valves*
■ *ventricular aneurysms*
■ *mural thrombi causing cerebral or pulmonary emboli*
■ *extensions of the original infarction*
■ *post-MI pericarditis (Dressler's syndrome), which occurs days to weeks after an MI and causes residual pain, malaise, and fever*
■ *psychological problems caused by fear of another MI or organic brain disorder from tissue hypoxia*
■ *personality changes.*

(Text continues on page 270.)

Understanding myocardial infarction

In myocardial infarction, the blood supply to the myocardium is interrupted. Here's what happens:

1. Injury to the endothelial lining of the coronary arteries causes platelets, white blood cells, fibrin, and lipids to converge at the injured site, as shown below. Foam cells, or resident macrophages, congregate under the damaged lining and absorb oxidized cholesterol, forming a fatty streak that narrows the arterial lumen.

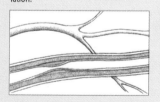

2. Because the arterial lumen narrows gradually, collateral circulation develops and helps maintain myocardial perfusion distal to the obstruction. The illustration below shows collateral circulation.

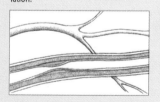

3. When myocardial demand for oxygen is more than the collateral circulation can supply, myocardial metabolism shifts from aerobic to anaerobic, producing lactic acid (represented

by **A**), which stimulates nerve endings, as shown below.

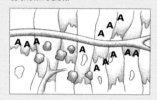

4. Lacking oxygen, the myocardial cells die (as shown below). This decreases contractility, stroke volume, and blood pressure.

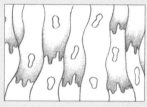

5. Hypoperfusion stimulates baroreceptors, which, in turn, stimulate the adrenal glands to release epinephrine and norepinephrine. This cycle is shown below. These catecholamines

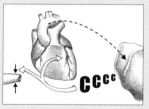

(represented by **C**) increase heart rate and cause peripheral vasoconstriction, further increasing myocardial oxygen demand.

6. Damaged cell membranes in the infarcted area allow intracellular contents into the vascular circulation, as shown below. Ventricular arrhythmias then develop with elevated serum levels of potassium (■), creatine kinase (CK), CK-MB (▲), cardiac troponin (●), aspartate aminotransferase, and lactate dehydrogenase (O).

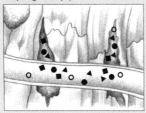

7. All myocardial cells are capable of spontaneous depolarization and repolarization, so the electrical conduction system may be affected by infarct, injury, and ischemia. The illustration below shows an injury site.

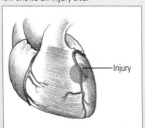

Injury

8. Extensive damage to the left ventricle may impair its ability to pump, allowing blood to back up into the left atrium and, eventually, into the pulmonary veins and capillaries, as shown below. Crackles may be heard in the lungs on auscultation. Pulmonary artery and capillary wedge pressures are increased.

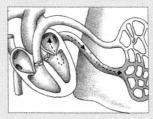

9. As back pressure rises, fluid crosses the alveolocapillary membrane, impeding diffusion of oxygen (O_2) and carbon dioxide (CO_2) (as shown below). Arterial blood gas analysis may show decreased partial pressure of arterial oxygen and arterial pH and increased partial pressure of arterial carbon dioxide.

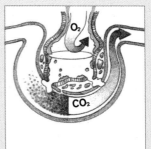

Signs and symptoms

The cardinal symptom of MI is persistent, crushing substernal pain that may radiate to the left arm, jaw, neck, or shoulder blades. The pain is commonly described as heavy, squeezing, or crushing and may persist for 12 hours or more.

In some patients — particularly the elderly or patients with diabetes — pain may not occur at all. In others, it may be mild and confused with indigestion. In patients with CAD, angina of increasing frequency, severity, or duration (especially if not provoked by exertion, a heavy meal, or cold and wind) may signal an impending infarction. Other effects include:

■ anxiety
■ cool extremities
■ diaphoresis
■ fatigue
■ feeling of impending doom
■ nausea
■ restlessness
■ shortness of breath
■ vomiting.

Fever is unusual at the onset of an MI, but a low-grade temperature may develop during the next few days. Blood pressure varies. Hypotension or hypertension may occur.

Test results

■ Serial 12-lead ECG may be normal or inconclusive during the first few hours after an MI. Abnormalities include serial ST-segment depression in a subendocardial MI and ST-segment elevation and Q waves, representing scarring and necrosis, in a Q-wave MI.
■ Serum creatine kinase (CK) level is elevated, especially the CK-MB isoenzyme, the cardiac muscle fraction of CK.
■ Echocardiography shows ventricular wall dyskinesia with a Q-wave MI and is used to evaluate the ejection fraction.
■ Radionuclide scans using I.V. technetium 99m can show acutely damaged muscle by picking up accumulations of radionuclide, which appear as a "hot spot" on the film. Myocardial perfusion imaging with thallium-201 reveals a "cold spot" in most patients during the first few hours after a Q-wave MI.
■ Cardiac troponin levels remain elevated for 4 to 6 hours after an MI.

TEACHING FOCUS

Myocardial infarction teaching topics

● Provide emotional support, and help the patient identify measures to reduce stress and anxiety. Explain procedures and answer questions. Explaining the intensive care unit environment and routine can ease anxiety. Involve the patient's family in his care as much as possible.

● Thoroughly explain dosages and therapy to promote compliance with the prescribed drug regimen and other treatment measures. Warn about adverse effects, and advise the patient to watch for and report signs of toxicity (anorexia, nausea, vomiting, and yellow vision, for example, if the patient is receiving digoxin [Lanoxin]).

● Review dietary restrictions with the patient. If he must follow a low-sodium or low-fat and low-choles-terol diet, provide a list of foods that he should avoid. Ask the dietitian to speak to the patient and his family.

● Counsel the patient to resume sexual activity gradually.

● Advise the patient to report typical or atypical chest pain. Postinfarction syndrome may develop, producing chest pain that must be differentiated from recurrent MI, pulmonary infarct, or heart failure.

● If the patient has a Holter monitor in place, explain its purpose and use.

● Stress the need to stop smoking.

● Encourage the patient to participate in a cardiac rehabilitation program.

● Review follow-up procedures, such as office visits and treadmill testing, with the patient.

Treatment

Treatment for MI aims to relieve chest pain, stabilize heart rhythm, and reduce cardiac workload. Arrhythmias, the most common problem during the first 48 hours after an MI, require antiarrhythmics, a pacemaker (possibly), and cardioversion (rarely). (See *Myocardial infarction teaching topics*.)

DRUG THERAPY

Drugs are the mainstay of therapy. Typical drugs include:

■ thrombolytic agents, such as tissue plasminogen activator (tPA, TNKase) and streptokinase (Streptase) to revascularize myocardial tissue

■ procainamide (Pronestyl) or another antiarrhythmic, such as lidocaine or amiodarone (Cordarone), or disopyramide (Norpace) for ventricular arrhythmias

■ I.V. atropine for heart block or bradycardia

- sublingual, topical, transdermal, or I.V. nitroglycerin and calcium channel blockers, such as diltiazem (Cardizem), given by mouth or I.V. to relieve angina
- I.V. morphine, drug of choice, or hydromorphone (Dilaudid) for pain and sedation
- drugs that increase myocardial contractility, such as dobutamine (Dobutrex), inamrinone, and milrinone (Primacor)
- beta blockers, such as propranolol (Inderal), metoprolol (Lopressor), and timolol (Blocadren), after an acute MI to help prevent reinfarction by decreasing myocardial workload and oxygen demand.

OTHER THERAPIES
The patient may need a temporary pacemaker for heart block or bradycardia. He may receive oxygen by face mask or nasal cannula at a modest flow rate for 24 to 48 hours, or at a lower concentration if he has chronic obstructive pulmonary disease. Maintain bed rest with a bedside commode to decrease the patient's cardiac workload. A few patients may need pulmonary artery catheterization to detect left-sided or right-sided heart failure and to monitor the response to treatment. Some patients may need IABP for cardiogenic shock. Some may need cardiac catheterization, PTCA, stent placement, or CABG.

REVASCULARIZATION THERAPY
Revascularization therapy may be performed on patients younger than age 70 who don't have a history of stroke, bleeding, GI ulcers, marked hypertension, recent surgery, or chest pain lasting longer than 6 hours. It must begin within 6 hours after the onset of symptoms, using I.V. intracoronary or systemic streptokinase or tPA. The best response occurs when treatment begins within 1 hour after symptoms first appear.

PERICARDITIS
Pericarditis is inflammation of the fibroserous sac that envelops, supports, and protects the heart. This condition occurs in acute and chronic forms. The acute form can be fibrinous or effusive, with serous, purulent, or hemorrhagic exudate. The chronic form, which is called *constrictive pericarditis,* is characterized by dense, fibrous pericardial thickening. The prognosis depends on the underlying cause but is typically good in acute pericarditis, unless constriction occurs.

Pathophysiology

Common causes of pericarditis include these:

■ bacterial, fungal, or viral infection (infectious pericarditis)
■ drugs, such as hydralazine (Apresoline) or procainamide (Pronestyl)
■ high-dose radiation to the chest
■ hypersensitivity or autoimmune disease, such as systemic lupus erythematosus, rheumatoid arthritis, or acute rheumatic fever (most common cause of pericarditis in children)
■ idiopathic factors (most common in acute pericarditis)
■ neoplasms (primary or metastatic from lungs, breasts, or other organs)
■ postcardiac injury, such as MI (which later causes an autoimmune reaction in the pericardium), trauma, and surgery that leaves the pericardium intact but allows blood to leak into the pericardial cavity
■ uremia
■ aortic aneurysm with pericardial leakage (less common)
■ myxedema with cholesterol deposits in the pericardium (less common).

As the pericardium becomes inflamed, it may become thickened and fibrotic. If it doesn't heal completely after an acute episode, it may calcify over a long period and form a firm scar around the heart. This scarring interferes with diastolic filling of the ventricles. (See *Understanding pericarditis*, page 274 and 275.)

🔖 **RED FLAG** *Pericardial effusion is the major complication of acute pericarditis. If fluid accumulates rapidly, cardiac tamponade may occur. This may lead to shock, cardiovascular collapse and, eventually, death.*

Signs and symptoms

In acute pericarditis, a sharp, sudden pain usually starts over the sternum and radiates to the neck, shoulders, back, and arms. However, unlike the pain of MI, this pain is commonly pleuritic, increasing with deep inspiration and decreasing when the patient sits up and leans forward, pulling the heart away from the diaphragmatic pleurae of the lungs. A friction rub (a distinct sound heard when two dry surfaces rub together) is audible on auscultation.

Pericardial effusion, the major complication of acute pericarditis, may produce effects of heart failure, such as dyspnea, orthopnea, and tachycardia. It also may produce ill-defined substernal chest pain and a feeling of chest fullness. If the fluid accumulates rapidly, cardiac tamponade may occur, causing pallor, clammy skin, hy-

Understanding pericarditis

Pericarditis occurs when a pathogen or other substance attacks the pericardium, leading to the events described here.

1. INFLAMMATION

Pericardial tissue damaged by bacteria or other substances releases chemical mediators of inflammation (such as prostaglandin, histamine, bradykinin, and serotonin) into the surrounding tissue, starting the inflammatory

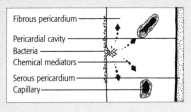

process. Friction occurs as the inflamed pericardial layers rub against each other.

2. VASODILATION AND CLOTTING

Histamine and other chemical mediators cause vasodilation and increased vessel permeability. Local blood flow (hyperemia) increases. Vessel walls leak fluids and proteins (including fibrinogen) into tissues, causing extracellular edema. Clots of fibrinogen and tissue fluid form a wall, blocking tissue spaces and lymph vessels in the injured area. This wall prevents the spread of bacteria and toxins to adjoining healthy tissues.

3. INITIAL PHAGOCYTOSIS

Macrophages already present in the tissues begin to phago-cytose the invading bacteria but usually fail to stop the in-fection.

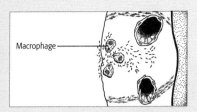

potension, pulsus paradoxus, jugular vein distention and, eventually, cardiovascular collapse and death.

Chronic constrictive pericarditis causes a gradual increase in systemic venous pressure and produces symptoms similar to those of chronic right-sided heart failure, including fluid retention, ascites, and hepatomegaly.

Test results

Laboratory test results reflect inflammation and may identify the disorder's cause.

4. ENHANCED PHAGOCYTOSIS

Substances released by the injured tissue stimulate neutrophil production in the bone marrow. Neutrophils then travel to the injury site through the bloodstream and join macrophages in destroying pathogens. Meanwhile, additional macrophages and monocytes migrate to the injured area and continue phagocytosis.

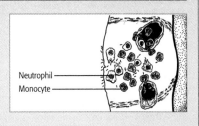

5. EXUDATION

After several days, the infected area fills with an exudate composed of necrotic tissue, dead and dying bacteria, neutrophils, and macrophages. Thinner than pus, this exudate forms until all infection ceases, creating a cavity that remains until tissue destruction stops. The contents of the cavity autolyze and are gradually reabsorbed into healthy tissue.

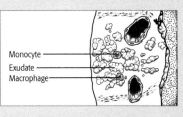

6. FIBROSIS AND SCARRING

As the end products of the infection slowly disappear, fibrosis and scar tissue may form. Scarring, which can be extensive, may ultimately cause heart failure if it restricts movement.

■ The WBC count may be normal or elevated, especially in infectious pericarditis.
■ The erythrocyte sedimentation rate (ESR) is elevated.
■ Serum CK-MB levels are slightly elevated with associated myocarditis.
■ Pericardial fluid culture obtained by open surgical drainage or pericardiocentesis sometimes identifies a causative organism in bacterial or fungal pericarditis.
■ BUN level detects uremia, antistreptolysin-O titer detects rheumatic fever, and purified protein derivative skin test detects tuberculosis.

◼ ECG shows characteristic changes in acute pericarditis. They include elevated ST segments in the limb leads and most precordial leads. QRS segments may be diminished when pericardial effusion is present. Rhythm changes also may occur, including atrial ectopic rhythms, such as atrial fibrillation and sinus arrhythmias.
◼ Echocardiography diagnoses pericardial effusion when it shows an echo-free space between the ventricular wall and the pericardium.

Treatment

Treatment for pericarditis strives to relieve symptoms, prevent or treat pericardial effusion and cardiac tamponade, and manage the underlying disease. (See *Pericarditis teaching topics.*)

In idiopathic pericarditis, post-MI pericarditis, and postthoracotomy pericarditis, treatment includes bed rest as long as fever and pain persist and nonsteroidal anti-inflammatory drugs, such as aspirin and indomethacin (Indocin), to relieve pain and reduce inflammation. If symptoms continue, the physician may prescribe corticosteroids. Although they provide rapid and effective relief, corticosteroids must be used cautiously because pericarditis may recur when drug therapy stops.

When infectious pericarditis results from disease of the left pleural space, mediastinal abscesses, or septicemia, the patient requires antibiotics, surgical drainage, or both.

If cardiac tamponade develops, the physician may perform emergency pericardiocentesis and may inject antibiotics directly into the pericardial sac.

Recurrent pericarditis may require partial pericardectomy, which creates a window that allows fluid to drain into the pleural space.

In constrictive pericarditis, total pericardectomy may be needed to permit the heart to fill and contract adequately.

RHEUMATIC FEVER AND RHEUMATIC HEART DISEASE

A systemic inflammatory disease of childhood, acute rheumatic fever develops after infection of the upper respiratory tract with group A beta-hemolytic streptococci. It mainly involves the heart, joints, central nervous system, skin, and subcutaneous tissues and commonly recurs. If rheumatic fever isn't treated, scarring deformity of the cardiac structures results in rheumatic heart disease.

Worldwide, 12 million new cases of rheumatic fever are reported each year. The disease strikes most often during cool, damp weather in the winter and early spring. In the United States, it's most common in the north. Rheumatic fever tends to run in families, suggesting a possible genetic predisposition. Environmental factors also seem to be significant. For example, in lower socioeconomic groups, the disease is most common in children ages 5 to 15, probably because of malnutrition and crowded living conditions.

Pathophysiology

Rheumatic fever appears to be a hypersensitivity reaction. For some reason, antibodies produced to combat streptococci react and produce characteristic lesions at specific tissue sites. Because only about 0.3% of people infected with *Streptococcus* bacteria contract rheumatic fever, an altered immune response probably is involved in its development or recurrence.

The extent of heart damage depends on where the infection strikes. Myocarditis produces characteristic lesions called Aschoff bodies in the interstitial tissue of the heart as well as cellular swelling and fragmentation of interstitial collagen. These lesions lead to the formation of progressively fibrotic nodules and interstitial scars.

Endocarditis causes valve leaflet swelling, erosion along the lines of leaflet closure, and blood, platelet, and fibrin deposits, which form beadlike vegetation. Endocarditis strikes the mitral valve most commonly in females and the aortic valve in males. It affects the tricuspid valves in both sexes and, rarely, affects the pulmonic valve.

RED FLAG The mitral and aortic valves are commonly destroyed by rheumatic fever's long-term effects. Their malfunction leads to severe heart inflammation (called carditis) and, occasionally, produces pericardial effusion and fatal heart failure. Of the patients who survive this complication, about 20% die within 10 years.

Carditis develops in up to 50% of patients with rheumatic fever and may affect the endocardium, myocardium, or pericardium during the early acute phase. Later, the heart valves may be damaged, causing chronic valvular disease.

Signs and symptoms

In 95% of patients, rheumatic fever follows a streptococcal infection that appeared a few days to 6 weeks earlier. A temperature of at least 100.4° F (38° C) occurs. Most patients complain of migratory joint pain or polyarthritis. Swelling, redness, and signs of effusion usually accompany such pain, which most commonly affects the knees, ankles, elbows, and hips.

About 5% of patients (usually those with carditis) develop a nonpruritic, macular, transient rash called *erythema marginatum*. This rash gives rise to red lesions with blanched centers. These same patients also may develop firm, movable, nontender subcutaneous nodules about 3 mm to 2 cm in diameter, usually near tendons or bony prominences of joints. These nodules persist for a few days to several weeks.

Test results

No specific laboratory tests can determine the presence of rheumatic fever, but some test results support the diagnosis.

- The WBC count and ESR may be elevated during the acute phase; blood studies show slight anemia caused by suppressed erythropoiesis during inflammation.
- C-reactive protein is positive, especially during the acute phase.
- Cardiac enzyme levels may be increased in severe myocarditis.
- Antistreptolysin-O titer is elevated in 95% of patients within 2 months of onset.
- Throat cultures may continue to show group A beta-hemolytic streptococci; however, they usually occur in small numbers, and isolating them is difficult.
- ECG reveals no diagnostic changes, but 20% of patients show a prolonged PR interval.
- Chest X-ray shows normal heart size, except with myocarditis, heart failure, and pericardial effusion.
- Echocardiography helps evaluate valvular damage, chamber size, ventricular function, and the presence of pericardial effusion.
- Cardiac catheterization evaluates valvular damage and left ventricular function in severe cardiac dysfunction.

Treatment

Effective treatment for rheumatic fever and rheumatic heart disease aims to eradicate the streptococcal infection, relieve symptoms, and

TEACHING FOCUS

Rheumatic fever and rheumatic heart disease teaching topics

● Teach the patient and his family about the disease and its treatment. Warn parents to watch for and immediately report signs of recurrent streptococcal infection: sudden sore throat, diffuse throat redness and oropharyngeal exudate, swollen and tender cervical lymph glands, pain on swallowing, temperature of 101° to 104° F (38.3° to 40° C), headache, and nausea. Urge them to keep their child away from people with respiratory tract infections.

● Warn that a hypersensitivity reaction to penicillin is possible. Tell the patient and his family to stop the drug and call the physician immediately if the patient develops a rash, fever, chills, or other signs of allergy at any time during penicillin therapy.

● Instruct the patient and his family to watch for and report early signs of heart failure, such as dyspnea and a hacking, nonproductive cough.

● Stress the need for bed rest during the acute phase and suggest appropriate, physically undemanding diversions. After the acute phase, encourage family members and friends to spend as much time as possible with the patient to minimize boredom. Advise parents to secure tutorial services to help the child keep up with schoolwork during the long convalescence.

● Promote good dental hygiene to prevent gingival infection. Make sure that the patient and his family understand the need to comply with prolonged antibiotic therapy and follow-up care and the need for additional antibiotics during dental surgery or procedures.

● Teach the patient to follow current recommendations of the American Heart Association to prevent bacterial endocarditis.

prevent recurrence, thus reducing the chance of permanent cardiac damage. (See *Rheumatic fever and rheumatic heart disease teaching topics*.)

ACUTE PHASE

During the acute phase, treatment includes penicillin or erythromycin (E-Mycin) for patients with penicillin hypersensitivity. Salicylates, such as aspirin, relieve fever and minimize joint swelling and pain. If the patient has carditis or if salicylates fail to relieve pain and inflammation, the physician may prescribe corticosteroids. Patients with active carditis require strict bed rest for about 5 weeks during the acute phase, followed by a progressive increase in physical activity. The increase depends on clinical and laboratory findings and the patient's response to treatment.

After the acute phase subsides, a monthly I.M. injection of penicillin G benzathine (Permapen) or daily doses of oral sulfadiazine or penicillin G may be used to prevent recurrence. This treatment usually continues for at least 5 years or until age 25.

The patient may need additional treatment if complications develop. Heart failure requires continued bed rest and diuretics. Severe mitral or aortic valvular dysfunction that causes persistent heart failure requires corrective surgery, such as commissurotomy (separation of the adherent, thickened leaflets of the mitral valve), valvuloplasty (inflation of a balloon within a valve), or valve replacement (with a prosthetic valve). However, this surgery is seldom needed before late adolescence.

9

NEUROLOGIC SYSTEM

Understanding the neurologic system

The neurologic, or nervous, system is the body's communication network. It coordinates and organizes the functions of all other body systems. This intricate network has two main divisions.

- The central nervous system (CNS), made up of the brain and spinal cord, is the body's control center.
- The peripheral nervous system (PNS), containing cranial and spinal nerves, provides communication between the CNS and remote body parts.

The neuron, or nerve cell, is the nervous system's fundamental unit. This highly specialized conductor cell receives and transmits electrochemical nerve impulses. Delicate, threadlike nerve fibers called *axons* and *dendrites* extend from the central cell body and transmit signals. Axons carry impulses away from the cell body; dendrites carry impulses to the cell body. Most neurons have multiple dendrites but only one axon. Neuroglial cells, which outnumber neurons, provide support, nourishment, and protection for neurons.

This intricate network of receptors and transmitters, along with the brain and spinal cord, forms a living computer that controls and regulates every mental and physical function. From birth to death, the nervous system efficiently organizes the body's affairs, controlling the smallest actions, thoughts, and feelings.

CENTRAL NERVOUS SYSTEM

The CNS includes the brain and the spinal cord, which are protected by the bony skull and vertebrae, cerebrospinal fluid (CSF), and three membranes—dura mater, arachnoid mater, and pia mater.

The *dura mater*, which forms the outermost protective layer, is a tough, fibrous, leatherlike tissue composed of two layers, the endosteal dura and the meningeal dura. The endosteal dura forms the periosteum of the skull and is continuous with the lining of the vertebral canal, whereas the meningeal dura, a thick membrane, covers the brain, dipping between the brain tissue and providing support and protection.

The *arachnoid mater,* which forms the middle protective layer, is a thin, delicate, fibrous membrane that loosely hugs the brain and spinal cord. The arachnoid mater is avascular.

The *pia mater* is the innermost protective layer of connective tissue that covers and contours the spinal tissue and brain. The pia mater is vascular.

The epidural space lies between the skull and the dura mater. Between the dura mater and the arachnoid mater is the subdural space. Between the arachnoid mater and the pia mater is the subarachnoid space.

Inside the subarachnoid space and the brain's four ventricles is CSF, a liquid composed of water and traces of organic materials (especially protein), glucose, and minerals. This fluid protects the brain and spinal tissue from jolts and blows.

Cerebrum

The cerebrum, the largest part of the brain, houses the nerve center that controls sensory and motor activities and intelligence. The outer layer, the cerebral cortex, consists of neuron cell bodies (gray matter). The inner layer consists of axons (white matter) plus basal ganglia, which control motor coordination and steadiness.

HEMISPHERES

The cerebrum is divided into the right and left hemispheres. Because motor impulses descending from the brain cross in the medulla, the right hemisphere controls the left side of the body and the left hemisphere controls the right side of the body. Several fissures divide the cerebrum into lobes. Each lobe has a specific function. (See *A close look at lobes and fissures.*)

THALAMUS

The thalamus, a relay center in the cerebrum, further organizes cerebral function by transmitting impulses to and from appropriate areas of the cerebrum. The thalamus is also responsible for primitive emotional responses, such as fear, and for distinguishing pleasant stimuli from unpleasant ones.

A close look at lobes and fissures

Several fissures divide the cerebrum into hemispheres and lobes. Each lobe has a specific function.
● The frontal lobe controls voluntary muscle movements and contains motor areas such as the one for speech (Broca's area). It's the center for personality, behavioral functions, intellectual functions (such as judgment, memory, and problem solving), autonomic functions, and cardiac and emotional responses.
● The temporal lobe is the center for taste, hearing, smell, and interpretation of spoken language.

● The parietal lobe coordinates and interprets sensory information from the opposite side of the body.
● The occipital lobe interprets visual stimuli.
● The fissure of Sylvius, or the lateral sulcus, separates the temporal lobe from the frontal and parietal lobes.
● The fissure of Rolando, or the central sulcus, separates the frontal lobes from the parietal lobe.
● The parieto-occipital fissure separates the occipital lobe from the two parietal lobes.

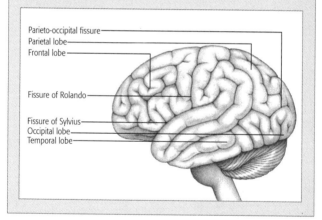

Parieto-occipital fissure
Parietal lobe
Frontal lobe
Fissure of Rolando
Fissure of Sylvius
Occipital lobe
Temporal lobe

HYPOTHALAMUS

The hypothalamus, located beneath the thalamus, is an autonomic center with connections to the brain, spinal cord, autonomic nervous system, and pituitary gland. It regulates temperature control, appetite, blood pressure, breathing, sleep patterns, and peripheral nerve discharges that occur with behavioral and emotional expression. It also partially controls pituitary gland secretion and stress reaction.

Cerebellum and brain stem

Other main parts of the brain are the cerebellum and the brain stem. The cerebellum lies beneath the cerebrum, at the base of the brain. It coordinates muscle movements, controls posture, and maintains equilibrium.

The brain stem includes the midbrain, pons, and medulla oblongata. It houses cell bodies for most of the cranial nerves. Along with the thalamus and hypothalamus, it makes up a nerve network called the *reticular formation,* which acts as an arousal mechanism.

The three parts of the brain stem provide two-way conduction between the spinal cord and the brain. They perform other functions as well. The midbrain is the reflex center for the third and fourth cranial nerves and mediates pupillary reflexes and eye movements. The pons helps regulate respirations. It's also the reflex center for the fifth through eighth cranial nerves and mediates chewing, taste, saliva secretion, hearing, and equilibrium. The medulla oblongata influences cardiac, respiratory, and vasomotor functions. It's the center for the vomiting, coughing, and hiccuping reflexes.

Spinal cord

The spinal cord extends downward from the brain to the second lumbar vertebra and functions as a two-way conductor between the brain stem and the PNS. (See *A look inside the spinal cord.*)

The spinal cord contains a mass of gray matter divided into horns consisting mostly of neuron cell bodies. Cell bodies in the posterior or dorsal horn mainly relay information. Those in the anterior or ventral horn are used for voluntary or reflex motor activity.

The outside of the horns is surrounded by white matter consisting of myelinated nerve fibers grouped in vertical columns called *tracts.* The sensory, or ascending, tracts carry sensory impulses up the spinal cord to the brain; the motor, or descending, tracts carry motor impulses down the spinal cord.

The brain's motor impulses reach a descending tract and continue to the PNS via upper motor neurons (also called *cranial motor neurons*). Upper motor neurons in the brain conduct impulses from the brain to the spinal cord. Upper motor neurons form two major systems. The pyramidal system, or corticospinal tract, is responsible for fine, skilled movements of skeletal muscle. The extrapyramidal system, or extracorticospinal tract, is responsible for the control of gross motor movements.

Lower motor neurons (also called *spinal motor neurons*) conduct impulses that originate in upper motor neurons to the muscles.

A look inside the spinal cord

This illustration shows the major components of the spinal cord.

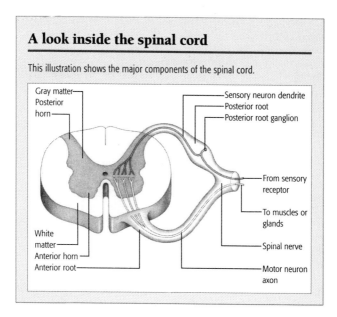

PERIPHERAL NERVOUS SYSTEM

Messages transmitted through the spinal cord reach outlying areas through the PNS. The PNS originates in 31 pairs of spinal nerves arranged in segments and attached to the spinal cord. Spinal nerves are numbered according to their point of origin in the spinal cord:

■ 8 cervical — C1 to C8
■ 12 thoracic — T1 to T12
■ 5 lumbar — L1 to L5
■ 5 sacral — S1 to S5
■ 1 coccygeal.

Spinal nerves are attached to the spinal cord by two roots. The anterior, or ventral, root consists of motor fibers that relay impulses from the spinal cord to the glands and muscles. The posterior, or dorsal, root consists of sensory fibers that relay information from receptors to the spinal cord. A swollen area of the posterior root, the posterior root ganglion, is made up of sensory neuron cell bodies.

After leaving the vertebral column, each spinal nerve separates into branches called *rami,* which distribute peripherally with extensive overlapping. This overlapping reduces the chance of lost sensory or motor function from interruption of a single spinal nerve.

The PNS can be divided into the autonomic nervous system and the somatic nervous system.

Autonomic nervous system
The autonomic nervous system helps regulate the body's internal environment through involuntary control of body functions, such as digestion, respirations, and cardiovascular function. It's usually divided into two antagonistic systems that balance each other to support homeostasis.

The sympathetic nervous system controls energy expenditure, especially under stress, by releasing the adrenergic catecholamine norepinephrine. The parasympathetic nervous system helps conserve energy by releasing the cholinergic neurohormone acetylcholine.

Somatic nervous system
The somatic nervous system, composed of somatic nerve fibers, regulates voluntary motor control. It conducts impulses from the CNS to skeletal muscles. It's typically referred to as the voluntary nervous system because it allows conscious control of skeletal muscles.

Neurologic disorders

In this section, you'll find information about these common neurologic disorders:
- Alzheimer's disease
- amyotrophic lateral sclerosis
- epilepsy
- Guillain-Barré syndrome
- meningitis
- multiple sclerosis
- myasthenia gravis
- Parkinson's disease
- stroke.

ALZHEIMER'S DISEASE
Alzheimer's disease is a progressive degenerative disorder of the cerebral cortex. It accounts for more than half of all cases of dementia. Cortical degeneration is most marked in the frontal lobes, but atrophy occurs in all areas of the cortex.

About 4.5 million Americans have Alzheimer's disease, a number that has more than doubled since 1980. One in 10 people older than age 65 and nearly half of those older than age 85 are affected. (See *Aging and Alzheimer's disease*.)

Aging and Alzheimer's disease

Although Alzheimer's disease isn't a normal part of aging, advancing age is the most important known risk factor. The number of people with the disease doubles every 5 years beyond age 65. Although the reasons for this haven't yet been fully explained, current research is focusing on some specific areas.

Low levels of the B vitamin folic acid may predispose people to Alzheimer's disease. As people age, the lining of the stomach becomes thinner, which decreases the production of hydrochloric acid. This acid is needed for absorption of folic acid from foods. Some research is now being directed at the use of folic acid supplements, which don't rely on hydrochloric acid for absorption, as a preventive measure against Alzheimer's disease.

Research is also evaluating the roles of physical, mental, and social activities in preventing Alzheimer's disease. As people age, the tendency to engage in these activities may decline. However, they may serve as protective factors against Alzheimer's disease by keeping the brain active and healthy. Doing puzzles, playing chess, learning a new foreign language, or taking dance classes may delay or prevent Alzheimer's disease.

Because this is a primary progressive dementia, the prognosis is poor. Most patients die 2 to 20 years after symptoms start. The average duration of the illness before death is 8 years.

Researchers recognize two forms of Alzheimer's disease. In familial Alzheimer's, genes directly cause the disease. These cases are very rare and have been identified in a relatively small number of families, with many people in multiple generations affected. (See *Genes and Alzheimer's disease,* page 288.)

In sporadic Alzheimer's, the most common form of the disease, genes don't cause the disease but may influence the risk of developing it. It's less predictable than the familial type and occurs in fewer family members.

Pathophysiology

The cause of Alzheimer's disease is unknown, but the four factors that probably contribute include:

■ neurochemical factors, such as deficiencies in the neurotransmitters acetylcholine, somatostatin, substance P, and norepinephrine
■ viral factors such as slow-growing central nervous system (CNS) viruses
■ trauma
■ genetic factors.

GENETIC CONNECTION

Genes and Alzheimer's disease

FAMILIAL ALZHEIMER'S DISEASE
According to the Alzheimer's Association, in this form of Alzheimer's disease, the affected person has inherited an abnormal mutation in one of three genes – PS1, PS2, or APP – all of which influence beta-amyloid production. A person who carries one of the mutated genes has a 50% chance of passing the gene to his children. Those who inherit the mutated gene will most likely develop Alzheimer's disease.

SPORADIC ALZHEIMER'S DISEASE
Sporadic Alzheimer's disease doesn't develop with a mutation in one gene. Instead, slight variations in genes may make someone more or less susceptible to the disease.

The most researched gene in sporadic Alzheimer's disease is APOE, which is responsible for production of a protein that transports cholesterol and other fats through the body. The protein may also be involved in the structure and function of the outer wall of a brain cell.

APOE has three common forms – APOE–epsilon 2, APOE–epsilon 3, and APOE–epsilon 4. A person inherits one form of the gene from each parent. The form linked with sporadic Alzheimer's disease is APOE–epsilon 4. People who carry at least one of this type of gene have a higher risk of developing Alzheimer's disease. About 35% to 50% of people with Alzheimer's disease have at least one copy of this form of the gene. Those who have two copies of the gene are at even higher risk and, when they develop the disease, typically show symptoms at a younger age.

The brain tissue of Alzheimer's patients has three distinguishing features: neurofibrillary tangles formed out of proteins in the neurons, beta-amyloid plaques, and granulovascular degeneration of neurons. The disease causes degeneration of neuropils (dense complexes of interwoven nerve cells and neuroglial cells), especially in the frontal, parietal, and occipital lobes. It also enlarges the ventricles (brain cavities filled with cerebral spinal fluid [CSF]).

Early cerebral changes include formation of microscopic plaques, consisting of a core surrounded by fibrous tissue. Later on, atrophy of the cerebral cortex becomes strikingly evident.

In a person with a large number of beta-amyloid plaques, the dementia will be more severe. The amyloid in the plaques may have neurotoxic effects, and plaques play an important part in bringing about the death of neurons.

Problems with neurotransmitters and the enzymes involved in their metabolism may play a role in the disease. The severity of dementia is directly related to reduced acetylcholine levels. On autopsy, the brains of Alzheimer's patients may contain as little as 10% of the normal amount of acetylcholine.

▨ *RED FLAG Because Alzheimer's disease may lead to violent behavior and wandering, complications may include injury to the patient or others. They also include pneumonia and other infections, especially if the patient doesn't receive enough exercise; malnutrition and dehydration, especially if the patient refuses or forgets to eat; and aspiration.*

Signs and symptoms
Alzheimer's disease starts insidiously. At first, changes are barely perceptible, but they gradually become serious. In fact, the patient's history almost always comes from a family member or caregiver. Early changes may include forgetfulness, subtle memory loss without loss of social skills or behavior patterns, trouble learning and retaining new information, trouble concentrating, and a decline in personal hygiene and appearance.

As the disease progresses, signs and symptoms indicate a degenerative disorder of the frontal lobe. They may include:
▨ trouble with abstract thinking and activities that take judgment
▨ progressive difficulty communicating
▨ severe decline of memory, language, and motor function progressing to loss of coordination and an inability to speak or write
▨ repetitive actions
▨ restlessness
▨ irritability, depression, mood swings, paranoia, hostility, and combativeness
▨ nocturnal awakenings
▨ disorientation.

Neurologic examination confirms many of the problems revealed during the history. In addition, it commonly reveals an impaired sense of smell (usually an early symptom), inability to recognize and understand the form and nature of objects by touching them, gait disorders, tremors, and a positive snout reflex (grimacing or puckering of the lips in response to a tap or stroke of the lips or the area just under the nose).

In the final stages, urinary or fecal incontinence, twitching, and seizures commonly occur.

Test results
Alzheimer's disease can't be confirmed until death, when an autopsy reveals changes. These tests help rule out other disorders.
▨ Positron emission tomography (PET) scan shows metabolic activity in the cerebral cortex and may help confirm early diagnosis.

TEACHING FOCUS

Alzheimer's disease teaching topics

● Teach the patient, family, and caregiver about the disease and its treatments, and refer them to social services and community resources for legal and financial advice and support.
● Explain the need for activity and exercise to maintain mobility and help prevent complications.

● Discuss dietary adjustments for patients with restlessness, dysphagia, or coordination problems.
● Emphasize the importance of establishing a daily routine, providing a safe environment, and avoiding over-stimulation.
● Instruct the patient, family, and caregiver about self-care, including the importance of adequate rest, good nutrition, and private time.

■ Computed tomography (CT) scan may show more brain atrophy than occurs in normal aging.
■ Magnetic resonance imaging (MRI) evaluates the condition of the brain and rules out intracranial lesions as the source of dementia.
■ EEG evaluates the brain's electrical activity and may show brain wave slowing late in the disease. It also identifies tumors, abscesses, and other intracranial lesions that might cause symptoms.
■ CSF analysis helps determine whether signs and symptoms stem from a chronic neurologic infection.
■ Cerebral blood flow studies may detect abnormalities in blood flow to the brain.

Treatment

There's no cure for the progressive loss of brain cells that characterizes Alzheimer's disease. The drugs listed below may help minimize or stabilize the symptoms. (See *Alzheimer's disease teaching topics*.)

Cholinesterase inhibitors prevent the breakdown of acetylcholine, a brain chemical that's important for memory and other thinking skills. These drugs keep acetylcholine levels high, even while the cells that produce it continue to become damaged or die. Cholinesterase inhibitors include donepezil (Aricept), rivastigmine (Exelon), and galantamine (Razadyne).

Memantine (Namenda), an uncompetitive low- to moderate-affinity N-methyl-D-aspartate receptor antagonist, may be prescribed. It appears to work by regulating glutamate, a brain chemical involved in processing, storing, and retrieving information.

Vitamin E supplements are commonly prescribed because they may help defend the brain against damage.

At least one of the many clinical trials under way for Alzheimer's disease treatments involves a vaccine that would stimulate the immune system to recognize and attack the beta-amyloid plaques characteristic of the disease.

AMYOTROPHIC LATERAL SCLEROSIS

Commonly called *Lou Gehrig disease,* after the New York Yankee first baseman who died of the disorder, amyotrophic lateral sclerosis (ALS) is the most common of the motor neuron diseases that cause muscular atrophy. Others include progressive muscular atrophy and progressive bulbar palsy. ALS typically starts between ages 40 and 70. A chronic, progressively debilitating disease, ALS is rapidly fatal.

More than 30,000 Americans have ALS. About 5,000 new cases are diagnosed each year, with men affected three times more than women. The exact cause of ALS is unknown, but 5% to 10% of ALS cases have a genetic component. In genetic cases, ALS is an autosomal dominant trait and affects men and women equally. (See *Breakthrough in amyotrophic lateral sclerosis,* page 292.)

ALS and other motor neuron diseases may result from a slow-acting virus, from nutritional deficiency caused by disturbed enzyme metabolism, from metabolic interference in nucleic acid production by the nerve fibers, or from autoimmune disorders that affect immune complexes in the renal glomerulus and basement membrane. Acute deterioration may be sparked by such factors as trauma, viral infection, and physical exhaustion.

Pathophysiology

In ALS, motor neurons (nerve cells that control muscles) are destroyed. These neurons are located in the anterior gray horns of the spinal column and the motor nuclei of the lower brain stem. Motor neurons may be lost in both the upper and lower motor neuron systems. As cells die, the muscle fibers that they supply atrophy. Signs and symptoms develop according to the affected motor neurons because specific neurons activate specific muscle fibers.

RED FLAG Common complications of ALS include respiratory tract infections, such as pneumonia; respiratory failure; aspiration; and complications of physical immobility, such as pressure ulcers and contractures.

Signs and symptoms

Patients with ALS develop fasciculations (involuntary twitching or contraction of muscles), accompanied by atrophy and weakness, es-

Breakthrough in amyotrophic lateral sclerosis

The first and most important breakthrough so far in amyotrophic lateral sclerosis (ALS) genetic research is the discovery of mutations in the SOD1 gene. This mutation is seen in about 20% of patients with familial ALS.

Although researchers are excited about this discovery, they're also perplexed. That's because the mutation is quite complex and involves the acquisition of a toxic property. This means that the gene gains a function rather than losing its normal function, leaving researchers confused about what that gain of function involves. Therefore, genetic studies continue.

pecially in the muscles of the forearms and hands. Other signs and symptoms include impaired speech, trouble chewing and swallowing, trouble breathing, choking, excessive drooling, depression, inappropriate laughing, and crying spells.

Test results
These tests help confirm the diagnosis.
■ Electromyography helps show nerve damage instead of muscle damage.
■ Muscle biopsy helps rule out muscle disease.
■ CSF analysis reveals increased protein content in one-third of patients.

Treatment
Treatment aims to control symptoms and provide emotional, psychological, and physical support. Patients who have trouble swallowing may need gastric feedings. If the patient wishes, tracheotomy and mechanical ventilation may be an option when hypoventilation develops. (See *Amyotrophic lateral sclerosis teaching topics*.)

DRUG THERAPY
Riluzole (Rilutek), a neuroprotector, slows the deterioration of motor neurons early in ALS. Baclofen (Kemstro), dantrolene (Dantrium), or diazepam (Valium) may be given to control spasticity. Quinine therapy may be prescribed for painful muscle cramps.

STEM CELL THERAPY
Stem cell therapy is now being studied and shows great promise in treating ALS.

TEACHING FOCUS

Amyotrophic lateral sclerosis teaching topics

- Teach the patient, family, and caregiver how motor neuron degeneration affects muscles and their motor function.
- Urge the patient to exercise to maintain strength in unaffected muscles.
- Describe dietary changes that ease swallowing.
- Demonstrate how to operate a wheelchair safely.
- Explain how to prevent and manage complications such as pressure ulcers.

- Help the patient develop alternative communication techniques.
- Teach the patient to suction himself if he's unable to handle an increased accumulation of secretions.
- If the patient has a gastrostomy tube, show the patient's family and caregiver (or the patient, if he can still feed himself) how to administer tube feedings.
- Discuss advance directives regarding health care decisions.

EPILEPSY

Also known as *seizure disorder,* epilepsy is a brain condition characterized by recurrent seizures. Seizures are caused by abnormal electrical discharge by neurons in the brain. The discharge may trigger a convulsive movement, an interruption of sensation, an alteration in level of consciousness (LOC), or a combination of these events. In most patients, epilepsy doesn't affect intelligence.

This condition affects people of all ages, races, and ethnic backgrounds. More than 2.5 million Americans are living with epilepsy. Every year, 181,000 Americans develop seizures for the first time. The condition appears most commonly in early childhood or old age. With strict adherence to treatment, about 80% of patients have good seizure control.

Pathophysiology

In about half of patients with epilepsy, no cause can be identified and the patient has no other neurologic abnormality. In other patients, possible causes of epilepsy include:
- brain tumors or other space-occupying lesions of the cortex
- fever
- genetic abnormalities, such as tuberous sclerosis (tumors and sclerotic patches in the brain) and phenylketonuria (inability to convert phenylalanine into tyrosine)
- hereditary abnormalities (some seizure disorders run in families)
- infections, such as meningitis, encephalitis, or brain abscess
- ingestion of toxins, such as mercury, lead, or carbon monoxide

Understanding status epilepticus

Status epilepticus is a continuous seizure state that must be interrupted by emergency measures. It can occur during all types of seizures. For example, generalized tonic-clonic status epilepticus is a continuous generalized tonic-clonic seizure without an intervening return of consciousness.

Status epilepticus can result from withdrawal of antiepileptic drugs, hypoxic or metabolic encephalopathy,

acute head trauma, or septicemia caused by encephalitis or meningitis.

Emergency treatment usually includes lorazepam (Ativan), phenytoin (Dilantin), or phenobarbital (Luminal); I.V. dextrose 50% when seizures are caused by hypoglycemia; and I.V. thiamine in patients with chronic alcoholism or who are undergoing withdrawal.

■ metabolic abnormalities, such as hyponatremia, hypocalcemia, hypoglycemia, and pyridoxine deficiency
■ perinatal injuries
■ stroke
■ traumatic injury, especially if the dura mater has been penetrated.

During a seizure, the electrical balance at the neuronal level is altered, causing the neuronal membrane to become overly susceptible to activation. This alteration may occur when certain neurons lose their ability to transmit impulses from the periphery toward the CNS, creating an epileptogenic focus. Increased permeability of the cytoplasmic membranes helps hypersensitive neurons fire abnormally. Abnormal firing may be activated by hyperthermia, hypoglycemia, hyponatremia, hypoxia, or repeated sensory stimulation.

When the intensity of a seizure discharge has progressed sufficiently, it spreads to adjacent brain areas. The midbrain, thalamus, and cerebral cortex are most likely to become epileptogenic. Excitement feeds back from the primary focus to other parts of the brain. The discharges become less frequent until they stop.

RED FLAG Depending on the type of seizure the patient has, the risk of falls and injury may increase, either from confusion or from rapid, jerking movements that occur during or after a seizure. Anoxia may result from airway occlusion by the tongue, aspiration of vomit, or traumatic injury. Status epilepticus can cause respiratory distress and even death.(See Understanding status epilepticus.*)*

Signs and symptoms

Signs and symptoms of epilepsy vary with the type and cause of the seizure. (See *Understanding types of seizures.*)

Understanding types of seizures

Use these guidelines to understand different seizure types. Remember that patients may be affected by more than one type of seizure.

PARTIAL SEIZURES

These seizures start in a localized area in the brain and may spread to the entire brain (generalized seizure). Partial seizures include simple (jacksonian and sensory), complex, and secondarily generalized.

Jacksonian seizure

This localized motor seizure spreads to adjacent areas of the brain, causing tingling and stiffening or jerking in one limb. The patient seldom loses consciousness, but the seizure may generalize to tonic-clonic.

Sensory seizure

Symptoms include hallucinations, flashing lights, tingling, vertigo, déjà vu, and smelling a foul odor.

Complex partial seizure

Signs and symptoms vary but may start with an aura and usually include purposeless behavior, including a glassy stare, picking at clothes, aimless wandering, lip-smacking or chewing motions, and unintelligible speech. The seizure may last a few seconds to 20 minutes. After, confusion may last several minutes and make the person look intoxicated or psychotic. The patient has no memory of his actions during the seizure.

Secondarily generalized seizure

This seizure can be simple or complex and can generalize. An aura may occur first, with loss of consciousness immediately or 1 to 2 minutes later.

GENERALIZED SEIZURES

These seizures cause a generalized electrical abnormality in the brain.

Absence seizure

Most common in children, this seizure usually causes a mild change consciousness (blinking or rolling the eyes, blank stare, slight mouth movements) and lasts 1 to 10 seconds. Untreated, these seizures can recur up to 100 times a day and become generalized tonic-clonic seizures.

Myoclonic seizure

Also called *bilateral massive epileptic myoclonus,* this seizure is marked by brief, involuntary, possibly rhythmic muscular jerks of the body or limbs and a brief loss of consciousness.

Generalized tonic-clonic seizure

This seizure usually starts with a loud cry. The person loses consciousness and falls to the ground, first stiff (tonic) and then alternating spasm and relaxation (clonic). He may have tongue biting, incontinence, labored breathing, apnea, and cyanosis. After 2 to 5 minutes abnormal electrical discharge stops and the person regains consciousness but is confused, drowsy, fatigued, sore, or weak. He may have a headache and fall asleep.

Akinetic seizure

This seizure affects young children and may be called a drop attack. It causes a loss of postural tone and temporary loss of consciousness.

Physical findings may be normal if the cause is idiopathic and the patient doesn't have a seizure during assessment. If the seizure is caused by an underlying problem, the patient's history and physical examination should uncover related signs and symptoms.

In many cases, the patient's history shows that seizures are unpredictable and unrelated to activities. Some patients may report precipitating factors. For example, the seizures may always take place at a certain time, such as during sleep, or after a particular circumstance, such as lack of sleep or emotional stress. Or they may cause nonspecific symptoms, such as headache, mood changes, lethargy, and myoclonic jerking up to several hours beforehand.

Some patients report an aura a few seconds or minutes before a generalized seizure. An aura signals the start of abnormal electrical discharge in a focal area of the brain. Typical auras include a pungent smell, nausea or indigestion, a rising or sinking feeling in the stomach, a dreamy feeling, an unusual taste, or a visual disturbance such as a flashing light.

Test results
These tests are used to diagnose epilepsy.
- EEG showing paroxysmal abnormalities may confirm the diagnosis by showing continuing seizure tendency. A negative EEG doesn't rule out epilepsy, because paroxysmal abnormalities occur intermittently. An EEG also helps determine the prognosis and can help classify the disorder.
- CT scan and MRI provide density readings of the brain and may show abnormalities in internal structures.
- Other tests include serum glucose and calcium studies, skull X-rays, lumbar puncture, brain scan, and cerebral angiography.

Treatment
Treatment seeks to reduce the frequency of seizures or to prevent them. (See *Epilepsy teaching topics.*) Drug therapy is specific to the type of seizure. For generalized tonic-clonic and complex partial seizures, the most common drugs, given individually, include phenytoin (Dilantin), carbamazepine (Tegretol), phenobarbital (Luminal), and primidone (Mysoline). Also for partial seizures, lamotrigine (Lamictal) may be given as adjunct therapy.

For absence seizures, common drugs include valproic acid (Depakene), clonazepam (Klonopin), and ethosuximide (Zarontin).

If drug therapy fails, treatment may include surgical removal of a focal lesion to try to stop seizures. Surgery may also be used when epilepsy results from an underlying problem, such as an intracranial tumor, a brain abscess or cyst, or vascular abnormalities.

GUILLAIN-BARRÉ SYNDROME

Also known as *acute demyelinating polyneuropathy,* Guillain-Barré syndrome results from segmented demyelination of peripheral nerves. This syndrome arises equally in both sexes, usually between ages 30 and 50. It affects about 1 in 100,000 people. It's acute, rapidly progressive, and possibly fatal. However, thanks to improved symptom management, 80% to 90% of patients recover with few or no residual symptoms.

Pathophysiology

The clinical course of Guillain-Barré syndrome has three phases. The acute phase begins when the first definitive symptom develops and ends 1 to 3 weeks later, when no further deterioration is noted. The plateau phase lasts for several days to 2 weeks. The recovery phase, believed to coincide with remyelination and axonal process regrowth, can last from 4 months to 3 years.

The precise cause of Guillain-Barré syndrome is unknown, but it's probably a cell-mediated, immunologic attack on peripheral nerves in response to a virus. Risk factors include surgery, rabies or swine influenza vaccination, viral illness, Hodgkin's disease or another malignant disease, and lupus erythematosus.

An immunologic reaction causes segmental demyelination of the peripheral nerves, which prevents normal transmission of electrical impulses along the sensorimotor nerve roots.

The myelin sheath, which covers the nerve axons and conducts electrical impulses along the nerve pathways, degenerates for unknown reasons. With degeneration comes inflammation, swelling, and patchy demyelination.

As myelin is destroyed, the nodes of Ranvier, located at the junctures of the myelin sheaths, widen. This delays and impairs impulse transmission along the dorsal and ventral nerve roots.

RED FLAG Guillain-Barré syndrome commonly affects respiratory muscles. If the patient dies, it's usually from respiratory complications. Paralysis of internal and external intercostal muscles reduces the patient's ability to breathe. Also, vagus nerve paralysis impairs the protective mechanisms that respond to bronchial irritation and foreign bodies; it also leads to a reduced or absent gag reflex.

Signs and symptoms

Symptoms usually follow an ascending pattern, beginning in the legs and progressing to the arms, trunk, and face. Impairment of dorsal nerve roots affects sensory function, causing tingling and numbness. Impairment of ventral nerve roots affects motor function, causing muscle weakness, immobility, and paralysis. In mild forms, only cranial nerves may be affected. Some patients may have no muscle weakness. Other signs and symptoms include muscle stiffness and pain, sensory loss, loss of position sense, and diminished or absent deep tendon reflexes.

Test results

These tests are used to diagnose Guillain-Barré syndrome.
- CSF analysis may show a normal white blood cell (WBC) count, an elevated protein count and, in severe disease, increased CSF pressure. The CSF protein level begins to rise several days after signs and symptoms start and peaks in 4 to 6 weeks, probably because of widespread inflammatory disease of the nerve roots.
- Electromyography may show repeated firing of the same motor unit instead of widespread sectional stimulation.
- Electrophysiologic testing may reveal marked slowing of nerve conduction.

Treatment

Treatment is mainly supportive. If the patient has trouble clearing secretions, it may involve endotracheal intubation or tracheotomy; if

Guillain-Barré syndrome teaching topics

● Explain the disease and its signs and symptoms to the patient and family members. Explain the diagnostic tests that will be performed.

● If the patient loses his gag reflex, tell him tube feeding will be needed to maintain nutritional status.

● Advise family members to help the patient maintain mental alertness, fight boredom, and avoid depression. Suggest that they plan frequent visits, read books to the patient, or borrow library books on tape for him.

● Before discharge, teach the patient how to transfer from bed to wheelchair and from wheelchair to toilet or tub and how to walk short distances with a walker or a cane.

● Instruct family members on how to help the patient eat, compensating for facial weakness, and how to help him avoid skin breakdown.

● Emphasize the importance of establishing a regular bowel and bladder elimination routine.

● Refer the patient for physical therapy, occupational therapy, and speech therapy, as needed.

he has respiratory problems, it may include mechanical ventilation. (See *Guillain-Barré syndrome teaching topics.*)

■ Continuous electrocardiographic (ECG) monitoring is needed to identify autonomic symptoms such as cardiac arrhythmias.

■ Atropine may be given for bradycardia.

■ Marked hypotension may require volume replacement and administration of vasopressors, such as dopamine (Inotropin), phenylephrine (Neo-Synephrine), or norepinephrine (Levophed).

Most patients recover spontaneously. To prevent muscle and joint contractures, intensive physical therapy starts as soon as voluntary movement returns. However, a small percentage of patients are left with some residual disability.

ALTERNATIVE APPROACHES

High-dose I.V. immune globulin (Gamimune) and plasmapheresis may shorten recovery time. Plasmapheresis temporarily reduces circulating antibodies by removing the patient's blood, using a centrifuge to remove plasma, and reinfusing the blood. It's most effective during the first few weeks of the disease, and patients need less ventilatory support if treatment begins within 2 weeks of onset. They may receive three to five plasma exchanges.

MENINGITIS

In meningitis, the brain and spinal cord meninges become inflamed. The inflammation may involve all three meningeal membranes: dura mater, arachnoid mater, and pia mater with underlying cortex. Blood flow to the brain is reduced. Tissues swell, causing increased intracranial pressure (ICP).

The prognosis for patients with meningitis is good, and complications are rare, especially if the disease is recognized early and the infecting organism responds to antibiotics. However, mortality in untreated meningitis is 70% to 100%. The prognosis is poorer for infants and elderly people.

Pathophysiology

The origin of meningeal inflammation may be bacterial, viral, protozoal, or fungal. The most common causes of meningitis are bacterial and viral.

Bacterial meningitis is one of the most serious infections that may affect infants and children. It occurs when an organism, such as *Neisseria meningitidis, Haemophilus influenzae, Streptococcus pneumoniae,* or *Escherichia coli,* enters the subarachnoid space and causes an inflammatory response. The organisms gain access to the subarachnoid space and the CSF, where they cause irritation of the tissues bathed by the fluid.

In most patients, the infection that causes meningitis is secondary to another bacterial infection, such as bacteremia (especially from pneumonia, empyema, osteomyelitis, or endocarditis), sinusitis, otitis media, encephalitis, myelitis, or brain abscess. Respiratory infections increase the risk of bacterial meningitis. Meningitis may also follow a skull fracture, a penetrating head wound, lumbar puncture, ventricular shunting, or other neurosurgical procedures.

Meningitis caused by a virus is called *aseptic viral meningitis.* It may result from a direct infection or be secondary to disease, such as mumps, herpes, measles, or leukemia. Usually, symptoms are mild and the disease is self-limiting. (See *Understanding aseptic viral meningitis.*)

Infants, children, and elderly people have the highest risk of meningitis. Other risk factors include malnourishment, immunosuppression (from radiation therapy, for example), and CNS trauma.

RED FLAG Complications of meningitis may include vision impairment, optic neuritis, cranial nerve palsies, deafness, personality changes, headache, paresis or paralysis, endocarditis, coma, vasculitis, and cerebral infarction. Complications in infants and children may include sensory hearing loss, epilepsy, mental retardation, hydrocephalus, and subdural effusion.

Understanding aseptic viral meningitis

A benign syndrome, aseptic viral meningitis results from infection with enterovirus (most common), arbovirus, herpes simplex virus, mumps virus, or lymphocytic choriomeningitis virus.

Signs and symptoms usually begin suddenly with a temperature up to 104° F (40° C), drowsiness, confusion, stupor, and slight neck or spine stiffness when the patient bends forward. The patient history may reveal a recent illness.

Other signs and symptoms include headache, nausea, vomiting, abdominal pain, poorly defined chest pain, and sore throat.

A complete patient history and knowledge of seasonal epidemics are key to differentiating among the many forms of aseptic viral meningitis. Negative bacteriologic cultures and cerebrospinal fluid (CSF) analysis showing pleocytosis (increased number of cells in the CSF) and increased protein suggest the diagnosis. Isolation of the virus from CSF confirms it.

Treatment for aseptic viral meningitis includes bed rest, maintenance of fluid and electrolyte balance, analgesics for pain, and exercises to combat residual weakness. Careful handling of excretions and good handwashing technique prevent the spread of the disease.

Signs and symptoms

The cardinal signs and symptoms of meningitis are those of infection and increased ICP, including:

■ altered LOC, such as confusion or delirium
■ chills
■ fever
■ headache
■ malaise
■ photophobia
■ seizures
■ stiff neck and back
■ twitching
■ vomiting.

Signs and symptoms in infants and children also may include fretfulness, bulging of the fontanels (infants), and refusal to eat. (See *Important signs of meningitis*, page 302.)

Findings vary with the type and severity of meningitis. In pneumococcal meningitis, the patient's history may include a recent lung, ear, or sinus infection or endocarditis. It may also reveal alcoholism, sickle cell disease, basal skull fracture, recent splenectomy, or organ transplant. In meningitis caused by *H. influenzae*, the history may reveal a recent respiratory tract or ear infection. In meningococcal

Important signs of meningitis

A positive response to the following tests helps diagnose meningitis.

BRUDZINSKI'S SIGN
Place the patient in a dorsal recumbent position; then put your hands behind his neck and bend it forward. Pain and resistance may indicate neck injury or arthritis. But if the patient also involuntarily flexes the hips and knees, chances are he has meningeal irritation and inflammation, a sign of meningitis.

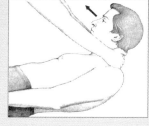

KERNIG'S SIGN
Place the patient in a supine position. Flex his leg at the hip and knee; then straighten the knee. Pain or resistance suggests meningitis.

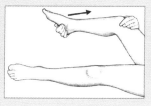

meningitis, you may see a petechial, purpuric, or ecchymotic rash on the patient's lower body.

Signs of meningeal irritation include nuchal rigidity, exaggerated and symmetrical deep tendon reflexes, opisthotonos (a spasm in which the back and limbs arch backward so the body rests on the head and heels), and positive Brudzinski's and Kernig's signs.

Test results
These tests are used to diagnose meningitis.
- Vision tests may show diplopia and other vision problems.
- Lumbar puncture shows elevated CSF pressure, cloudy or milky CSF, a high protein level, a positive Gram's stain and culture that usually identifies the infecting organism (unless it's a virus), and decreased CSF glucose level.
- Chest X-rays may reveal pneumonitis or lung abscess, tubercular lesions, or granulomas caused by fungal infection.
- Sinus and skull X-rays may reveal cranial osteomyelitis, paranasal sinusitis, or skull fracture.

TEACHING FOCUS

Meningitis teaching topics

● Teach the patient and his family about meningitis and its signs and symptoms, including its effects on behavior. Reassure the family that the delirium and behavior changes caused by meningitis usually disappear.
● Urge the patient take drugs exactly as prescribed.
● To help prevent meningitis, teach patients with chronic sinusitis or other chronic infections – as well as those exposed to people with meningitis – the importance of quick and proper medical treatment.

■ WBC count usually indicates leukocytosis and abnormal serum electrolyte levels.
■ CT scan rules out cerebral hematoma, hemorrhage, and tumor.

Treatment

Treatment for meningitis includes drugs, vigorous supportive care, and treatment of existing conditions, such as pneumonia and endocarditis. (See *Meningitis teaching topics.*)

DRUG THERAPY

Usually, I.V. antibiotics are given for at least 2 weeks, followed by oral antibiotics. The most commonly used antibiotics are penicillin G (Permapen), ampicillin, and nafcillin.

For patients allergic to penicillin, antibiotics include tetracycline (Sumycin), chloramphenicol (Chloromycetin), and kanamycin (Kantrex). Prophylactic antibiotics also may be used after ventricular shunting procedures, skull fractures, or penetrating head wounds, but this use is controversial.

Other drugs used in treatment include digoxin (Lanoxin) to control arrhythmias, mannitol (Osmitrol) to decrease cerebral edema, an I.V. anticonvulsant to prevent seizures, a sedative to reduce restlessness, and aspirin or acetaminophen to relieve headache and fever.

SUPPORTIVE MEASURES

Supportive measures include bed rest, fever reduction, and fluid therapy to prevent dehydration. If nasal cultures are positive, the patient will need isolation.

MULTIPLE SCLEROSIS

Multiple sclerosis (MS) results from progressive demyelination of the white matter of the brain and spinal cord, leading to widespread neurologic dysfunction. Usually, MS affects the optic and oculomotor nerves and the spinal nerve tracts. It doesn't affect the peripheral nervous system.

Characterized by exacerbations and remissions, MS is a major cause of chronic disability in people ages 18 to 40. It's most common in women, in northern urban areas, in higher socioeconomic groups, and in people with a family history of the disease.

The prognosis varies. The disease may progress rapidly, causing death in a few months or disability by early adulthood. However, about 70% of patients lead active, productive lives with prolonged remissions.

Pathophysiology

The exact cause of MS is unknown but may include factors that help destroy axons and the myelin sheath, such as a slow-acting viral infection, an autoimmune response of the nervous system, an allergic response, trauma, anoxia, toxins, nutritional deficiencies, vascular lesions, and anorexia nervosa. Emotional stress, overwork, fatigue, pregnancy, or an acute respiratory tract infection may precede the onset of this illness. Genetic factors may also play a part.

MS affects the white matter of brain and spinal cord by causing scattered demyelinated lesions that prevent normal conduction of nerve impulses. After myelin is destroyed, neuroglial tissue in the white matter of the CNS proliferates, forming hard yellow plaques of scar tissue. Proliferation of neuroglial tissue is called *gliosis*.

Scar tissue damages the underlying axon fiber and disrupts nerve conduction. Symptoms caused by demyelination become irreversible as the disease progresses. However, remission may result from healing of demyelinated areas by sclerotic tissue.

RED FLAG Complications include injuries from falls, urinary tract infections, constipation, joint contractures, pressure ulcers, rectal distention, and pneumonia.

Signs and symptoms

Signs and symptoms of MS depend on four factors, including the extent of myelin destruction, the site of myelin destruction, the extent of remyelination, and the adequacy of subsequent restored synaptic transmission.

Symptoms may be unpredictable and difficult for the patient to describe. They may be transient or may last for hours or weeks.

Usually, the history reveals two initial symptoms: vision problems (caused by an optic neuritis) and sensory impairment (such as paresthesia). After the initial episode, findings may vary. They may include blurred vision or diplopia, emotional lability (from involvement of the white matter of the frontal lobes), and dysphagia.

Other signs and symptoms include poorly articulated speech (caused by cerebellar involvement), muscle weakness and spasticity (caused by lesions in the corticospinal tracts), hyperreflexia, urinary problems, intention tremor, gait ataxia, paralysis ranging from monoplegia to quadriplegia, and vision problems, such as scotoma (an area of lost vision in the visual field), optic neuritis, and ophthalmoplegia (paralysis of the eye muscles).

Test results

Remissions may delay a diagnosis of MS for years. These tests help diagnose the disease.

- ◾ EEG shows abnormalities in one-third of patients.
- ◾ CSF analysis reveals elevated immunoglobulin G levels but normal total protein levels. This elevation is significant only when serum gamma globulin levels are normal, and it reflects hyperactivity of the immune system from chronic demyelination. The WBC count may be slightly increased.
- ◾ Evoked potential studies show slowed conduction of nerve impulses in 80% of patients.
- ◾ CT scan may reveal lesions in the brain's white matter.
- ◾ MRI is the most sensitive method of detecting lesions and is also used to evaluate disease progression. More than 90% of patients show lesions.
- ◾ Neuropsychological tests may help rule out other disorders.

Treatment

Treatment for MS aims to shorten exacerbations and, if possible, to relieve neurologic deficits so the patient can resume a near-normal lifestyle. (See *Multiple sclerosis teaching topics,* page 306.)

DRUG OPTIONS

Because MS may have allergic and inflammatory causes, prednisone or dexamethasone (Decadron) may be used to reduce edema of the myelin sheath during exacerbations, relieving symptoms and hastening remissions. However, these drugs don't prevent relapses.

Currently, the preferred treatment during an acute attack is a short course of methylprednisolone (Medrol), with or without a short prednisone taper. Interferon beta-1a (Avonex) or interferon beta-1b (Betaseron) also may be given to decrease the frequency of

TEACHING FOCUS

Multiple sclerosis teaching topics

● Teach the patient and family about the disease process, including its symptoms, complications, and treatments.

● Teach about prescribed drugs, including their names, indications, dosages, adverse effects, and special considerations.

● Discuss the chronic course of multiple sclerosis (MS), including that exacerbations are unpredictable and demand physical and emotional adjustments.

● Emphasize the need to avoid temperature extremes, stress, fatigue, and infections and other illnesses, all of which can trigger an MS attack.

● Advise the patient to maintain independence by developing new ways of performing daily activities.

● Stress the importance of eating a nutritious, well-balanced diet that contains sufficient roughage and adequate fluids to prevent constipation.

● Teach correct use of suppositories to help attain a regular bowel schedule.

● Discuss methods to relieve urinary incontinence and urine retention, including Credé's maneuver and self-catheterization.

● Encourage daily physical exercise and regular rest periods to prevent fatigue.

● Discuss sexual dysfunction and childbearing concerns.

relapses. How these drugs work isn't clear. Interferon beta-1b, a naturally occurring antiviral and immunoregulatory agent derived from human fibroblasts, probably attaches to membrane receptors to cause cellular changes, including increased protein synthesis.

Other useful drugs include chlordiazepoxide (Librium) to mitigate mood swings, baclofen (Lioresal) or dantrolene (Dantrium) to relieve spasticity, and bethanechol (Urecholine) or oxybutynin (Ditropan) to relieve urine retention and minimize urinary frequency and urgency.

SUPPORTIVE MEASURES

During acute exacerbations, supportive measures include bed rest, massage, prevention of fatigue and pressure ulcers, bowel and bladder training, treatment of bladder infections with antibiotics, physical therapy, and counseling.

MYASTHENIA GRAVIS

Myasthenia gravis produces sporadic, progressive weakness and abnormal fatigue of voluntary skeletal muscles. It usually affects muscles in the face, lips, tongue, neck, and throat, which are innervated by the cranial nerves — however, it can affect any muscle group.

These effects are worsened by exercise and repeated movement. Eventually, muscle fibers may degenerate, and weakness (especially of the head, neck, trunk, and limb muscles) may become irreversible. When the disease involves the respiratory system, it may be life-threatening.

Myasthenia gravis affects 14 people per 100,000 and occurs at any age. The most common age of onset in women is 20 to 30; in men, ages 70 to 80. In the past, the disease affected more women than men, but now, because of their increasing life span, men are affected more commonly than women.

The disease follows an unpredictable course with periodic exacerbations and remissions. Spontaneous remissions occur in about 25% of patients. There's no known cure, but drug therapy can help patients lead relatively normal lives except during exacerbations.

Pathophysiology

The cause of myasthenia gravis is unknown. It commonly accompanies autoimmune and thyroid disorders. In fact, 15% of patients with myasthenia gravis have thymomas.

For some reason, the patient's blood cells and thymus gland produce antibodies that block, destroy, or weaken the neuroreceptors that transmit nerve impulses, causing a failure in transmission of nerve impulses at the neuromuscular junction. (See *What happens in myasthenia gravis,* page 308.)

RED FLAG Complications of myasthenia gravis include respiratory difficulty, pneumonia, and problems with chewing and swallowing, possibly leading to choking and aspiration. Progressive weakness of the diaphragm and intercostal muscles may eventually lead to myasthenic crisis, which causes severe respiratory distress.

Signs and symptoms

Signs and symptoms of myasthenia gravis vary with the muscles involved and the severity of the disease. However, in all cases, muscle weakness is progressive and, eventually, some muscles may lose function entirely.

Common signs and symptoms include extreme muscle weakness, fatigue, ptosis, diplopia, trouble chewing and swallowing, a sleepy masklike expression, a drooping jaw, a bobbing head, and arm or hand weakness. The patient may report needing to tilt her head back to see properly. She usually notes that symptoms are milder on awakening and worsen as the day progresses and that short rest periods temporarily restore muscle function. She also may report that symptoms become more intense during menses and after stress, prolonged exposure to sunlight or cold, or infection.

What happens in myasthenia gravis

During normal neuromuscular transmission, a motor nerve impulse travels to a motor nerve terminal, stimulating the release of a chemical neurotransmitter called *acetylcholine*. When acetylcholine diffuses across the synapse, receptor sites in the motor end plate react and depolarize the muscle fiber. The depolarization spreads through the muscle fiber, causing muscle contraction.

In myasthenia gravis, antibodies attach to the acetylcholine receptor sites. They block, destroy, and weaken these sites, leaving them insensitive to acetylcholine, thereby blocking neuromuscular transmission.

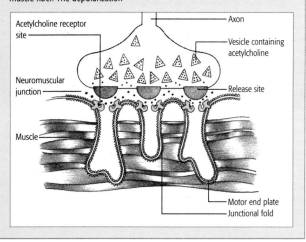

Auscultation may reveal hypoventilation if the respiratory muscles are involved. This may lead to decreased tidal volume, making breathing difficult and predisposing the patient to pneumonia and other respiratory tract infections.

Test results

These tests are used to diagnose myasthenia gravis.

■ Tensilon test confirms diagnosis by temporarily improving muscle function after an I.V. injection of edrophonium (Tensilon) or, occasionally, neostigmine (Prostigmin). However, long-standing ocular muscle dysfunction may not respond. This test also differentiates myasthenic crisis from cholinergic crisis.

■ Electromyography measures the electrical potential of muscle cells and helps differentiate nerve disorders from muscle disor-

Myasthenia gravis teaching topics

● Teach the patient and family about the disease process, including its symptoms, complications, and treatments.

● Teach about prescribed drugs, including their names, indications, dosages, adverse effects, and special considerations.

● Help the patient plan daily activities to coincide with energy peaks.

● Stress the need for frequent rest periods throughout the day.

● Explain that remissions, exacerbations, and daily fluctuations are common.

● Teach the patient how to recognize adverse effects and evidence of toxicity from anticholinesterase drugs (headaches, weakness, sweating, abdominal cramps, nausea, vomiting, diarrhea, excessive salivation, and bronchospasm) and corticosteroids (euphoria, insomnia, edema, and increased appetite).

● Warn the patient to avoid strenuous exercise, stress, infection, and needless exposure to the sun or cold, which can worsen signs and symptoms.

● Teach the patient about thymectomy, if indicated.

ders. In myasthenia gravis, the amplitude of motor unit potential falls off with continued use. Muscle contractions decrease with each test, reflecting fatigue.

■ Nerve conduction studies measure the speed at which electrical impulses travel along a nerve and also help distinguish nerve disorders from muscle disorders.

■ Chest X-ray or CT scan may identify a thymoma.

Treatment

The main treatment for myasthenia gravis is anticholinesterase drugs, such as neostigmine and pyridostigmine (Mestinon). These drugs counteract fatigue and muscle weakness and restore about 80% of muscle function. However, they become less effective as the disease worsens. Corticosteroids also may help relieve symptoms. (See *Myasthenia gravis teaching topics*.)

If drugs aren't effective, some patients undergo plasmapheresis to remove acetylcholine-receptor antibodies and temporarily lessen the severity of symptoms. Patients with thymomas need thymectomy, which leads to remission in adult-onset disease in about 40% of patients if done within 2 years after diagnosis.

Myasthenic crisis requires immediate hospitalization. Endotracheal intubation, mechanical ventilation, and vigorous suctioning to remove secretions usually bring improvement in a few days. Because anticholinesterase drugs aren't effective in myasthenic crisis, they're stopped until respiratory function improves.

PARKINSON'S DISEASE

Parkinson's disease produces progressive muscle rigidity, loss of muscle movement (*akinesia*), and involuntary tremors. The patient's condition may deteriorate for more than 10 years. Eventually, aspiration pneumonia or some other infection causes death.

One of the most common crippling diseases in the United States, Parkinson's disease affects more men than women and usually occurs in middle age or later, affecting 1 in every 100 people over age 60.

Pathophysiology

In Parkinson's disease, a dopamine deficiency occurs in the basal ganglia, the dopamine-releasing pathway that connects the substantia nigra to the corpus striatum. Reduction of dopamine in the corpus striatum upsets the normal balance between the inhibitory dopamine and excitatory acetylcholine neurotransmitters. This prevents affected brain cells from performing their normal inhibitory function in the CNS and causes most parkinsonian symptoms.

In most cases, the cause of Parkinson's disease is unknown. However, some cases result from exposure to toxins, such as manganese dust or carbon monoxide, that destroy cells in the substantia nigra of the brain.

Parkinson's disease affects the extrapyramidal system, which influences the initiation, modulation, and completion of movement. The extrapyramidal system includes the corpus striatum, globus pallidus, and substantia nigra.

RED FLAG *Common complications of Parkinson's disease include injury from falls, aspiration from impaired swallowing, urinary tract infections, and skin breakdown from increased immobility.*

Signs and symptoms

Important signs of Parkinson's disease include muscle rigidity, akinesia, and a unilateral "pill-roll" tremor. Muscle rigidity results in resistance to passive muscle stretching, which may be uniform (lead-pipe rigidity) or jerky (cogwheel rigidity).

Akinesia causes gait and movement disturbances. The patient walks bent forward, takes a long time initiating purposeful movement, pivots with difficulty, and easily loses his balance. Akinesia also may cause other signs, including a masklike facial expression and blepharospasm, in which the eyelids stay closed.

The pill-roll tremor is insidious. It begins in the fingers, increases during stress or anxiety, and decreases with purposeful movement and sleep.

Other signs and symptoms of Parkinson's disease include:

TEACHING FOCUS

Parkinson's disease teaching topics

- Teach the patient and family about the disorder, including its progressive symptoms, complications, and treatments.
- Discuss warning signs of complications that require immediate attention.
- Teach the patient about prescribed drugs, including their names, indications, dosages, adverse effects, and special considerations (such as dietary restrictions and the need to stand up slowly if the patient takes levodopa).
- Reinforce the importance of range-of-motion exercises, routine daily activities, walking, and baths and massage to help relax muscles.
- Explain to the patient and family how to prevent pressure ulcers and contractures by proper positioning.
- Explain household safety measures to prevent accidents.
- Reinforce a swallowing therapy regimen to prevent aspiration.

- drooling
- dysarthria (impaired speech from a disturbance in muscle control)
- dysphagia (trouble swallowing)
- fatigue
- high-pitched, monotone voice
- increased perspiration
- insomnia
- mood changes
- muscle cramps in the legs, neck, and trunk
- oily skin.

Test results

Diagnosis of Parkinson's disease is based on the patient's age, history, and signs and symptoms. Laboratory tests usually have little value. Urinalysis may reveal decreased dopamine levels, and CT scan or MRI may rule out other disorders such as intracranial tumors.

Treatment

Treatment for Parkinson's disease aims to relieve symptoms and keep the patient functional for as long as possible. It includes drugs, physical therapy, and stereotactic neurosurgery (in extreme cases). (See *Parkinson's disease teaching topics*.)

DRUG THERAPY

Drug therapy usually includes levodopa (Larodopa), a dopamine replacement that's most effective in the first few years it's used. It's given in increasing doses until signs and symptoms are relieved or adverse effects develop. Because adverse effects can be serious, levodopa commonly is given with carbidopa (Sinemet) to halt peripheral dopamine synthesis. Bromocriptine (Parlodel) may be given as an additive to reduce the levodopa dose.

Stalevo combines carbidopa, levodopa, and entacapone (Comtan) and may be used when carbidopa and levodopa are no longer effective throughout the dosage interval. The added component entacapone prolongs the time that levodopa is active in the brain.

When levodopa is ineffective or too toxic, anticholinergics and antihistamines may be given. Anticholinergics, such as trihexyphenidyl (Artane) and benztropine (Cogentin), may be used to control tremors and rigidity. They also may be used with levodopa. Antihistamines such as diphenhydramine (Benadryl) may help decrease tremors through central anticholinergic and sedative effects.

Amantadine (Symmetrel), an antiviral, is used early in treatment to reduce rigidity, tremors, and akinesia. Patients with mild disease are given selegiline (Carbex) to slow the disease and ease symptoms. Tricyclic antidepressants may be given for depression.

DEEP BRAIN STIMULATION

Deep brain stimulation is now the preferred surgical option over pallidotomy and thalamotomy. Electrodes are implanted into the targeted brain area. These electrodes are connected to wires attached to an impulse generator that's implanted under the collarbone. The electrodes control symptoms on the opposite side of the body by sending electrical impulses to the brain.

PHYSICAL THERAPY

Physical therapy helps maintain normal muscle tone and function. It includes active and passive range-of-motion exercises, routine daily activities, walking, and baths and massage to help relax muscles.

STROKE

Previously known as *cerebrovascular accident,* stroke is a sudden impairment of cerebral circulation in one or more of the blood vessels supplying the brain. It interrupts or reduces oxygen supply, causing serious damage or necrosis in brain tissues. Although it mostly affects older adults, it can strike people of any age. Black men have a higher risk than other population groups.

Stroke is the third leading cause of death in the United States and the most common cause of neurologic disability. It affects about 700,000 people each year, and half of them die as a result. About half of those who survive remain permanently disabled and have

Understanding transient ischemic attack

A transient ischemic attack (TIA) is a neurologic deficit that lasts seconds to hours and clears in 12 to 24 hours. It's usually considered a warning sign of an impending thrombotic stroke; 50% to 80% of patients who've had a cerebral infarction from thrombosis have also had a TIA. The age of onset varies, but occurrence rises dramatically after age 50 and is highest among blacks and men.

In a TIA, microemboli released from a thrombus may temporarily interrupt blood flow, especially in the small distal branches of the brain's arterial tree. Small spasms in those arterioles may precede TIA and also impair blood flow.

The most distinctive characteristics of TIAs are the transient nature of the neurologic deficits and the complete return of normal function. Signs and symptoms correlate with the location of the affected artery. They include double vision, unilateral blindness, staggering or uncoordinated gait, unilateral weakness or numbness, falling because of weakness in the legs, dizziness, and speech deficits, such as slurring or thickness.

During a TIA, treatment aims to prevent a completed stroke and consists of aspirin or anticoagulants to minimize the risk of thrombosis. After or between attacks, preventive treatment includes carotid endarterectomy or cerebral microvascular bypass.

another stroke within weeks, months, or years. The sooner circulation returns to normal, the better the chance of complete recovery.

Stroke is classified according to how it progresses.

■ Transient ischemic attack (TIA), the least severe type, is caused by temporarily stopped blood flow, usually in carotid and vertebrobasilar arteries. (See *Understanding transient ischemic attack.*)
■ Progressive stroke, also called *stroke-in-evolution* or *thrombus-in-evolution,* begins with a slight neurologic deficit and worsens in a day or two.
■ Completed stroke, the most severe type, causes maximum neurologic deficits at the onset.

Pathophysiology
Factors that increase the risk of stroke include:
■ arrhythmias, especially atrial fibrillation
■ atherosclerosis
■ cardiac enlargement
■ diabetes mellitus
■ drug abuse
■ electrocardiogram changes
■ family history of cerebrovascular disease
■ gout

- high serum triglyceride levels
- history of TIA
- hypertension
- lack of exercise
- orthostatic hypotension
- rheumatic heart disease
- sickle cell disease
- smoking
- use of hormonal contraceptives.

Major causes of stroke include thrombosis, embolism, and hemorrhage.

THROMBOSIS

Thrombosis is the most common cause of stroke in middle-aged and elderly people. It causes congestion and edema in the affected vessel as well as ischemia in the brain tissue supplied by the vessel. Thrombosis usually results from an obstruction in the extracerebral vessels, but sometimes it's intracerebral. The risk increases with obesity, smoking, hormonal contraceptive use, and surgery.

EMBOLISM

An embolism is a blood vessel occlusion caused by a fragmented clot, a tumor, fat, bacteria, or air. An embolus cuts off circulation in the cerebral vasculature by lodging in a narrow portion of the artery, causing necrosis and edema. If the embolus is septic and the infection extends beyond the vessel wall, encephalitis may develop. If the infection stays within the vessel wall, an aneurysm may form, which could lead to the sudden rupture of an artery, or cerebral hemorrhage. (See *Common sites of aneurysm.*)

An embolus can occur at any age, especially in patients with a history of rheumatic heart disease, endocarditis, posttraumatic valvular disease, or atrial fibrillation or other cardiac arrhythmia. It also can occur after open-heart surgery. Embolism usually develops rapidly — in 10 to 20 seconds — and without warning. The left middle cerebral artery is usually the embolus site.

HEMORRHAGE

Hemorrhage, the third most common cause of stroke, also may occur suddenly at any age. A brain artery bursts, reducing blood supply to the area served by the artery. Blood also accumulates deep in the brain, further damaging neural tissue.

Hemorrhagic stroke commonly arises from chronic hypertension or aneurysms. Cocaine use also increases the risk of hemorrhagic stroke because it causes severe hypertension.

Common sites of aneurysm

Cerebral aneurysms usually arise at an arterial junction in the circle of Willis (shown in color below), a circular anastomosis forming the major cerebral arteries at the base of the brain. Cerebral aneurysms commonly rupture and cause subarachnoid hemorrhage.

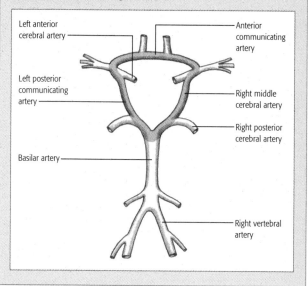

Left anterior cerebral artery

Left posterior communicating artery

Basilar artery

Anterior communicating artery

Right middle cerebral artery

Right posterior cerebral artery

Right vertebral artery

RED FLAG *Among many complications of stroke are unstable blood pressure from loss of vasomotor control, fluid imbalances, malnutrition, infections (such as pneumonia), and sensory impairment, including vision problems. Altered level of consciousness, aspiration, contractures, and pulmonary emboli also may occur.*

Signs and symptoms

When taking the patient's history, you may uncover risk factors for stroke. You may observe loss of consciousness, dizziness, or seizures. Obtain information from a family member or friend, if needed. Neurologic examination provides most of the information about the physical effects of stroke.

Physical findings depend on artery affected and the portion of the brain it supplies (see *Neurologic deficits in stroke,* pages 316 and 317),

Neurologic deficits in stroke

In stroke, functional loss reflects damage to the brain area normally perfused by the occluded or ruptured artery. Whereas one patient may experience only mild hand weakness, another may develop unilateral paralysis. Hypoxia and ischemia may produce edema that affects distal parts of the brain, causing further neurologic deficits. The signs and symptoms that accompany stroke at different sites are described below.

SITE	SIGNS AND SYMPTOMS
ANTERIOR CEREBRAL ARTERY	• Confusion • Impaired motor and sensory functions • Incontinence • Numbness on the affected side (especially in the arm) • Paralysis of the contralateral foot and leg with accompanying footdrop • Personality changes, such as flat affect and distractibility • Poor coordination • Weakness
INTERNAL CAROTID ARTERY	• Altered level of consciousness • Aphasia • Bruits over the carotid artery • Dysphasia • Headaches • Numbness • Paralysis • Ptosis • Sensory changes • Vision disturbances such as blurring on the affected side • Weakness
MIDDLE CEREBRAL ARTERY	• Aphasia • Dysgraphia (inability to write) • Dyslexia (reading problems) • Dysphasia • Hemiparesis on the affected side that's more severe in the face and arm than in the leg • Visual field cuts

Neurologic deficits in stroke (*continued*)

SITE	SIGNS AND SYMPTOMS
POSTERIOR CEREBRAL ARTERY	● Blindness from ischemia in the occipital area ● Coma ● Dyslexia ● Sensory impairment ● Visual field cuts
VERTEBRAL OR BASILAR ARTERY	● Amnesia ● Ataxia ● Dizziness ● Dysphagia ● Mouth and lip numbness ● Poor coordination ● Slurred speech ● Vision deficits, such as color blindness, lack of depth perception, and diplopia ● Weakness on the affected side

the severity of the damage, and the extent of collateral circulation that develops to help the brain compensate for a decreased blood supply.

If the stroke occurs in the brain's left hemisphere, it produces signs and symptoms on the right side of the body. If it occurs in the right hemisphere, signs and symptoms appear on the left side. However, a stroke that damages cranial nerves produces signs on the same side as the damage.

Assessment of motor function and muscle strength commonly shows a loss of voluntary muscle control and hemiparesis or hemiplegia. In the initial phase, the patient may have flaccid paralysis with decreased deep tendon reflexes. These reflexes return to normal after the initial phase, accompanied by an increase in muscle tone and, in some cases, muscle spasticity on the affected side.

Vision testing usually reveals reduced vision or blindness on the affected side of the body and, in patients with left-sided hemiplegia, problems with visual-spatial relations. Sensory assessment may reveal sensory losses ranging from slight impairment of touch to an inability to perceive the position and motion of body parts. The patient may also have trouble interpreting visual, tactile, and auditory stimuli.

Test results

These tests are used to diagnose stroke.

■ Cerebral angiography shows disruption or displacement of the cerebral circulation by occlusion or hemorrhage. It's the test of choice for examining the entire cerebral circulation.

■ Digital subtraction angiography evaluates the patency of cerebral vessels and identifies their position in the head and neck. It also detects and evaluates lesions and vascular abnormalities.

■ CT scan detects structural abnormalities, edema, and lesions, such as nonhemorrhagic infarction and aneurysms. It differentiates stroke from other disorders, such as primary metastatic tumor and subdural, intracerebral, or epidural hematoma. Patients with TIA commonly have a normal CT scan.

■ PET scan provides data on cerebral metabolism and cerebral blood flow changes, especially in ischemic stroke.

■ Single-photon emission tomography identifies cerebral blood flow and helps diagnose cerebral infarction.

■ MRI and magnetic resonance angiography evaluate the lesion's location and size. MRI doesn't distinguish hemorrhage, tumor, or infarction as well as a CT scan does, but it provides better images of the cerebellum and brain stem.

■ Transcranial Doppler studies evaluate the velocity of blood flow through major intracranial vessels, an indication of diameter.

■ Cerebral blood flow studies measure blood flow to the brain and help detect abnormalities.

■ Ophthalmoscopy may show signs of hypertension and atherosclerotic changes in the retinal arteries.

■ EEG may detect reduced electrical activity in an area of cortical infarction and is especially useful when CT scan results are inconclusive. It can also differentiate seizure activity from stroke.

■ Oculoplethysmography indirectly measures ophthalmic blood flow and carotid artery blood flow.

Treatment

Treatment for stroke commonly includes physical rehabilitation, diet and drugs to help decrease risk factors, and measures to help the patient adapt to specific deficits, such as speech impairment and paralysis. (See *Stroke teaching topics.*)

Drugs commonly used for stroke therapy include:

■ thrombolytic therapy such as recombinant tissue plasminogen activator (TNKase) given within the first 3 hours of an ischemic stroke to restore circulation to the affected brain tissue and limit the extent of brain injury

TEACHING FOCUS

Stroke teaching topics

- Teach the patient and family about the disease process, including types of strokes and their signs and symptoms and treatments.
- Teach about prescribed drugs, including their names, indications, dosages, adverse effects, and special considerations.
- Discuss warning signs of complications that require immediate medical attention.
- Discuss risk factors for stroke, and help the patient identify those he can alter to reduce his risk of further stroke.
- If the patient is having surgery, explain the procedure and what he can expect before and after.
- Teach the importance of following a low-cholesterol, low-salt diet; achieving and maintaining an ideal

weight; increasing activity; avoiding smoking and prolonged bed rest; and minimizing stress.
- Warn the patient or his family to seek emergency medical attention for any premonitory signs of a stroke, such as severe headache, drowsiness, confusion, and dizziness.
- Emphasize the importance of regular follow-up visits.
- Stress the importance of continuing rehabilitation to minimize deficits.
- Discuss alternate communication techniques, if indicated.
- Review dietary adjustments, such as semisoft foods for dysphagia and the use of assistive feeding devices.
- Review the safe use of a cane or walker and home safety tips.

■ anticonvulsants, such as phenytoin (Dilantin), to treat or prevent seizures

■ stool softeners, such as docusate (Colace), to prevent straining, which increases intracranial pressure

■ corticosteroids, such as dexamethasone (Decadron), to minimize cerebral edema

■ anticoagulants, such as heparin, warfarin (Coumadin), and ticlopidine (Ticlid), to reduce the risk of thrombotic stroke

■ analgesics, such as acetaminophen (Tylenol), to relieve headache that may follow hemorrhagic stroke.

Depending on the stroke's cause and extent, the patient also may need surgery. A craniotomy may be done to remove a hematoma, an endarterectomy to remove atherosclerotic plaque from the inner arterial wall, or extracranial-intracranial bypass to circumvent an artery that's blocked by occlusion or stenosis. Ventricular shunts may be needed to drain cerebrospinal fluid if hydrocephalus develops.

10

GASTROINTESTINAL SYSTEM

The digestive system is the body's food processing complex. It performs the critical task of supplying essential nutrients to fuel the other organs and body systems. The digestive system has two major components. They include the GI tract, or alimentary canal, and the accessory glands and organs.

A malfunction along the GI tract or in one of the accessory glands or organs can produce far-reaching metabolic effects, which may become life-threatening. (See *A close look at the digestive system*.)

GI TRACT

The GI tract is basically a hollow, muscular tube that begins in the mouth and ends at the anus. It includes the mouth, esophagus, stomach, small intestine, and large intestine.

Mouth and esophagus

The digestive process begins in the mouth. Chewing and salivation soften food, making it easy to swallow. An enzyme in saliva, called *ptyalin*, starts converting starches to sugars before food is swallowed.

When a person swallows, the upper esophageal sphincter relaxes, allowing food to enter the esophagus. In the esophagus, peristaltic waves activated by the glossopharyngeal nerve propel food toward the stomach.

Stomach

Digestion occurs in two phases: the cephalic phase and the gastric phase. By the time food is traveling through the esophagus on its way to the stomach, the cephalic phase of digestion has begun. In

A close look at the digestive system

This illustration shows the organs of the GI tract and several accessory organs.

Parotid gland —
Epiglottis —
Submandibular gland —
Esophagus —
Liver —
Duodenum —
Gallbladder —
Ascending colon —
Jejunum —
Cecum —
Vermiform appendix —

— Mouth
— Sublingual gland
— Pharynx
— Spleen
— Stomach
— Pancreas
— Transverse colon
— Descending colon
— Ileum
— Sigmoid colon
— Rectum

this phase, the stomach secretes hydrochloric acid and pepsin, which are digestive juices that help break down food.

The gastric phase of digestion begins when food passes the cardiac sphincter, a circle of muscle at the end of the esophagus. The food exits the esophagus and enters the stomach, causing the stomach wall to distend. This stimulates the mucosal lining of the stomach to release the hormone gastrin. Gastrin serves two purposes. It stimulates secretion of gastric juice. And it stimulates the stomach's motor functions.

Gastric secretions are highly acidic, with a pH of 0.9 to 1.5. In addition to hydrochloric acid and pepsin, the gastric juices contain intrinsic factor (which helps the body absorb vitamin B_{12}) and proteolytic enzymes (which help the body use protein). The gastric juices mix with the food, which becomes a thick, gruel-like material called *chyme*.

The stomach has three major motor functions. It holds food. It mixes food by peristaltic contractions with gastric juices. And it slowly releases chyme into the small intestine for further digestion and absorption.

Small intestine

Nearly all digestion takes place in the small intestine, which is about 20′ (6 m) long. Chyme passes through the small intestine propelled by peristaltic contractions. The small intestine has three major sections, including the duodenum, the jejunum, and the ileum.

The duodenum is a 10′ (25.4-cm) long, C-shaped curve of the small intestine that extends from the stomach. Food passes from the stomach to the duodenum through a narrow opening called the *pylorus*. The duodenum also has an opening through which bile and pancreatic enzymes enter the intestine to neutralize acidic chyme and aid digestion. This opening is called the *sphincter of Oddi*.

The jejunum extends from the duodenum and forms the longest portion of the small intestine. The jejunum leads to the ileum, the narrowest portion of the small intestine.

Digestive secretions convert carbohydrates, proteins, and fats into sugars, amino acids, fatty acids, and glycerin. Along with water and electrolytes, these nutrients are absorbed through the intestinal mucosa into the bloodstream for use by the body. Nonnutrients, such as vegetable fibers, are carried through the intestine.

The small intestine ends at the ileocecal valve, located in the lower right part of the abdomen. The ileocecal valve is a sphincter that empties nutrient-depleted chyme into the large intestine.

Large intestine

After chyme passes through the small intestine, it enters the ascending colon at the cecum, the pouchlike beginning of the large intestine. By this time, chyme consists of mostly indigestible material. From the ascending colon, chyme passes through the transverse colon and then down through the descending colon to the rectum and anal canal, where it's finally expelled.

The large intestine produces no hormones or digestive enzymes. Rather, it's where absorption takes place. The large intestine absorbs nearly all of the water remaining in the chyme plus large amounts of sodium and chloride.

The large intestine also harbors the bacteria *Escherichia coli, Enterobacter aerogenes, Clostridium welchii,* and *Lactobacillus bifidus,* which help produce vitamin K and break down cellulose into usable carbohydrates. In the lower part of the descending colon, long, relatively sluggish contractions cause propulsive waves known as *mass movements.* These movements propel the intestinal contents into the rectum and produce the urge to defecate.

ACCESSORY GLANDS AND ORGANS

The liver, gallbladder, and pancreas contribute several substances, such as enzymes, bile, and hormones that are vital to digestion. These structures deliver their secretions to the duodenum through the ampulla of Vater.

Liver

A large, highly vascular organ, the liver is enclosed in a fibrous capsule in the upper right area of the abdomen. The liver performs many complex and important functions, many of which are related to digestion and nutrition.
- It filters and detoxifies blood, removing foreign substances, such as drugs, alcohol, and other toxins.
- It removes naturally occurring ammonia from body fluids, converting it to urea for excretion in urine.
- It produces plasma proteins, nonessential amino acids, and vitamin A.
- It stores essential nutrients, such as iron and vitamins K, D, and B_{12}.
- It produces bile to aid digestion.
- It converts glucose to glycogen and stores it as fuel for muscles.
- It stores fats and converts excess sugars to fats for storage in other parts of the body.

Gallbladder

The gallbladder is a small, pear-shaped organ nestled under the liver and joined to the larger organ by the cystic duct. The gallbladder's job is to store and concentrate bile produced by the liver. Bile is a clear, yellowish liquid that helps break down fats and neutralize gastric secretions in the chyme.

Secretion of the hormone cholecystokinin causes the gallbladder to contract and the ampulla of Vater to relax. This allows the release of bile into the common bile duct for delivery to the duodenum. When the ampulla of Vater closes, bile shunts to the gallbladder for storage.

Pancreas

The pancreas lies behind the stomach, with its head and neck extending into the curve of the duodenum and its tail lying against the spleen. The pancreas is made up exocrine and endocrine tissue.

Exocrine tissue secretes enzymes through ducts to the digestive system. Small, scattered glands — called *acini* — secrete more than 1,000 ml of digestive enzymes daily. These lobules release secretions into small ducts that merge to form the pancreatic duct, which runs the length of the pancreas and joins the bile duct from the gallbladder before entering the duodenum. Vagus nerve stimulation and the release of two hormones (secretin and cholecystokinin) control the rate and amount of pancreatic secretion.

Endocrine tissue secretes hormones into the blood.Endocrine function involves the islets of Langerhans, microscopic structures scattered throughout the pancreas. More than 1 million islets house two major cell types: alpha and beta. Alpha cells secrete glucagon, a hormone that stimulates glucose formation in the liver. Beta cells secrete insulin to promote carbohydrate metabolism. Both hormones flow directly into the blood; their release is mediated by blood glucose levels.

Digestive disorders

The disorders discussed in this section include:

- appendicitis
- cholecystitis
- cirrhosis
- Crohn's disease
- diverticular disease
- gastroesophageal reflux disease
- hiatal hernia
- irritable bowel syndrome
- pancreatitis
- peptic ulcer
- ulcerative colitis
- viral hepatitis.

APPENDICITIS

Appendicitis is an inflammation of the vermiform appendix, a small, fingerlike projection attached to the cecum just below the ileocecal valve. Appendectomy the most common major surgical emergency. Appendicitis may occur at any age and affects both sexes equally; however, between puberty and age 25, it's more prevalent in men.

Pathophysiology

Although the appendix has no known function, it does regularly fill and empty itself of food. Until recently, appendicitis was thought to result from an obstruction by a fecal mass, a stricture, barium ingestion, or viral infection. Obstruction does sometimes occur, but mucosal ulceration usually happens first. Although the exact cause of the ulceration is unknown, it may be viral.

After ulceration occurs, inflammation may develop and temporarily obstruct the appendix. A physical obstruction, if present, is usually caused by stool accumulation around vegetable fibers (called a *fecalith*). Then mucus outflow is blocked, which distends the organ and increases its internal pressure; the appendix contracts. Bacteria multiply, and inflammation and pressure continue to increase, affecting blood flow to the organ and causing severe abdominal pain.

RED FLAG Inflammation can lead to infection, clotting, tissue decay, and perforation of the appendix. If the appendix ruptures or perforates, the infected contents spill into the abdominal cavity, causing peritonitis, the most common and dangerous complication.

Signs and symptoms

The history and sequence of pain is important in diagnosing appendicitis. The first symptom is almost always vague epigastric pain, sometimes described as a cramping sensation. Over time, the pain becomes more localized and moves to the right lower abdominal area. If the appendix is behind the cecum or in the pelvis, the patient may have flank tenderness instead of abdominal tenderness. Other signs and symptoms include anorexia, a low-grade fever, and nausea or vomiting.

In cases of rupture, spasm will occur, and abdominal pain may stop briefly. Untreated appendicitis is invariably fatal.

Test results

These tests are sometimes helpful in diagnosis, but normal findings don't rule out appendicitis.

■ White blood cell (WBC) count is moderately high with an increased number of immature cells.

■ X-ray with a radiographic contrast agent aids diagnosis. Failure of the organ to fill with contrast agent indicates appendicitis.

Differential diagnosis rules out illnesses with similar symptoms, such as bladder infection, diverticulitis, gastritis, ovarian cyst, pancreatitis, renal colic, and uterine disease.

TEACHING FOCUS

Appendicitis teaching topics

- Explain to the patient and family what happens in appendicitis. Help them understand the required surgery and its possible complications. If time allows, provide preoperative teaching.
- Teach the patient to cough, breathe deeply, and turn frequently to prevent postoperative pulmonary complications.
- Review the proper use of all prescribed drugs. Make sure the patient knows how to take each drug and understands the desired effects and possible adverse effects.

Treatment

Appendectomy is the only effective treatment. Laparoscopic appendectomies, which decrease the recovery time and facility stay, are now performed. If peritonitis develops, treatment involves gastric intubation, parenteral replacement of fluids and electrolytes, and antibiotic administration. (See *Appendicitis teaching topics*.)

CHOLECYSTITIS

In cholecystitis, the gallbladder becomes inflamed, usually after a gallstone lodges in the cystic duct, causing painful gallbladder distention. Cholecystitis may be acute or chronic. The former is most common during middle age; the latter, among elderly people.

Pathophysiology

The cause of gallstone formation isn't entirely clear, although abnormal metabolism of cholesterol and bile salts plays an important role. Bile is made continuously by the liver and is concentrated and stored in the gallbladder until the duodenum needs it to help digest fat. Certain conditions, such as age, obesity, and estrogen imbalance, cause the liver to secrete bile that's abnormally high in cholesterol or lacking the proper concentration of bile salts.

When the gallbladder concentrates this bile, inflammation may occur. Excessive water and bile salts are reabsorbed, making the bile less soluble. Cholesterol, calcium, and bilirubin precipitate into gallstones. Fat entering the duodenum causes the intestinal mucosa to secrete the hormone cholecystokinin, which stimulates the gallbladder to contract and empty. If a stone lodges in the cystic duct, the gallbladder contracts but can't empty. If a stone lodges in the common bile duct, bile flow into the duodenum is obstructed. Bilirubin is absorbed into the blood, causing jaundice.

Biliary narrowing and swelling of the tissue around the stone also may cause irritation and inflammation of the common bile duct. Inflammation can progress up the biliary tree and cause infection of any of the bile ducts. This causes scar tissue, fluid accumulation, cirrhosis, portal hypertension, and bleeding.

Risk factors that predispose a person to gallstones include obesity; a high-calorie, high-cholesterol diet; increased estrogen levels from hormonal contraceptives, hormone replacement therapy, or pregnancy; use of clofibrate, an antilipemic drug; diabetes mellitus; ileal disease; blood disorders; liver disease; and pancreatitis.

In acute cholecystitis, inflammation of the gallbladder wall usually develops after a gallstone lodges in the cystic duct. When bile flow is blocked, the gallbladder becomes inflamed and distended. Bacterial growth, usually *Escherichia coli,* may contribute to the inflammation. Acute cholecystitis also may result from poor or absent blood flow to the gallbladder.

Edema affects the gallbladder and sometimes the cystic duct. It obstructs bile flow, which chemically irritates the gallbladder. Cells in the gallbladder wall may become oxygen starved and die as the distended organ presses on vessels and impairs blood flow. Those dead cells then slough off. An exudate covers ulcerated areas, causing the gallbladder to adhere to surrounding structures.

RED FLAG Cholecystitis may lead to a number of complications. For example, pus or fluid (hydrops) may accumulate in the gallbladder. The gallbladder may become distended with mucus (mucocele). Gangrene may develop, causing perforation, peritonitis, abnormal passages in the tissues (fistulas), and pancreatitis. Or chronic cholecystitis or cholangitis (bile duct infection) may develop.

Signs and symptoms

Acute cholecystitis usually strikes after a meal that's rich in fats and may occur at night, awakening the person suddenly. Signs and symptoms include:

- acute abdominal pain in the right upper quadrant that may radiate to the back, between the shoulders, or to the chest
- belching
- chills
- colic from passage of gallstones along the bile duct (biliary colic)
- flatulence
- indigestion
- jaundice and clay-colored stools (if a stone obstructs the common bile duct)
- light-headedness
- low-grade fever

■ nausea
■ vomiting.

Cholecystitis accounts for 10% to 25% of all patients requiring gallbladder surgery. The prognosis is good with treatment.

Test results

These tests are used to diagnose cholecystitis.

■ X-rays reveal gallstones if they contain enough calcium to be radiopaque and also help disclose porcelain gallbladder, limy bile, and gallstone ileus.
■ Ultrasonography confirms gallstones as small as 2 mm and distinguishes between obstructive and nonobstructive jaundice.
■ Oral cholecystography confirms the presence of gallstones, although this test is gradually being replaced by ultrasonography.
■ Technetium-labeled scan indicates cystic duct obstruction and acute or chronic cholecystitis if the gallbladder can't be seen.
■ Percutaneous transhepatic cholangiography, performed with fluoroscopy, supports the diagnosis of obstructive jaundice and reveals calculi in the ducts.
■ Blood studies may reveal high levels of serum alkaline phosphatase, lactate dehydrogenase, aspartate aminotransferase, and total bilirubin. The icteric index, a measure of bilirubin in the blood, is elevated.
■ WBC count is slightly elevated during a cholecystitis attack.

Treatment

Surgery is the most common treatment for gallbladder and bile duct disease. It may involve removal of the gallbladder (cholecystectomy), with or without X-ray of the bile ducts (operative cholangiography); creation of an opening into the common bile duct for drainage (choledochostomy); or exploration of the common bile duct. Other invasive procedures include:

■ insertion of a flexible catheter through a sinus tract into the common bile duct and removal of stones using a basket-shaped tool guided by fluoroscopy
■ endoscopic retrograde cholangiopancreatography, which removes stones with a balloon or basket-shaped tool passed through an endoscope
■ lithotripsy, which breaks up gallstones with ultrasonic waves (contraindicated in patients with pacemakers or implantable defibrillators)
■ stone dissolution with oral chenodeoxycholic acid or ursodeoxycholic acid (of limited use). (See *Cholecystitis teaching topics.*)

TEACHING FOCUS

Cholecystitis teaching topics

● Explain the disease process and its treatments to the patient and his family.
● If the patient is having surgery, tell him what to expect before and after it.
● If the patient will be discharged with a T tube, teach him how to perform dressing changes and routine skin care.
● At discharge, advise the patient who has had surgery against heavy lifting or straining for 6 weeks.
● Discuss evidence of biliary colic, such as pain, belching, and nausea.

● Instruct the patient about cholelithiasis and other complications that require medical attention.
● Explain that food restrictions aren't needed unless the patient has an intolerance to a specific food or some underlying condition (such as diabetes, atherosclerosis, or obesity) that requires such restriction.
● Teach about drugs the patient will be taking, including their dosages, adverse effects, and special considerations.
● Reinforce the importance of follow-up care to detect recurrent gallstones.

The patient may receive other treatments as well. They include a low-fat diet with replacement of vitamins A, D, E, and K and administration of bile salts to facilitate digestion and vitamin absorption. The patient may receive opioids to relieve pain during an acute attack, antispasmodics and anticholinergics to relax smooth muscles and decrease ductal tone and spasm, and antiemetics to reduce nausea and vomiting.

A nasogastric tube connected to intermittent low-pressure suction may relieve vomiting. Cholestyramine (Questran) may be given if the patient has obstructive jaundice with severe itching from accumulation of bile salts in the skin. Aromatherapy, usually using a few drops of rosemary oil in a warm bath, may help improve gallbladder function.

CIRRHOSIS

Cirrhosis, a chronic liver disease, is characterized by widespread destruction of hepatic cells, which are replaced by fibrous cells. This process is called *fibrotic regeneration*. Cirrhosis is a common cause of death in the United States and, among people ages 35 to 55, the fourth leading cause of death. It can occur at any age.

Pathophysiology

There are many types of cirrhosis, each with a different cause. The most common include the following.

- Laënnec's cirrhosis, also called *portal, nutritional,* or *alcoholic cirrhosis,* stems from chronic alcoholism and malnutrition. It's most prevalent among malnourished alcoholic men and accounts for more than half of all cirrhosis cases in the United States. Many alcoholics never develop the disease; others develop it even with adequate nutrition.
- Postnecrotic cirrhosis is usually a complication of viral hepatitis (inflammation of the liver), but it may occur after exposure to liver toxins, such as arsenic, carbon tetrachloride, or phosphorus. This form is more common in women and is the most common type of cirrhosis worldwide.
- Biliary cirrhosis results from prolonged bile duct obstruction or inflammation.
- Cardiac cirrhosis is caused by prolonged venous congestion in the liver from right-sided heart failure.
- Idiopathic cirrhosis may develop with no known cause.

Cirrhosis is characterized by irreversible chronic injury of the liver, extensive fibrosis, and nodular tissue growth. These changes result from liver cell death (hepatocyte necrosis), collapse of the liver's supporting structure (the reticulin network), distortion of the vascular bed (blood vessels throughout the liver), and nodular regeneration of remaining liver tissue.

RED FLAG When the liver begins to malfunction, blood clotting disorders (coagulopathies), jaundice, edema, and various metabolic problems develop. Fibrosis and the distortion of blood vessels may impede blood flow in the capillary branches of the portal vein and hepatic artery, leading to portal hypertension (elevated pressure in the portal vein). Increased pressure may lead to the development of esophageal varices — enlarged, tortuous veins in the lower part of the esophagus, the area where it meets the stomach. Esophageal varices may easily rupture and leak large amounts of blood into the upper GI tract.

Signs and symptoms

Early signs and symptoms of cirrhosis are vague but usually include loss of appetite, indigestion, nausea, vomiting, constipation, diarrhea, dull abdominal ache, and jaundice. The patient may report bruising easily.

Late-stage signs and symptoms affect several body systems and include:

- respiratory effects — fluid in the lungs and weak chest expansion, leading to hypoxia

- central nervous system effects — lethargy, mental changes, slurred speech, asterixis (a motor disturbance marked by intermittent lapses in posture), and peripheral nerve damage
- hematologic effects — nosebleeds, easy bruising, bleeding gums, and anemia
- endocrine effects — testicular atrophy, menstrual irregularities, gynecomastia, and loss of chest and axillary hair
- skin effects — severe itching and dryness, poor tissue turgor, abnormal pigmentation, and spider veins
- hepatic effects — jaundice, enlarged liver (hepatomegaly), fluid in the abdomen (ascites), and edema
- renal effects — insufficiency that may progress to failure
- miscellaneous effects — musty breath, enlarged superficial abdominal veins, muscle atrophy, pain in the upper right abdominal quadrant that worsens when the patient sits up or leans forward, palpable liver or spleen, temperature of 101° to 103° F (38.3° to 39.4° C), and bleeding from esophageal varices.

Test results
These tests help confirm cirrhosis.
- Liver biopsy, the definitive test, reveals tissue destruction (necrosis) and fibrosis.
- Abdominal X-ray shows liver size, cysts or gas in the biliary tract or liver, liver calcification, and massive fluid accumulation (ascites).
- Computed tomography (CT) and liver scans show liver size, abnormal masses, and hepatic blood flow and obstruction.
- Esophagogastroduodenoscopy reveals bleeding esophageal varices, stomach irritation or ulceration, or duodenal bleeding and irritation.
- Blood studies show elevated liver enzyme, total serum bilirubin, and indirect bilirubin levels. Total serum albumin and protein levels decrease; prothrombin time (PT) is prolonged; hemoglobin and serum electrolyte levels and hematocrit decrease; and vitamins A, C, and K are deficient.
- Urine studies show increased bilirubin and urobilinogen levels.
- Fecal studies show decreased fecal urobilinogen levels.

Treatment
Therapy for cirrhosis aims to remove or alleviate the underlying cause, prevent further liver damage, and prevent or treat complications. (See *Cirrhosis teaching topics,* page 332.)

Cirrhosis teaching topics

- Explain the disease process and its treatments to the patient and family.
- Discuss measures to reduce the risk of bleeding, such as warning the patient against taking nonsteroidal anti-inflammatory drugs, straining while defecating, and blowing his nose or sneezing too vigorously. Suggest using an electric razor and a soft toothbrush.
- Tell the patient that rest and good nutrition will conserve energy and decrease metabolic demands on the liver.
- Urge the patient to eat small, frequent, high-calorie meals.
- Stress the need to avoid infections and abstain from alcohol. If needed, refer the patient to Alcoholics Anonymous.
- Explain the need to avoid sedatives and acetaminophen (Tylenol).

DRUG THERAPY

Drug therapy requires special caution because a cirrhotic liver can't detoxify harmful substances efficiently. The patient may receive vitamins and nutritional supplements to help heal damaged liver cells and improve nutritional status. Treatment also may include antacids to reduce gastric distress and decrease the risk of GI bleeding; potassium-sparing diuretics, such as furosemide (Lasix), to reduce fluid accumulation; and vasopressin (Pitressin) for esophageal varices.

NONINVASIVE PROCEDURES

To control bleeding from esophageal varices or other GI hemorrhage, two measures are attempted first. In gastric intubation, the stomach is lavaged until the contents are clear. Antacids and histamine antagonists are then administered if the bleeding is caused by a gastric ulcer. In esophageal balloon tamponade, bleeding vessels are compressed to stop blood loss from esophageal varices.

SURGERY

In patients with ascites, paracentesis may be used to relieve abdominal pressure. A shunt may be inserted to divert ascites into venous circulation. This treatment causes weight loss, decreased abdominal girth, increased renal sodium excretion, and improved urine output.

SCLEROTHERAPY

If conservative treatment fails to stop hemorrhaging, a sclerosing agent is injected into the oozing vessels to cause clotting and sclerosis. If bleeding from the varices doesn't stop in 2 to 5 minutes, a second injection is given below the bleeding site. Sclerotherapy may also be performed on nonbleeding varices to prevent hemorrhaging.

RADIOLOGIC INTERVENTION

A radiologic procedure known as *transjugular intrahepatic portosystemic shunt* may be performed. During this procedure, a shunt is placed between the portal vein and the hepatic vein. The procedure reduces pressure in the varices, preventing them from bleeding.

LAST RESORT

As a last resort, portosystemic shunts may be inserted during surgery to control bleeding from esophageal varices and decrease portal hypertension. These shunts divert some portal vein blood flow away from the liver. This procedure is seldom performed because it can cause bleeding, infection, and shunt thrombosis. Massive hemorrhage requires blood transfusions to maintain blood pressure.

CROHN'S DISEASE

Crohn's disease is an inflammatory bowel disease that may affect any part of the GI tract. Inflammation extends through all layers of the intestinal wall and may involve lymph nodes and supporting membranes in the area. Ulcers form as the inflammation extends into the peritoneum.

Crohn's disease is most common in adults ages 20 to 40. It affects men and women equally and tends to run in families — up to 20% of patients have a positive family history.

When Crohn's disease affects only the small bowel, it's known as *regional enteritis.* When it includes the colon or affects only the colon, it's known as *Crohn's disease of the colon.* Crohn's disease of the colon is sometimes called *granulomatous colitis;* however, not all patients develop granulomas (tumorlike masses of granulation tissue).

Pathophysiology

Although researchers are still studying Crohn's disease, possible causes include lymphatic obstruction, infection, allergies, genetic factors (see *Nod$_2$ mutation,* page 334), and immune disorders, such as altered immunoglobulin A production and increased suppressor T-cell activity.

In Crohn's disease, inflammation spreads slowly and progressively. Lymph nodes enlarge, and lymph flow in the submucosa is blocked. Lymphatic obstruction causes edema, mucosal ulceration, fissures, abscesses, and sometimes granulomas. Mucosal ulcerations are called *skipping lesions* because they aren't continuous, as in ulcerative colitis.

Oval, elevated patches of closely packed lymph follicles — called *Peyer's patches* — develop on the lining of the small intestine. Fibrosis occurs, thickening the bowel wall and causing stenosis, or narrowing of the lumen. Stenosis can occur in any part of the intestine and cause varying degrees of intestinal obstruction. At first, the mucosa may appear normal but, as the disease progresses, it takes on a cobblestone appearance.

Inflammation of the serous membrane (serositis) develops, inflamed bowel loops adhere to other diseased or normal loops, and diseased bowel segments become interspersed with healthy ones. Eventually, diseased parts of the bowel become thicker, narrower, and shorter.

RED FLAG Severe diarrhea and corrosion of the perineal area by enzymes can cause anal fistula, the most common complication. Perineal abscess also may develop during the active inflammatory state. Fistulas may develop to the bladder, vagina, or even skin in an old scar area. Other complications include intestinal obstruction, nutrient deficiencies from malabsorption of bile salts and vitamin B_{12} and by poor digestion, fluid imbalances and, rarely, inflammation of abdominal linings (peritonitis).

Signs and symptoms

Initially, the patient has malaise and diarrhea, usually with pain in the right lower quadrant or generalized abdominal pain and fever. Chronic diarrhea results from bile salt malabsorption, loss of healthy intestinal surface area, and bacterial growth. Weight loss, nausea, and vomiting also occur. Stools may be bloody.

TEACHING FOCUS

Crohn's disease teaching topics

- Teach the patient and his family about the disease process, including its symptoms, complications, and treatments.
- Explain the importance of adequate rest.
- Stress the need for a severely restricted diet.
- Help the patient identify sources of stress and stress-reducing practices.
- Teach about prescribed drugs, including their names, dosages, frequencies, adverse effects, and special considerations.
- Discuss complications that require immediate medical attention.
- If the patient is having surgery, explain surgical procedures and refer him to an enterostomal therapist.
- Explain postileostomy self-care and lifestyle modifications.
- Refer the patient to a support group such as the Crohn's and Colitis Foundation of America.

Test results

These tests and results support a diagnosis of Crohn's disease.

- Fecal occult test shows minute amounts of blood in stools.
- Small-bowel X-ray shows irregular mucosa, ulceration, and stiffening.
- Barium enema reveals the string sign (segments of stricture separated by normal bowel) and may also show fissures and narrowing of the bowel.
- Sigmoidoscopy and colonoscopy show patchy areas of inflammation, which helps rule out ulcerative colitis. The mucosal surface has a cobblestone appearance. When the colon is involved, ulcers may appear.
- Biopsy performed during sigmoidoscopy or colonoscopy reveals granulomas in up to one-half of all specimens.
- Laboratory tests indicate increased WBC count and erythrocyte sedimentation rate (ESR). Other findings include decreased potassium, calcium, magnesium, and hemoglobin levels in the blood.

Treatment

Treatment for Crohn's disease requires drug therapy, lifestyle changes and, sometimes, surgery. During acute attacks, maintaining fluid and electrolyte balance is the key. Debilitated patients need total parenteral nutrition to provide adequate calories and nutrition while resting the bowel. (See *Crohn's disease teaching topics*.)

DRUG THERAPY

Drug therapy aims to combat inflammation and relieve symptoms. Corticosteroids, such as prednisone, reduce diarrhea, pain, and bleeding by decreasing inflammation. Immunosuppressants, such as azathioprine (Imuran), methotrexate (Trexall), and mercaptopurine (Purinethol), suppress the body's response to antigens. Aminosalicylates, such as sulfasalazine (Azulfidine) and mesalamine (Pentasa), reduce inflammation. Metronidazole (Flagyl) treats perianal complications. Antidiarrheals, such as diphenoxylate and atropine (Lomotil), combat diarrhea but aren't used in patients with significant bowel obstruction. Opioids control pain and diarrhea. The antitumor necrosis factor agent infliximab (Remicade) treats moderate to severe disease that doesn't respond to conventional therapy.

LIFESTYLE CHANGES

Stress reduction and reduced physical activity rest the bowel and allow it to heal. Vitamin supplements compensate for the bowel's inability to absorb vitamins. Dietary changes decrease bowel activity while still providing adequate nutrition. The foods usually eliminated include high-fiber foods, such as fruits and vegetables; foods and liquids that irritate the mucosa, such as dairy products and spicy and fatty foods; and foods or liquids that stimulate excessive intestinal activity, such as carbonated or caffeinated beverages.

SURGERY

Surgery is needed if bowel perforation, massive hemorrhage, fistulas, or acute intestinal obstruction develop. Colectomy with ileostomy is commonly performed in patients with extensive disease of the large intestine and rectum.

DIVERTICULAR DISEASE

Diverticular disease is a common problem that affects men and women equally. The risk increases with age. Diverticular disease occurs throughout the world but is more common in developed countries, where its occurrence has increased. This suggests that environmental and lifestyle factors may play a role in its development.

One contributing factor may be low intake of dietary fiber. High-fiber diets increase stool bulk, thereby decreasing the wall tension in the colon. High wall tension is thought to increase the risk of developing diverticula.

In diverticular disease, bulging pouches (diverticula) in the GI wall push the mucosal lining through the surrounding muscle. Although the most common site of diverticula is in the sigmoid colon, they may develop anywhere, from the proximal end of the pharynx to the anus. Other typical sites include the duodenum, near the pancreatic border or the ampulla of Vater, and the jejunum.

Diverticular disease has two clinical forms: diverticulosis, in which diverticula are present but don't cause symptoms; and diverticulitis, in which diverticula are inflamed and may cause potentially fatal obstruction, infection, or hemorrhage.

Pathophysiology

Diverticula probably result from high intraluminal pressure on an area of weakness in the GI wall where blood vessels enter. Diet may be a contributing factor because insufficient fiber reduces fecal residue, narrows the bowel lumen, and increases intra-abdominal pressure during defecation.

RED FLAG In diverticulitis, retained undigested food and bacteria accumulate in the diverticular sac. This hard mass cuts off the blood supply to the thin walls of the sac, making them more susceptible to attack by colonic bacteria. Inflammation follows and may lead to perforation, abscess, peritonitis, obstruction, or hemor-rhage. Occasionally, the inflamed colon segment may adhere to the bladder or other organs and cause a fistula.

Signs and symptoms

Typically, a patient with diverticulosis is asymptomatic and will remain so unless diverticulitis develops.

Mild diverticulitis

In mild diverticulitis, signs and symptoms include moderate left lower quadrant pain from inflamed diverticula and a low-grade fever and leukocytosis from trapping of bacteria-rich stool in the diverticula.

Severe diverticulitis

In severe diverticulitis, signs and symptoms include:
- abdominal rigidity from diverticula rupture, abscesses, and peritonitis
- left lower quadrant pain secondary to rupture of the diverticula and subsequent inflammation and infection
- high fever, chills, hypotension from sepsis, and shock from the release of fecal material from the rupture site
- microscopic or massive hemorrhage from rupture of diverticulum near a vessel.

TEACHING FOCUS

Diverticular disease teaching topics

- Teach the patient and family about the disease process, including its symptoms, complications, and treatments.
- Reinforce the importance of dietary fiber and the harmful effects of constipation and straining during defecation.
- Encourage increased intake of foods high in indigestible fiber, including fresh fruits and vegetables, whole-grain bread, and wheat or bran cereals.
- Warn that a high-fiber diet may temporarily cause flatulence and discomfort.

- Advise the patient to relieve constipation with stool softeners or bulk-forming cathartics.
- Teach about prescribed drugs, including their names, indications, dosages, adverse effects, and special considerations.
- Discuss warning signs of complications, such as obstruction, infection, and hemorrhage, and the need to seek immediate medical attention if they occur.
- If the patient is having surgery, explain what to expect before and after it, and refer him to an enterostomal therapist.

CHRONIC DIVERTICULITIS

In chronic diverticulitis, signs and symptoms include constipation, ribbonlike stools, intermittent diarrhea, and abdominal distention from intestinal obstruction (possible when fibrosis and adhesions narrow the bowel's lumen). The patient also may have abdominal rigidity and pain, diminishing or absent bowel sounds, nausea, and vomiting from intestinal obstruction.

Test results

These tests help to diagnose and confirm diverticular disease.
- Upper GI series confirms or rules out diverticulosis of the esophagus and upper bowel.
- Barium enema reveals filling of diverticula, confirming diagnosis.
- Biopsy reveals evidence of benign disease, ruling out cancer.
- Blood studies show an elevated ESR in diverticulitis.

Treatment

Treatment for diverticular disease may include:
- liquid or bland diet, stool softeners, and occasional doses of mineral oil to relieve symptoms, minimize irritation, and lessen the risk of progression to diverticulitis
- high-residue diet for diverticulosis after pain has subsided, to help decrease intra-abdominal pressure during defecation

- exercise to increase the rate of stool passage
- antibiotics to treat infection of the diverticula
- analgesics, such as morphine, to control pain and relax smooth muscle
- antispasmodics to control muscle spasms
- colon resection with removal of involved segment to correct cases refractory to medical treatment
- temporary colostomy, if needed, to drain abscesses and rest the colon in diverticulitis with perforation, peritonitis, obstruction, or fistula
- blood transfusions, if needed, for blood loss from hemorrhage
- fluid replacement as needed. (See *Diverticular disease teaching topics.*)

GASTROESOPHAGEAL REFLUX DISEASE

Popularly known as *heartburn,* gastroesophageal reflux disease (GERD) involves the backflow of gastric or duodenal contents or both into the esophagus and past the lower esophageal sphincter (LES) without belching or vomiting. The reflux of gastric contents causes acute epigastric pain, usually after a meal. The pain may radiate to the chest or arms.

Up to 36% of otherwise healthy Americans have heartburn at least once monthly, and about 7% have heartburn at least once daily. About 2% of adults have GERD. It's much more common after age 40, and it's common in pregnant or obese people.

Pathophysiology

Various factors can lead to GERD, including:

- a weakened esophageal sphincter
- increased abdominal pressure, as with obesity or pregnancy
- hiatal hernia
- drugs, such as morphine, diazepam (Valium), calcium channel blockers, meperidine (Demerol), and anticholinergics
- alcohol ingestion or cigarette smoking, which lower LES pressure
- eating foods that lower LES pressure, such as high-fat meals
- nasogastric intubation for more than 4 days.

Normally, the LES maintains enough pressure around the lower end of the esophagus to close it and prevent reflux. It relaxes after each swallow to let food into the stomach. In GERD, the sphincter doesn't remain closed (usually because of deficient LES pressure or stomach pressure that exceeds LES pressure), and pressure in the stomach pushes its contents into the esophagus. The acidity of stomach contents causes pain and irritation in the esophagus.

RED FLAG *Reflux esophagitis, the main complication of GERD, can lead to other problems, including esophageal stricture, esophageal ulcer, and replacement of normal squamous epithelium with columnar epithelium (Barrett's epithelium). A patient with severe reflux esophagitis also may develop anemia from chronic low-grade bleeding of inflamed mucosa.*

Pulmonary complications may develop if the patient has reflux of gastric contents into the throat and subsequent aspiration. Reflux aspiration can lead to chronic pulmonary disease.

Signs and symptoms

A patient with GERD typically complains of a burning pain in the epigastric area; it's caused by reflux of gastric contents into the esophagus, which causes irritation and esophageal spasm. The pain may radiate to the arms and chest. Pain usually occurs after meals or when the patient lies down, when increased abdominal pressure more easily leads to reflux.

The patient also may complain of a feeling of fluid accumulating in the throat. The fluid doesn't have a sour or bitter taste because of the hypersecretion of saliva.

Test results

Diagnostic tests are aimed at determining the underlying cause of GERD.

- Esophageal acidity test evaluates the competence of the LES and provides an objective measure of reflux.
- Acid perfusion test confirms esophagitis and distinguishes it from cardiac disorders.
- Esophagoscopy allows visual examination of the lining of the esophagus to reveal the extent of the disease and confirm pathologic changes in mucosa.
- Barium swallow identifies hiatal hernia as the cause.
- Upper GI series detects hiatal hernia or motility problems.
- Esophageal manometry evaluates the resting pressure of LES and determines sphincter competence.

Treatment

Treatment of GERD is multifaceted and may include:

- diet therapy with frequent, small meals and avoidance of eating before bedtime to reduce abdominal pressure and reflux
- positioning—sitting up during and after meals and sleeping with the head of the bed elevated—to reduce abdominal pressure and prevent reflux

TEACHING FOCUS

Gastroesophageal reflux disease teaching topics

- Teach the patient and family about the disease process, including its symptoms, complications, and treatments.
- Explain what causes reflux, how to follow an antireflux regimen (drug, diet, and positional therapy), and what symptoms to watch for and report.
- Tell the patient that he shouldn't eat for 2 hours before going to bed.
- Urge the patient to sit upright, particularly after meals, and to eat small, frequent meals. Advise raising the head of the bed 6″ to 8″ (15 to 20 cm).
- Instruct the patient to avoid circumstances that increase intra-abdominal pressure (such as bending, coughing, vigorous exercise, tight clothing, constipation, and obesity)

as well as substances that reduce sphincter control (cigarettes, alcohol, fatty foods, and caffeine).
- Tell the patient to avoid highly seasoned food, acidic juices, alcoholic drinks, bedtime snacks, and foods high in fat or carbohydrates, which reduce pressure in the lower esophageal sphincter.
- Teach about prescribed drugs, including their names, dosages, frequencies, adverse effects, and special considerations.
- Discuss warning signs of complications that require immediate medical attention, such as coughing, choking, and difficulty breathing and swallowing.
- Tell the patient to take antacids as ordered (usually 1 hour before or 3 hours after meals and at bedtime).

- increased fluid intake to wash gastric contents from the esophagus
- antacids to neutralize acidic content of the stomach and minimize irritation
- histamine$_2$ receptor antagonists to inhibit gastric acid secretion
- proton pump inhibitors to reduce gastric acidity
- cholinergic agents to increase LES pressure
- smoking cessation to increase LES pressure
- surgery if hiatal hernia is the cause or if the patient has refractory symptoms. (See *Gastroesophageal reflux disease teaching topics*.)

HIATAL HERNIA

Hiatal hernia occurs when a defect in the diaphragm permits a portion of the stomach to pass through the diaphragmatic opening (the esophageal hiatus) into the chest cavity. Some people remain asymptomatic, whereas others experience reflux, heartburn, and chest pain. Hiatal hernia is more common in women than in men.

Pathophysiology

Usually, hiatal hernia results from muscle weakening that's common with aging. It also may be secondary to esophageal cancer, kyphoscoliosis, trauma, and certain surgical procedures. It also may result from diaphragmatic malformations that cause congenital weakness.

In hiatal hernia, the muscular collar around the esophageal and diaphragmatic junction loosens, and the lower portion of the esophagus and the stomach rise into the chest when intra-abdominal pressure increases (possibly causing esophageal reflux). Such increased intra-abdominal pressure may result from ascites, pregnancy, obesity, constrictive clothing, bending, straining, coughing, Valsalva's maneuver, or extreme physical exertion.

Two types of hiatal hernia include sliding and paraesophageal. (See *Two types of hiatal hernia.*) A third may include features of both.

RED FLAG If the hiatal hernia is related to GERD, the esophageal mucosa may become irritated, leading to esophagitis, esophageal ulceration, hemorrhage, peritonitis, and mediastinitis. Aspiration of refluxed fluids may lead to respiratory distress, aspiration pneumonia, or cardiac dysfunction from pressure on the heart and lungs. Other complications include esophageal stricture and incarceration, in which a large portion of the stomach is caught above the diaphragm. Incarceration may lead to perforation, gastric ulcer, strangulation, and gangrene of the herniated stomach portion.

Signs and symptoms

Typically, a paraesophageal hernia produces no symptoms; it's usually an incidental finding on barium swallow.

A sliding hernia without an incompetent sphincter produces no reflux or symptoms and, consequently, doesn't need treatment. When a sliding hernia does cause symptoms, they're typical of gastric reflux and may include:

■ heartburn (pyrosis) occurring 1 to 4 hours after eating, aggravated by reclining and belching and possibly accompanied by regurgitation or vomiting

■ retrosternal or substernal chest pain occurring usually after meals or at bedtime, aggravated by reclining, belching, and increased intra-abdominal pressure.

Other signs or symptoms that reflect possible complications include dysphagia (trouble swallowing), bleeding from esophagitis, and severe pain and shock if the hernia becomes strangulated.

Test results

A diagnosis of hiatal hernia is based on typical clinical findings as well as the results of these laboratory studies and procedures.

Two types of hiatal hernia

These illustrations show structural differences between a normal stomach and defects caused by a sliding hiatal hernia and a paraesophageal or rolling hernia.

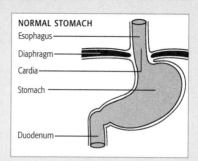

NORMAL STOMACH
Esophagus
Diaphragm
Cardia
Stomach
Duodenum

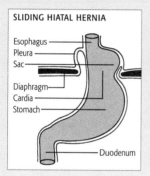

SLIDING HIATAL HERNIA
Esophagus
Pleura
Sac
Diaphragm
Cardia
Stomach
Duodenum

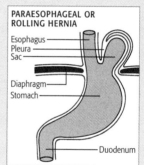

PARAESOPHAGEAL OR ROLLING HERNIA
Esophagus
Pleura
Sac
Diaphragm
Stomach
Duodenum

- Chest X-rays occasionally show an air shadow behind the heart (with a large hernia) and infiltrates in the lower lobes, if the patient has aspirated.
- In a barium study, the hernia may appear as an outpouching that contains barium at the lower end of the esophagus. (Small hernias are difficult to recognize.) This study also may reveal abnormalities in the diaphragm.
- Endoscopy and biopsy differentiate between hiatal hernia, varices, and other small gastroesophageal lesions.
- Esophageal motility studies assess the presence of esophageal motor abnormalities before surgical repair of the hernia.
- pH studies assess for reflux of gastric contents.

Hiatal hernia teaching topics

- Explain the disease process and its treatments to the patient and family.
- Teach about drugs the patient will be taking, including their dosages, adverse effects, and special considerations.
- Instruct the patient about signs and symptoms of complications to watch for and report.

■ An acid perfusion test indicates that heartburn results from esophageal reflux.

Treatment

The main goal of treatment for hiatal hernia is to relieve symptoms and to prevent or manage complications. (See *Hiatal hernia teaching topics*.)

DRUG THERAPY

Anticholinergics, such as bethanechol (Urecholine), are given to strengthen cardiac sphincter tone. Metoclopramide (Reglan) may be used to stimulate smooth-muscle contractions and decrease reflux. Antiemetics may be given for vomiting. Antitussives and antidiarrheals may be given, if appropriate. Antacids are prescribed to decrease the acidity of gastric contents.

NONINVASIVE INTERVENTIONS

Activity that increases intra-abdominal pressure (coughing, straining, bending) should be restricted. Tell the patient to eat small, frequent, bland meals at least 2 hours before lying down. Also tell him to eat slowly and to avoid spicy foods, fruit juices, alcoholic beverages, and coffee.

To reduce reflux, encourage an overweight patient to lose weight to help decrease intra-abdominal pressure. Raising the head of the bed about 6″ (15 cm) reduces gastric reflux by gravity.

SURGERY

If symptoms can't be controlled medically or if complications — such as bleeding, stricture, pulmonary aspiration, strangulation, or incarceration (constriction) — occur, surgical repair is needed. The procedure involves creating an artificial closing mechanism at the gastroesophageal junction to strengthen the esophageal hiatus. A transabdominal fundoplication is performed by wrapping the fundus of the stomach around the lower esophagus to prevent reflux of stomach contents. Although an abdominal or thoracic approach may be used, hiatal hernia is typically repaired by laparoscopy.

IRRITABLE BOWEL SYNDROME

Irritable bowel syndrome (IBS) is characterized by chronic abdominal pain, alternating constipation and diarrhea, and abdominal distention. This disorder is common, although about 20% of patients never seek medical care. It is twice as common in women as in men.

IBS is a functional GI disorder of unknown cause. It may be influenced by psychological stress, diverticular disease, ingestion of irritants (such as coffee, raw vegetables, or fruits), abuse of laxatives, food poisoning, or colon cancer.

Pathophysiology

Typically, a patient with IBS has a normal-appearing GI tract. However, careful examination of the colon may reveal functional irritability—an abnormality in colonic smooth-muscle function marked by excessive peristalsis and spasms, even during remission.

To understand what happens in IBS, consider how smooth muscle controls bowel function. Normally, segmental muscle contractions mix intestinal contents and peristalsis propels the contents through the GI tract. Motor activity is most propulsive in the proximal (stomach) and the distal (sigmoid) portions of the intestine. Activity in the rest of the intestines is slower, permitting nutrient and water absorption.

In IBS, the autonomic nervous system, which innervates the large intestine, doesn't cause the alternating contractions and relaxations that propel stools smoothly toward the rectum. The result is constipation, diarrhea, or both.

Some people have spasmodic intestinal contractions that cause partial obstruction by trapping gas and stools. This causes distention, bloating, gas pain, and constipation. Others have dramatically increased intestinal motility. With eating or cholinergic stimulation, the small intestine's contents rush into the large intestine, dumping watery stools and irritating the mucosa. The result is diarrhea.

If further spasms trap liquid stools, the intestinal mucosa adsorbs water from the stools, leaving them dry, hard, and difficult to pass. The result is a pattern of alternating diarrhea and constipation.

RED FLAG *Complications of IBS may include chronic inflammatory bowel disease, colon cancer, diverticular disease, and malnutrition.*

Signs and symptoms

The most commonly reported symptom is intermittent, crampy, lower abdominal pain, usually relieved by defecation or passage of flatus. It usually occurs during the day and intensifies with stress or 1 to 2 hours after meals. The patient may experience constipation alternating with diarrhea, with one being the dominant problem. Mucus is usually passed through the rectum. Abdominal distention and bloating are common.

Test results

No tests are specific for diagnosing IBS. Other disorders, such as diverticulitis, colon cancer, and lactose intolerance, should be ruled out by these tests.

■ Stool samples for ova, parasites, bacteria, and blood rule out infection.
■ Lactose intolerance test rules out lactose intolerance.
■ Barium enema may reveal colon spasm and tubular appearance of descending colon without evidence of cancer or diverticulosis.
■ Sigmoidoscopy or colonoscopy may reveal spastic contractions without evidence of colon cancer or inflammatory bowel disease.
■ Rectal biopsy rules out malignancy.

Treatment

Treatment for IBS aims to relieve symptoms. (See *Irritable bowel syndrome teaching topics.*)

MEDICAL THERAPY

Therapy aims to relieve symptoms and includes counseling to help the patient understand the relationship between stress and his illness. Dietary restrictions haven't proven effective, but the patient is encouraged to be aware of foods that worsen symptoms. Rest and heat applied to the abdomen are usually helpful. In the case of laxative overuse, bowel training is sometimes recommended.

DRUG THERAPY

Antispasmodics, such as propantheline (Pro-Banthine) or diphenoxylate with atropine (Lomotil), are commonly prescribed. A mild barbiturate, such as phenobarbital (Luminal), in judicious doses is sometimes helpful.

The 5-HT$_4$ receptor partial agonist tegaserod (Zelnorm) may be prescribed for short-term treatment of women with IBS whose primary symptom is constipation. It also relieves abdominal discomfort and bloating. The 5-HT$_3$ receptor antagonist alosetron (Lotronex) is a selective antagonist used for short-term treatment of women with

TEACHING FOCUS

Irritable bowel syndrome teaching topics

● Explain the disease process, its treatments, and possible complications to the patient and family.
● Teach about drugs the patient will be taking, including their indications, dosages, adverse effects, and special considerations.
● Tell the patient to avoid irritating foods and to drink 8 to 10 glasses of water each day.
● Encourage the patient to develop regular bowel habits.

● Help the patient deal with stress. Warn against dependence on sedatives or antispasmodics.
● Encourage regular checkups because the risk of diverticulitis and colon cancer may be higher than normal. For patients older than age 40, emphasize the need for an annual sigmoidoscopy and rectal examination.

IBS who have severe diarrhea. It's available through a restricted marketing program because of serious GI adverse effects; only practitioners enrolled in the program can prescribe it.

PANCREATITIS

Pancreatitis is an inflammation of the pancreas. It occurs in acute and chronic forms. In men, the disorder is commonly linked to alcoholism, trauma, or peptic ulcer; in women, to biliary tract disease.

The prognosis is good when pancreatitis follows biliary tract disease but poor when related to alcoholism. Mortality reaches 60% when pancreatitis causes tissue destruction or hemorrhage.

Pathophysiology

Besides biliary tract disease and alcoholism, pancreatitis may result from:

■ abnormal organ structure
■ blunt trauma or surgical trauma
■ drugs, such as glucocorticoids, sulfonamides, thiazides, and hormonal contraceptives
■ endoscopic examination of the bile ducts and pancreas
■ kidney failure or transplantation
■ metabolic or endocrine disorders, such as high cholesterol levels or overactive thyroid
■ pancreatic cysts or tumors
■ penetrating peptic ulcers.

In addition, heredity may predispose a patient to pancreatitis. In some patients, emotional or neurogenic factors play a part.

Chronic pancreatitis is a persistent inflammation that produces irreversible changes in pancreatic structure and function. It sometimes follows an episode of acute pancreatitis. It probably happens when protein precipitates block the pancreatic duct and eventually harden or calcify. Structural changes lead to fibrosis and atrophy of the glands. Growths called *pseudocysts,* containing pancreatic enzymes and tissue debris, form. Abscess results if these growths become infected.

Acute pancreatitis occurs in two forms: edematous (interstitial), which causes fluid accumulation and swelling; and necrotizing, which causes cell death and tissue damage. The inflammation that occurs with both types is caused by premature activation of enzymes, which causes tissue damage. Normally, the acini in the pancreas secrete enzymes in an inactive form.

Two theories explain why enzymes become prematurely activated. In the first, a toxic agent such as alcohol alters the way the pancreas secretes enzymes. Alcohol probably increases pancreatic secretion, alters the metabolism of the acinar cells, and encourages duct obstruction by causing pancreatic secretory proteins to precipitate. In the second, a reflux of duodenal contents containing activated enzymes enters the pancreatic duct, activating other enzymes and setting up a cycle of more pancreatic damage.

Pain can be caused by several factors, including escape of inflammatory exudate and enzymes into the back of the peritoneum, edema and distention of the pancreatic capsule, and obstruction of the biliary tract.

RED FLAG If pancreatitis damages the islets of Langerhans, *diabetes mellitus may result. Sudden, severe pancreatitis causes massive hemorrhage and total destruction of the pancreas. This may lead to diabetic acidosis, shock, or coma.*

Signs and symptoms

In many patients, the only symptom of mild pancreatitis is steady epigastric pain centered close to the navel, unrelieved by vomiting.

Acute pancreatitis causes severe, persistent, piercing abdominal pain, usually in the midepigastric region, although it may be generalized or occur in the left upper quadrant radiating to the back. The pain usually begins suddenly after eating a large meal or drinking alcohol. It increases when the patient lies on his back and is relieved when he rests on his knees and upper chest.

Test results

These tests are used to diagnose pancreatitis.

▪ Dramatically elevated serum amylase and lipase levels confirm acute pancreatitis. Dramatically elevated amylase levels are also found in urine, ascites, and pleural fluid.
▪ Blood and urine glucose tests may reveal transient glycosuria and hyperglycemia. In chronic pancreatitis, serum glucose levels may be transiently elevated.
▪ WBC count is elevated.
▪ Serum bilirubin levels are elevated in both acute and chronic pancreatitis.
▪ Blood calcium levels may be decreased.
▪ Stool analysis shows elevated lipid and trypsin levels in chronic pancreatitis.
▪ Abdominal and chest X-rays detect pleural effusions and differentiate pancreatitis from diseases that cause similar symptoms.
▪ CT scan and ultrasonography show an enlarged pancreas and pancreatic cysts and pseudocysts.
▪ Endoscopic retrograde cholangiopancreatography shows the anatomy of the pancreas; identifies ductal system abnormalities, such as calcification or strictures; and differentiates pancreatitis from other disorders such as pancreatic cancer.

Treatment

The goals of treatment for pancreatitis are to maintain circulation and fluid volume, relieve pain, and decrease pancreatic secretions. (See *Pancreatitis teaching topics,* page 350.)

ACUTE PANCREATITIS

Shock is the most common cause of death in the early stages of acute pancreatitis, so I.V. replacement of electrolytes and proteins is needed. Metabolic acidosis requires fluid volume replacement. Blood transfusions may be needed. Food and fluids are withheld to let the pancreas rest and to reduce pancreatic enzyme secretion. Nasogastric tube suctioning decreases stomach distention and suppresses pancreatic secretions. Positioning the patient for comfort in the knee-to-chest position has been helpful in reducing pain.

Drugs given for acute pancreatitis include:

▪ opioids, such as morphine or hydromorphone (Dilaudid), to relieve abdominal pain (morphine was previously thought to cause pancreatic complications; now it's the analgesic of choice for pancreatitis)
▪ antacids to neutralize gastric secretions

TEACHING FOCUS

Pancreatitis teaching topics

- Teach the patient and family about the disorder, including its causes, symptoms, and treatments.
- Discuss warning signs and symptoms of complications, such as diabetes and variceal bleeding, that require immediate medical attention.
- If the patient is having surgery, explain the surgical procedures and what to expect before and after it.
- Teach about prescribed drugs, including their names, indications,

dosages, adverse effects, and special considerations.
- Explain dietary changes and the need to take pancreatic enzymes.
- Discuss the importance of avoiding alcoholic beverages and joining a support group such as Alcoholics Anonymous, if needed.
- Talk about drug and nondrug measures to relieve pain.

- histamine antagonists, such as cimetidine (Tagamet), famotidine (Pepcid), or ranitidine (Zantac), to decrease hydrochloric acid production
- antibiotics, such as clindamycin (Cleocin) or gentamicin (Garamycin), to fight bacterial infections
- anticholinergics to reduce vagal stimulation, decrease GI motility, and inhibit pancreatic enzyme secretion
- insulin to correct hyperglycemia.

Surgical drainage is needed for a pancreatic abscess or pseudocyst. A laparotomy may be needed if biliary tract obstruction causes acute pancreatitis.

CHRONIC PANCREATITIS

Pain control measures are similar to those for acute pancreatitis. Morphine is the drug of choice. Some patients need only over-the-counter analgesics. Tricyclic antidepressants may be effective in low doses; they suppress the nervous system's reaction to inflammation.

Other treatment depends on the cause. Surgery relieves abdominal pain, restores pancreatic drainage, and reduces the frequency of attacks. Surgery also may help relieve obstruction. Patients with an abscess or pseudocyst, biliary tract disease, or a fibrotic pancreatic sphincter may undergo surgery.

PEPTIC ULCER

A peptic ulcer is a circumscribed lesion in the mucosal membrane of the upper GI tract. Peptic ulcers can develop in the lower esopha-

A close look at peptic ulcers

This illustration shows different degrees of peptic ulceration. Lesions that don't extend below the mucosal lining (epithelium) are called *erosions*. Lesions of acute and chronic ulcers can extend through the epithelium and may perforate the stomach wall. Chronic ulcers also have scar tissue at the base. Note that acute and chronic ulcers extend beyond the mucosal lining.

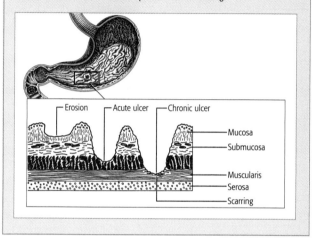

gus, stomach, duodenum, or jejunum. (See *A close look at peptic ulcers.*) More than 25 million United States residents will have an ulcer at some time in their life.

The two major forms of peptic ulcer are duodenal and gastric. Both are chronic conditions.

Duodenal ulcers affect the upper part of the small intestine. This type of ulcer accounts for about 80% of peptic ulcers, occurs mostly in men between ages 20 and 50, and follows a chronic course of remissions and exacerbations. About 5% to 10% of patients develop complications that warrant surgery.

Gastric ulcers affect the stomach lining (mucosa). They're most common in middle-aged and elderly men, especially poor and undernourished men. These ulcers commonly occur in chronic users of aspirin or alcohol.

Pathophysiology

There are three major causes of peptic ulcers: bacterial infection with *Helicobacter pylori*, the cause of 90% of peptic ulcers; use of nonsteroidal anti-inflammatory drugs; and hypersecretory states such as Zollinger-Ellison syndrome.

Researchers are still discovering the exact mechanisms of ulcer formation. Predisposing factors include blood types A (common in those with gastric ulcers) and O (common in those with duodenal ulcers), genetic factors, exposure to irritants, trauma, stress and anxiety, and normal aging.

In a peptic ulcer caused by *H. pylori*, acid adds to the effects of the bacterial infection. *H. pylori* releases a toxin that destroys the stomach's mucus coat, reducing the epithelium's resistance to acid digestion and causing gastritis and ulcer disease.

RED FLAG A possible complication of severe ulceration is erosion of the mucosa. This can cause GI hemorrhage, which can progress to hypovolemic shock, perforation, and obstruction. Obstruction of the pylorus may cause the stomach to distend with food and fluid, block blood flow, and cause tissue damage. The ulcer crater may extend beyond the duodenal wall into nearby structures, such as the pancreas or liver. This phenomenon is called penetration *and is a fairly common complication of duodenal ulcer.*

Signs and symptoms

A patient with a gastric ulcer may report recent loss of weight or appetite, pain, heartburn, indigestion, a feeling of abdominal fullness or distention, and pain triggered or aggravated by eating.

A patient with a duodenal ulcer may describe the pain as sharp, gnawing, burning, boring, aching, or hard to define. He may liken it to hunger, abdominal pressure, or fullness. Typically, pain occurs 90 minutes to 3 hours after eating. However, eating usually reduces the pain, so the patient may report a recent weight gain. The patient also may have pale skin from anemia caused by blood loss.

Test results

These tests are used to diagnose peptic ulcer.

■ Endoscopy is the major test for peptic ulcers. Upper GI endoscopy or esophagogastroduodenoscopy confirms an ulcer and allows cytologic studies and biopsy to rule out *H. pylori* or cancer.
■ Barium swallow and upper GI or small-bowel series may pinpoint the ulcer in a patient whose symptoms aren't severe.
■ Upper GI tract X-ray reveals mucosal abnormalities.
■ Stool analysis may detect occult blood in stools.

TEACHING FOCUS

Peptic ulcer teaching topics

● Teach the patient and family about the disorder, including its causes, symptoms, and treatments.
● Teach about prescribed drugs, including their names, indications, dosages, adverse effects, and special considerations.
● Educate the patient about the potential adverse effects of antibiotic therapy in treating *Helicobacter py-* *lori*, which include nausea, vomiting, and diarrhea.
● Advise the patient to avoid taking nonsteroidal anti-inflammatory drugs.
● Warn the patient to avoid stressful situations, excessive intake of coffee, and ingestion of alcoholic beverages during exacerbations of peptic ulcer disease.
● As appropriate, suggest a smoking cessation program.

■ WBC count is elevated; other blood tests may disclose signs of infection.
■ Gastric secretory studies show excess hydrochloric acid.
■ Carbon-13 urea breath test reflects *H. pylori* activity.

Treatment

Drug therapy for *H. pylori* infection consists of 1 to 2 weeks of antibiotic therapy using amoxicillin (Amoxil), tetracycline (Sumycin), metronidazole (Flagyl), or clarithromycin (Biaxin). Antibiotics should be used with ranitidine (Zantac), bismuth subsalicylate (Pepto-Bismol), or a proton pump inhibitor. According to the Centers for Disease Control and Prevention, duodenal and gastric ulcers recur in up to 80% of patients who receive drugs that reduce gastric acid but don't receive antibiotics. In those treated with antibiotics, the recurrence rate is 6%. (See *Peptic ulcer teaching topics*.)

Gastroscopy allows visualization of the bleeding site and coagulation by laser or cautery to control bleeding.

Surgery is performed if the patient doesn't respond to other treatment or has a perforation, suspected cancer, or other complications.

ULCERATIVE COLITIS

This inflammatory disease causes ulcerations of the mucosa in the colon. It commonly occurs as a chronic condition. As many as 1 in 1,000 people may have ulcerative colitis. Peak occurrence is between ages 15 and 30 and between ages 50 and 70. Ulcerative colitis is equally common among men and women.

Pathophysiology

Although the cause of ulcerative colitis is unknown, it may be related to an abnormal immune response in the GI tract, possibly related to genetic factors. Lymphocytes (T cells) in people with ulcerative colitis may have cytotoxic effects on the epithelial cells of the colon.

Stress doesn't cause the disorder, but it can increase the severity of an attack. Although no specific organism has been linked to ulcerative colitis, infection hasn't been ruled out.

Ulcerative colitis damages the large intestine's mucosal and submucosal layers. Usually, it originates in the rectum and lower colon. Then it spreads to the entire colon. The mucosa develops diffuse ulceration, with hemorrhage, congestion, edema, and exudative inflammation. Unlike in Crohn's disease, ulcerations are continuous. Abscesses formed in the mucosa drain pus, become necrotic, and ulcerate. Sloughing causes bloody, mucus-filled stools.

As ulcerative colitis progresses, the colon changes. Initially, the mucosal surface becomes dark, red, and velvety. Abscesses form and coalesce into ulcers and then into necrosis of the mucosa. As abscesses heal, scarring and thickening may appear in the bowel's inner muscle layer. As granulation tissue replaces the muscle layer, the colon narrows, shortens, and loses its characteristic pouches (haustral folds).

RED FLAG *Progression of ulcerative colitis may lead to intestinal obstruction, dehydration, and fluid and electrolyte imbalances. Malabsorption is common, and chronic anemia may result from loss of blood in the stools.*

Signs and symptoms

The hallmark of ulcerative colitis is recurrent bloody diarrhea—usually containing pus and mucus—alternating with symptom-free remissions. Accumulation of blood and mucus in the bowel causes cramping abdominal pain, rectal urgency, and diarrhea. Other symptoms include irritability, weight loss, weakness, anorexia, nausea, and vomiting.

Test results

These tests are used to diagnose ulcerative colitis.

- Sigmoidoscopy confirms rectal involvement by showing mucosal friability (vulnerability to breakdown) and flattening as well as thick, inflammatory exudate.
- Colonoscopy shows the extent of the disease, strictured areas, and pseudopolyps. It isn't performed when the patient has active signs and symptoms.
- Biopsy during colonoscopy can help confirm the diagnosis.

TEACHING FOCUS

Ulcerative colitis teaching topics

● Teach the patient and family about the disorder, including its causes, symptoms, and treatments.
● Discuss warning signs and symptoms of complications, such as intestinal obstruction and anemia, that require immediate medical attention.
● Teach about prescribed drugs, including their names, indications, dosages, adverse effects, and special considerations.
● Advise against GI stimulants, such as caffeine, alcohol, and smoking.
● If the patient will have a colostomy, teach him and his family about the procedure and proper care of a colostomy bag and the surrounding skin.
● If the patient will have a pouch ileostomy, teach him to insert the catheter and care for the stoma.
● Explain to the patient's family the importance of their positive reactions to the patient's adjustment.
● Discuss any dietary changes or restrictions.
● Tell the patient to avoid heavy lifting.
● Recommend a structured, gradually progressive exercise program to strengthen abdominal muscles.
● Reinforce the importance of yearly screening for colorectal cancer.

■ Barium enema shows the extent of the disease, detects complications, and identifies cancer. It isn't done in a patient with active signs and symptoms.
■ Stool specimen analysis reveals blood, pus, and mucus but no disease-causing organisms.
■ Other laboratory tests show decreased serum potassium, magnesium, and albumin levels; decreased WBC count; decreased hemoglobin level; and prolonged PT. Increased ESR correlates with the severity of the attack.

Treatment

The goals of treatment for ulcerative colitis are to control inflammation, replace lost nutrients and blood, and prevent complications. Supportive measures include bed rest, I.V. fluid replacement, and blood transfusions. (See *Ulcerative colitis teaching topics*.)

DRUG THERAPY

Corticosteroids, such as prednisone (Predicort) and hydrocortisone (Hydrocortone), may be prescribed for inflammation. Aminosalicylates also help control inflammation. Examples include sulfasalazine

(Azulfidine), olsalazine (Dipentum), mesalamine (Pentasa), and balsalazide (Colazal).

Antidiarrheals, such as diphenoxylate with atropine (Lomotil), may be helpful for patients with frequent, troublesome diarrhea whose ulcerative colitis is otherwise under control. Immunomodulators, such as 6-mercaptopurine (Purinethol) and azathioprine (Imuran), help reduce inflammation by acting on the immune system. And iron supplements can correct anemia.

DIET THERAPY
Patients with severe disease usually need total parenteral nutrition (TPN) and are allowed nothing by mouth. TPN is also used for patients awaiting surgery or those dehydrated or debilitated from excessive diarrhea. This treatment rests the intestinal tract, decreases stool volume, and restores nitrogen balance.

Patients with moderate signs and symptoms may receive supplemental drinks and elemental feedings. A low-residue diet may be ordered for the patient with mild disease.

SURGERY
Surgery is performed if the patient has massive dilation of the colon (toxic megacolon), if he doesn't respond to drugs and supportive measures, or if he finds the symptoms unbearable. The most common surgical technique is proctocolectomy with ileostomy, although pouch ileostomy and ileoanal reservoir are also done.

VIRAL HEPATITIS
Viral hepatitis is a common infection of the liver. In most patients, damaged liver cells eventually regenerate with little or no permanent damage. However, old age and serious underlying disorders make complications more likely. More than 70,000 cases are reported annually in the United States.

Pathophysiology
Viral hepatitis is marked by liver cell destruction, tissue death (necrosis), and self-destruction of cells (autolysis). It leads to anorexia, jaundice, and hepatomegaly.

Five types of viral hepatitis are recognized, each caused by a different virus. (See *Viral hepatitis from A to E,* pages 358 and 359.) Type A is transmitted almost exclusively by the fecal-oral route, and outbreaks are common in areas of overcrowding and poor sanitation. Day-care centers and other institutional settings are common sources of outbreaks. Infection is increasing among homosexuals and in people with human immunodeficiency virus (HIV).

Type B, also increasing among HIV-positive people, accounts for 5% to 10% of posttransfusion hepatitis cases in the United States. Vaccinations are available and are now required for health care workers and school children in many states.

Type C accounts for about 20% of all viral hepatitis as well as most cases that follow transfusion.

Type D, in the United States, is confined to people frequently exposed to blood and blood products, such as I.V. drug users and hemophiliacs.

Type E was formerly grouped with type C under the name *non-A, non-B hepatitis*. In the United States, this type mainly occurs in people who have visited an endemic area, such as India, Africa, Asia, or Central America.

Despite the different causes, changes to the liver are usually similar in each type of viral hepatitis. Varying degrees of liver cell injury and necrosis occur. These changes in the liver are completely reversible when the acute phase of the disease subsides.

RED FLAG A fairly common complication is chronic persistent hepatitis, which lengthens the recovery up to 8 months. Some patients also have relapses. A few may develop chronic active hepatitis, which destroys part of the liver and causes cirrhosis. In rare cases, severe and sudden (fulminant) hepatic failure and death may result from massive tissue loss. Primary hepatocellular carcinoma is a late complication that can cause death within 5 years, but it's rare in the United States.

Signs and symptoms

Signs and symptoms of viral hepatitis progress in three stages: prodromal, clinical, and recovery.

PRODROMAL STAGE

In this stage, when the infection is highly transmissible, signs and symptoms may be caused by circulating immune complexes:

- anorexia
- changes in the senses of taste and smell
- depression
- fatigue
- generalized malaise
- headache
- intolerance of light (photophobia)
- joint pain (arthralgia)
- mild weight loss
- muscle pain (myalgia)

Viral hepatitis from A to E

This table compares the features of each type of viral hepatitis.

FEATURE	HEPATITIS A	HEPATITIS B
INCUBATION	15 to 45 days	30 to 180 days
ONSET	Acute	Insidious
AGE-GROUP MOST AFFECTED	Children, young adults	Any age
TRANSMISSION	Fecal-oral, sexual (especially oral-anal contact), nonpercutaneous (sexual, maternal-neonatal), percutaneous (rare)	Blood-borne; parenteral route, sexual, maternal-neonatal; virus is shed in all body fluids
SEVERITY	Mild	Usually severe
PROGNOSIS	Generally good	Worsens with age and debility
PROGRESSION TO CHRONICITY	None	Occasional

■ nausea and vomiting
■ right upper quadrant tenderness, dark-colored urine, and clay-colored stools (1 to 5 days before the onset of the clinical jaundice stage)
■ temperature of 100° to 102° F (37.8° to 38.9° C)
■ weakness

CLINICAL STAGE

Also called the *icteric stage,* the clinical stage begins 1 to 2 weeks after the prodromal stage. It's the phase of actual illness. If the patient progresses to this stage, he may have these signs and symptoms:
■ abdominal pain or tenderness

HEPATITIS C	HEPATITIS D	HEPATITIS E
15 to 160 days	14 to 64 days	14 to 60 days
Insidious	Acute	Acute
More common in adults	Any age	Ages 20 to 40
Blood-borne; parenteral route	Parenteral route (most people infected with hepatitis D are also infected with hepatitis B)	Mainly fecal-oral
Moderate	Can be severe and lead to fulminant hepatitis	Highly virulent with common progression to fulminant hepatitis and hepatic failure, especially in pregnant patients
Moderate	Fair; worsens in chronic cases; can lead to chronic hepatitis D and chronic liver disease	Good unless pregnant
10% to 50% of cases	Occasional	None

- appetite loss (in early clinical stage)
- indigestion
- itching
- jaundice.

Jaundice lasts 1 to 2 weeks. It indicates that the damaged liver can't remove bilirubin from the blood, but it doesn't indicate disease severity and, occasionally, hepatitis occurs without jaundice.

RECOVERY STAGE
Recovery begins with the resolution of jaundice and lasts 2 to 6 weeks in uncomplicated cases. The prognosis is poor if edema and hepatic encephalopathy develop.

Test results

These tests are used to diagnose viral hepatitis.

- Hepatitis profile establishes the type of hepatitis.
- Liver function studies show disease stage.
- PT is prolonged.
- WBC count is elevated.
- Liver biopsy may be performed if chronic hepatitis is suspected.

Treatment

Hepatitis C has been treated somewhat successfully with interferon alfa (Intron A). No specific drug therapy has been developed for the other types of viral hepatitis. Instead, urge the patient to rest in the early stages of the illness and to combat anorexia by eating small, high-calorie, high-protein meals. (See *Hepatitis teaching topics*.)

Protein intake should be reduced if signs of precoma — lethargy, confusion, or mental changes — develop. Large meals are usually better tolerated in the morning because many patients have nausea late in the day.

In acute viral hepatitis, hospitalization is usually needed only for severe symptoms or complications. Parenteral nutrition may be needed if persistent vomiting keeps the patient from eating.

11

GENITOURINARY SYSTEM

Understanding the genitourinary system

The genitourinary system consists of the kidneys, ureters, bladder, and urethra. The kidneys are located on each side of the vertebral column in the upper abdomen outside the peritoneal cavity. These compact organs filter about 45 gallons of fluid each day. The by-product of this filtration is urine, which contains water, electrolytes, and waste products. (See *A close look at the kidney,* pages 362 and 363.)

After it's produced by the kidneys, urine passes through the urinary system and is expelled from the body. Other structures of the renal system, extending downward from the kidneys, include:

- ureters — 16″ to 18″ (40.5- to 45.5-cm) muscular tubes that contract rhythmically (peristaltic action) to transport urine from each kidney to the bladder
- urinary bladder — a sac with muscular walls that collects and holds urine (300 to 500 ml) that's expelled from the ureters every few seconds
- urethra — a narrow passageway, surrounded by the prostate gland in men, that leads from the bladder to the outside of the body and through which urine is excreted.

The kidneys' vital functions include:
- maintaining fluid and acid-base balance
- regulating electrolyte concentration
- detoxifying the blood and eliminating wastes
- regulating blood pressure
- aiding red blood cell (RBC) production (erythropoiesis)
- regulating vitamin D and calcium formation.

A close look at the kidney

Illustrated below is a kidney along with an enlargement of a nephron, the kidney's functional unit. Major structures of the kidney include:

● medulla, the inner portion of the kidney, which is made up of renal pyramids and tubular structures

● renal artery, which supplies blood to the kidney

● renal pyramid, which channels output to the renal pelvis for excretion

● renal calyx, which channels urine from the renal pyramids to the renal pelvis

● renal vein, through which about 99% of filtered blood is reabsorbed and circulated back to the general circulation (about 1%, which contains waste products, undergoes further processing in the kidney)

● renal pelvis, to which urine is channeled after blood that contains waste products is processed in the kidney

● ureter, the tube that terminates in the urethra, through which urine is excreted

● cortex, which is the outer layer of the kidney.

NOTE THE NEPHRON

The nephron is the functional and structural unit of the kidney. Each kidney contains about 1 million nephrons. The nephron has two main activities. One is selective reabsorption and secretion of ions. The other

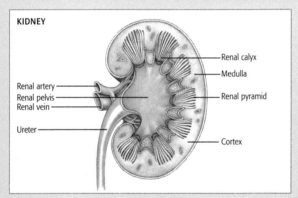

KIDNEY

Renal calyx
Medulla
Renal pyramid
Renal artery
Renal pelvis
Renal vein
Ureter
Cortex

MAINTAINING FLUID AND ACID-BASE BALANCE

Two important kidney functions are maintaining fluid balance and acid-base balance.

is mechanical filtration of fluids, wastes, electrolytes, and acids and bases.

Components of the nephron include:

● glomerulus, which is a network of twisted capillaries that filter and allow passage of protein-free and red blood cell–free filtrate to Bowman's capsule

● Bowman's capsule, which contains the glomerulus and acts as a reservoir for glomerular filtrate

● proximal convoluted tubule, which is the site of reabsorption of glucose, amino acids, metabolites, and electrolytes from filtrate and through which reabsorbed substances return to circulation

● loop of Henle, which is a U-shaped nephron tubule in the medulla that extends from the proximal convoluted tubule to the distal convoluted tubule and allows further concentration of filtrate through reabsorption

● distal convoluted tubule, from which filtrate enters the collecting tubule

● collecting tubule, which releases urine.

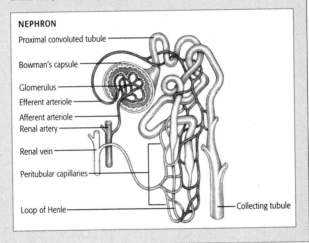

NEPHRON

- Proximal convoluted tubule
- Bowman's capsule
- Glomerulus
- Efferent arteriole
- Afferent arteriole
- Renal artery
- Renal vein
- Peritubular capillaries
- Loop of Henle
- Collecting tubule

Fluid balance

The kidneys maintain the body's fluid balance by regulating the amount and makeup of the fluids inside and around the cells. They maintain the volume and composition of extracellular fluid and, to a lesser extent, intracellular fluid by continuously exchanging water and solutes—such as hydrogen, sodium, potassium, chloride, bicarbonate, sulfate, and phosphate ions—across their cell membranes.

Hormones partially control the kidneys' role in fluid balance. This control depends on the response of specialized sensory nerve endings (osmoreceptors) to changes in osmolality (the ionic, or solute, concentration of a solution). The two hormones involved are:

■ antidiuretic hormone (ADH), produced by the pituitary gland
■ aldosterone, produced by the adrenal cortex.

Problems in hormone concentration may cause fluctuations in sodium and potassium concentrations that, in turn, may lead to hypertension. ADH alters the collecting tubules' permeability to water. When ADH concentration in plasma is high, the tubules are most permeable to water. This causes more water to be absorbed, creating a highly concentrated but small volume of urine that has a high specific gravity. If ADH concentration is low, the tubules are less permeable to water. This causes more water to be excreted, creating a larger volume of less concentrated urine with a low specific gravity.

Aldosterone regulates water reabsorption by the distal tubules and changes urine concentration by increasing sodium reabsorption. A high plasma aldosterone concentration increases sodium and water reabsorption by the tubules and decreases sodium and water excretion in urine. A low plasma aldosterone concentration promotes sodium and water excretion.

Aldosterone helps control potassium secretion by the distal tubules. A high aldosterone concentration increases potassium secretion. Other factors that affect potassium secretion include:

■ the amount of potassium ingested
■ the number of hydrogen ions secreted
■ potassium levels in the cells
■ the amount of sodium in the distal tubule
■ the glomerular filtration rate (GFR), the rate at which plasma is filtered as it flows through the glomerular capillary filtration membrane. Normal GFR is about 120 ml/minute.

The kidneys concentrate urine through the countercurrent exchange system. In this system, fluid flows in opposite directions through parallel tubes, up and down parallel sides of the loops of Henle. A concentration gradient causes fluid exchange; the longer the loop, the greater the concentration gradient.

Acid-base balance

To regulate acid-base balance, the kidneys secrete hydrogen ions, reabsorb sodium and bicarbonate ions, acidify phosphate salts, and produce ammonia. All of these regulating activities keep the blood at its normal pH of 7.35 to 7.45. Acidosis occurs when the pH falls below 7.35, and alkalosis occurs when the pH rises above 7.45.

WASTE COLLECTION

The kidneys collect and eliminate wastes from the body in a three-step process that includes glomerular filtration, tubular reabsorption, and tubular secretion.

In glomerular filtration, the glomeruli, a collection of nephron capillaries, filter blood flowing through them to form filtrate. In tubular reabsorption, the tubules (minute canals that make up the nephron) reabsorb the filtered fluid in surrounding blood vessels. And in tubular secretion, the filtered substance, known as *glomerular filtrate,* passes through the tubules to the collecting tubules and ducts.

Clearance is the complete removal of a substance from the blood — commonly described in terms of the amount of blood that can be cleared in a specific amount of time. For example, creatinine clearance is the volume of blood in milliliters that the kidneys can clear of creatinine in 1 minute. Some substances are filtered out of the blood by the glomeruli. Dissolved substances that remain in the fluid may be reabsorbed by the renal tubular cells.

In a patient whose kidneys have shrunk from disease, healthy nephrons (the filtering units of the kidney) enlarge to compensate. However, as nephron damage progresses, the enlargement can no longer adequately compensate, and the GFR slows.

BLOOD PRESSURE REGULATION

The kidneys help regulate blood pressure by producing and secreting an enzyme known as *renin* in response to an actual or perceived decline in extracellular fluid volume. Renin, in turn, forms angiotensin I, which is converted to the more potent vasopressor, angiotensin II.

Angiotensin II raises low arterial blood pressure levels by increasing peripheral vasoconstriction and stimulating aldosterone secretion. The increase in aldosterone promotes the reabsorption of sodium and water to correct the fluid deficit and inadequate blood flow (renal ischemia).

Hypertension can stem from a fluid and electrolyte imbalance as well as renin-angiotensin hyperactivity. High blood pressure can damage blood vessels as well as cause hardening of the kidneys (nephrosclerosis), one of the leading causes of chronic renal failure.

RED BLOOD CELL PRODUCTION

Erythropoietin is a hormone that prompts the bone marrow to increase RBC production. The kidneys secrete erythropoietin when the oxygen supply decreases in blood circulating through the tissues. Loss of renal function results in chronic anemia and insufficient calcium levels (hypocalcemia) because of a decrease in erythropoietin.

VITAMIN D REGULATION AND CALCIUM FORMATION

The kidneys help convert vitamin D to its active form. Active vitamin D helps regulate calcium and phosphorus balance and bone metabolism. When the kidneys fail, hypocalcemia and hypophosphatemia occur.

Genitourinary disorders

The genitourinary disorders discussed in this chapter include:
- acute tubular necrosis
- benign prostatic hyperplasia (BPH)
- glomerulonephritis
- hydronephrosis
- prostatitis
- renal calculi (kidney stones)
- renal failure (acute and chronic).

ACUTE TUBULAR NECROSIS

Acute tubular necrosis causes 75% of all cases of acute renal failure. Also called *acute tubulointerstitial nephritis,* this disorder destroys the tubular segment of the nephron, causing uremia (the excess accumulation of by-products of protein metabolism in the blood) and renal failure.

Pathophysiology

Usually, acute tubular necrosis follows an ischemic kidney injury. Sometimes it follows nephrotoxic injury; this is most likely in debilitated patients, such as the critically ill or those who have undergone extensive surgery. In ischemic injury, blood flow to the kidneys is disrupted. The longer it's disrupted, the worse the kidney damage. Blood flow to the kidneys may be disrupted by:
- anesthetics
- cardiogenic or septic shock
- circulatory collapse

- dehydration
- hemorrhage
- severe hypotension
- surgery
- transfusion reactions
- trauma.

Nephrotoxic injury may result from ingestion or inhalation of toxic chemicals, such as carbon tetrachloride, heavy metals, and methoxyflurane anesthetics. It also may result from a hypersensitivity reaction of the kidneys to such substances as antibiotics and radiographic contrast agents.

Specific causes of acute tubular necrosis and their effects may vary. For example, diseased tubular epithelium may allow glomerular filtrate that should be excreted to leak through the membranes and be reabsorbed into the blood. Urine flow may be obstructed by damaged cells, casts, red blood cells (RBCs), and other cellular debris in the tubular walls. Ischemic injury to glomerular epithelial cells may cause cellular collapse and poor glomerular capillary permeability. And ischemic injury to the vascular endothelium eventually may cause cellular swelling and tubular obstruction.

Deep or shallow lesions may occur in acute tubular necrosis. With ischemic injury, necrosis creates deep lesions, destroying the tubular epithelium and basement membrane (the delicate layer underlying the epithelium). Ischemic injury causes patches of necrosis in the tubules. Ischemia also can cause lesions in the connective tissue of the kidney.

With nephrotoxic injury, necrosis occurs only in the epithelium of the tubules, leaving the basement membrane of the nephrons intact. This type of damage may be reversible. (See *A close look at acute tubular necrosis,* page 368.)

Toxicity also may take a toll. Nephrotoxic agents can injure tubular cells by direct cellular toxic effects, by coagulation and destruction (lysis) of RBCs, by oxygen deprivation (hypoxia), and by crystal formation by solutes.

RED FLAG *Common complications of acute tubular necrosis include these.*

- *Infections (typically septicemia) complicate up to 70% of cases and are the leading cause of death.*
- *GI hemorrhage, fluid and electrolyte imbalance, and cardiovascular dysfunction may occur during the acute or recovery phase.*
- *Neurologic complications are common in elderly patients and occur occasionally in younger patients.*
- *Excess blood calcium (hypercalcemia) may occur during the recovery phase.*

A close look at acute tubular necrosis

In acute tubular necrosis caused by ischemia, patches of necrosis occur, usually in the straight portion of the proximal tubules, as shown. In areas without lesions, tubules are usually dilated.

In acute tubular necrosis caused by nephrotoxicity, the tubules have a more uniform appearance, as shown in the second illustration.

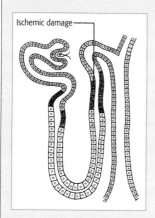

Ischemic damage

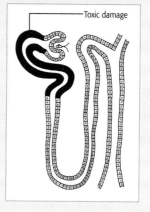

Toxic damage

Signs and symptoms

Early-stage acute tubular necrosis may be hard to spot because the patient's primary disease may obscure signs and symptoms. The first recognizable sign may be decreased urine output, usually less than 400 ml/24 hours. Other signs and symptoms depend on the severity of systemic involvement and may include:

■ agitation
■ bleeding abnormalities
■ confusion
■ dry skin and mucous membranes
■ edema
■ fluid and electrolyte imbalances
■ lethargy
■ muscle weakness with hyperkalemia
■ tachycardia and an irregular rhythm
■ vomiting of blood.

TEACHING FOCUS

Acute tubular necrosis teaching topics

● Teach the patient and his family about the disease process, including its signs and symptoms, complications, and treatments.
● Fully explain each procedure to the patient and his family as often as needed, and help them set goals that are realistic for the patient's progress.
● Teach about prescribed drugs, including their names, indications, dosages, intervals, and special considerations.

Mortality can be as high as 70%, depending on complications from underlying diseases. Nonoliguric forms of acute tubular necrosis have a better prognosis.

Test results
Acute tubular necrosis is hard to diagnose except in advanced stages. These tests are commonly performed.
■ Urinalysis shows dilute urine, low osmolality, high sodium level, and urine sediment containing RBCs and casts.
■ Blood studies reveal high blood urea nitrogen (BUN) and serum creatinine levels, low serum protein levels, anemia, platelet adherence defects, metabolic acidosis, and hyperkalemia.
■ Electrocardiogram (ECG) may show arrhythmias from electrolyte imbalances and, with hyperkalemia, a widening QRS complex, disappearing P waves, and tall, peaked T waves.

Treatment
Acute tubular necrosis requires vigorous supportive care during the acute phase until normal kidney function is restored. Initially, diuretics are given and fluids are infused to flush tubules of cellular casts and debris and replace lost fluids. Projected and calculated fluid losses require daily replacement. (See *Acute tubular necrosis teaching topics*.)

Packed RBCs are transfused for anemia. Nonnephrotoxic antibiotics are given for infection. Hyperkalemia requires an emergency I.V. infusion of 50% glucose and regular insulin. Sodium bicarbonate may be needed to combat metabolic acidosis. Sodium polystyrene sulfonate (Kayexalate) is given by mouth or by enema to reduce potassium level. Hemodialysis or peritoneal dialysis is used to prevent severe fluid and electrolyte imbalance and uremia.

BENIGN PROSTATIC HYPERPLASIA

Although most men older than age 50 have some prostate enlargement, in BPH, the prostate gland enlarges enough to compress the urethra and obstruct urine.

Pathophysiology

BPH may be linked to hormonal activity. As men age, production of hormones that stimulate male characteristics (androgens) decreases and estrogen production increases. This shift causes an androgen-estrogen imbalance and high levels of dihydrotestosterone, the main prostatic intracellular androgen. Other possible causes of prostate enlargement include a tumor, arteriosclerosis, inflammation, and metabolic or nutritional disturbances.

In BPH, increased estrogen levels prompt androgen receptors in the prostate gland to increase. This causes an overgrowth of normal cells (hyperplasia) that begins around the urethra. Growth eventually causes areas of poor blood flow and tissue damage (necrosis) in adjacent prostatic tissue. As the prostate enlarges, it may extend into the bladder and decrease urine flow by compressing or distorting the urethra.

RED FLAG *Urinary obstruction is a main complication that can lead to other complications. Enlargement that blocks the urethra and pushes up the bladder can stop urine flow and cause a urinary tract infection (UTI) or calculi. Bladder muscles may thicken and a pouch (diverticulum) may form in the bladder that retains urine when the rest of the bladder empties. Other complications include:*

- *formation of a fibrous cord of connective tissue in the bladder wall*
- *detrusor muscle enlargement*
- *narrowing of the urethra*
- *incontinence*
- *acute or chronic renal failure*
- *distention of the innermost area of the kidney — the renal pelvis and calices — with urine (hydronephrosis).*

Signs and symptoms

Signs and symptoms depend on the extent of the prostate's enlargement and the lobes affected. Symptoms include decreased size and force of the urine stream, an interrupted urine stream, and urinary hesitancy that causes straining and a feeling of incomplete voiding. As the obstruction increases, the patient may report frequent urination with nocturia, dribbling, urine retention, incontinence, and blood in the urine.

Benign prostatic hyperplasia teaching topics

- If the patient needs urinary catheterization, tell him that he may experience urinary frequency, dribbling and, occasionally, hematuria, after the catheter is removed. Reassure him and his family that he'll gradually regain urinary control.
- Teach the patient to recognize and report the signs and symptoms of urinary tract infection.

- Instruct the patient to follow the prescribed oral antibiotic regimen, and tell him the indications for using gentle laxatives.
- Urge the patient to seek immediate medical care if he can't void, passes bloody urine, or develops a fever.

An incompletely emptied and distended bladder is visible as a midline bulge, and an enlarged prostate is palpable with digital rectal examination.

Test results

These tests are used to diagnose BPH.
- Excretory urography may indicate urinary tract obstruction, hydronephrosis, calculi or tumors, and filling and emptying defects in the bladder.
- Elevated BUN and serum creatinine levels suggest impaired renal function.
- Urinalysis and urine culture show hematuria, pyuria, and a UTI.
- Cystourethroscopy can show prostate enlargement, bladder wall changes, calculi, and a raised bladder.
- Prostate-specific antigen test rules out prostate cancer.

Treatment

Depending on the size of the prostate, the patient's age and health, and the extent of obstruction, BPH may be treated surgically or symptomatically. Conservative treatments for relieving symptoms of an enlarged prostate include:
- short-term fluid restriction to prevent bladder distention
- antimicrobials if infection occurs
- regular sexual intercourse to relieve prostatic congestion
- terazosin (Hytrin) to improve urine flow rates
- finasteride (Proscar) to reduce prostate size. (See *Benign prostatic hyperplasia teaching topics*.)

Surgery is the only effective therapy for acute urine retention, kidney distention (hydronephrosis), severe hematuria, recurrent UTI, or other intolerable symptoms. A transurethral resection — in which tissue is removed with a wire loop and an electric current — may be performed if the prostate weighs less than 2 oz (56.7 g). Other transurethral procedures include vaporization of the prostate or a prostate incision with a scalpel or laser. Open surgical removal of the prostate is usually reserved for prostate cancer.

GLOMERULONEPHRITIS

Glomerulonephritis is a bilateral inflammation of the glomeruli, commonly following a streptococcal infection. Acute glomerulo-nephritis is most common in boys ages 3 to 7, but it can occur at any age. Up to 95% of children and 70% of adults recover fully; the rest, especially elderly patients, may progress to chronic renal failure within months.

Rapidly progressive glomerulonephritis usually occurs between ages 50 and 60. It may be idiopathic or linked to a proliferative glomerular disease such as poststreptococcal glomerulonephritis. Goodpasture's syndrome, a type of rapidly progressive glomerulo-nephritis, is rare but occurs most often in men ages 20 to 30.

Chronic glomerulonephritis is a slowly progressive disease characterized by inflammation, sclerosis, scarring, and eventual renal failure. It usually remains undetected until the progressive phase, which is irreversible.

Pathophysiology

In nearly all types of glomerulonephritis, the epithelial layer of the glomerular membrane is disturbed. Acute poststreptococcal glo-merulonephritis results from an immune response that occurs in the glomerulus. The antigen, group A beta-hemolytic streptococci, stim-ulates antibody formation. As an antigen-antibody complex forms, it lodges in the glomerular capillaries, causing an inflammatory re-sponse.

Glomerular injury occurs as a result of the inflammatory process when complexes prompt release of immunologic substances that break down cells and increase membrane permeability. The severity of glomerular damage and renal insufficiency is related to the size, number, location, duration of exposure to, and type of antigen-antibody complexes.

In Goodpasture's syndrome, antibodies are produced against the pulmonary capillaries and glomerular basement membrane. The glomerular filtration rate (GFR) becomes reduced, and renal failure occurs within weeks or months.

RED FLAG Progressive deterioration of renal function may occur as a result of acute glomerulonephritis, commonly in the form of glomerulosclerosis accompanied by hypertension. The more severe the disorder, the more likely it is that complications will follow. Chronic glomerulonephritis can cause contracted, granular kidneys and lead to end-stage renal failure. It can also produce severe hypertension, leading to cardiovascular complications, including cardiac hypertrophy and heart failure, which may speed the development of advanced renal failure and the need for dialysis or kidney transplantation.

Signs and symptoms

Signs and symptoms of glomerulonephritis may include:

■ arthralgia
■ bibasilar crackles on lung auscultation
■ decreased urination or oliguria
■ malaise
■ mild to severe hypertension
■ nausea
■ orthopnea
■ periorbital edema
■ shortness of breath
■ smoky or coffee-colored urine.

Test results

These tests aid in the diagnosis of glomerulonephritis.

■ BUN and creatinine levels are elevated.
■ Serum protein level is decreased.
■ Hemoglobin level may be decreased in chronic glomerulonephritis.
■ Antistreptolysin-O titers are elevated in 80% of patients.
■ Urinalysis reveals RBCs, white blood cells, mixed cell casts, and protein, indicating renal failure.
■ Kidney-ureter-bladder (KUB) radiography reveals bilateral kidney enlargement (acute glomerulonephritis).
■ Renal biopsy confirms the diagnosis.

Treatment

Treatment focuses on the underlying disease. (See *Glomerulonephritis teaching topics,* page 374.) Drugs used to treat glomerulonephritis include antibiotics (7 to 10 days) for infections that support an ongoing antigen-antibody response; diuretics, such as metolazone (Zaroxolyn) or furosemide (Lasix), to reduce fluid overload; va-

TEACHING FOCUS

Glomerulonephritis teaching topics

- Instruct the patient to take prescribed medications as scheduled, even if he feels better. Advise him to take diuretics in the morning so that his sleep won't be disturbed.
- Teach the patient the signs of infection, particularly those of a urinary tract infection, and warn him to report them immediately. Tell him to avoid contact with people who have communicable illnesses.
- Stress the importance of keeping all follow-up examinations.
- If the patient needs dialysis, explain the procedure fully.

sodilators, such as hydralazine (Apresoline), to control hypertension; and corticosteroids to decrease antibody synthesis and suppress inflammation.

In rapidly progressive glomerulonephritis, the patient may need plasmapheresis to suppress rebound antibody production. This procedure may be combined with corticosteroids and cyclophosphamide (Cytoxan). Dialysis or kidney transplantation also may be needed.

HYDRONEPHROSIS

An abnormal dilation of the renal pelvis and the calyces of one or both kidneys, hydronephrosis is caused by an obstruction of urine flow in the genitourinary tract.

Pathophysiology

Almost any type of disease that results from urinary tract obstruction can result in hydronephrosis. The most common causes are BPH, stenosis of the ureter or bladder outlet, and urethral strictures. Less common causes include abdominal tumors, blood clots, congenital abnormalities, neurogenic bladder, and tumors of the ureter and bladder.

If the obstruction is in the urethra or bladder, hydronephrosis usually affects both kidneys; if the obstruction is in a ureter, it usually affects one kidney. Obstructions distal to the bladder cause it to dilate and act as a buffer zone, delaying hydronephrosis. Total obstruction of urine flow with dilation of the collecting system ultimately causes complete atrophy of the cortex (the outer portion of the kidney) and cessation of glomerular filtration.

RED FLAG Untreated hydronephrosis can result in infection (pyelonephritis) from stasis that worsens renal damage and

TEACHING FOCUS

Hydronephrosis teaching topics

● Explain hydronephrosis to the patient and his family. Also explain the purpose of diagnostic tests and how they're performed.
● If the patient is scheduled for surgery, explain the procedure and postoperative care.
● If the patient will be discharged with a nephrostomy tube, teach him how to care for it, including how to thoroughly clean the skin around the insertion site.
● If the patient must take antibiotics after discharge, tell him to complete the prescription, even if he feels better before it's finished.
● Teach him to recognize and report symptoms of hydronephrosis, such as colicky pain or hematuria, and urinary tract infection.

may create a life-threatening crisis. Paralytic ileus commonly accompanies acute obstructive disease of the urinary tract.

Signs and symptoms

Signs and symptoms depend on the cause of the obstruction. In mild cases, hydronephrosis produces either no symptoms or mild pain and slightly decreased urine flow. In more severe cases, it may produce severe, colicky renal pain or dull flank pain that may radiate to the groin and gross urinary abnormalities, such as hematuria, pyuria, dysuria, alternating polyuria and oliguria, and anuria.

Other symptoms of hydronephrosis are more general and include abdominal fullness, dribbling, nausea and vomiting, and urinary hesitancy.

Test results

These tests are essential to the diagnosis of hydronephrosis.
■ Excretory urography confirms hydronephrosis.
■ Retrograde pyelography reveals hydronephrosis.
■ Renal ultrasonography reveals an obstruction and confirms hydronephrosis.
■ Renal function studies demonstrate hydronephrosis.

Treatment

Treatment for hydronephrosis aims to preserve the patient's renal function and prevent infection. (See *Hydronephrosis teaching topics.*)

Surgical removal of the obstruction is commonly needed as soon as the patient is medically stable. Procedures include dilatation for strictures of the urethra and prostatectomy for BPH. Inoperable obstructions may require decompression and drainage of the kidney using a nephrostomy tube placed temporarily or permanently in the renal pelvis.

If renal function has already been affected, therapy may include a diet low in protein, sodium, and potassium. This is designed to stop the progression of renal failure before surgery. If the patient has an infection, antibiotics typically are prescribed.

PROSTATITIS

Prostatitis is an inflammation of the prostate gland. Prostatic inflammation without infection is the most common type of prostatitis. Acute bacterial prostatitis is an ascending infection of the urinary tract. Chronic bacterial prostatitis is marked by recurrent UTI and persistent pathogenic bacteria.

Pathophysiology

About 80% of bacterial prostatitis cases result from *Escherichia coli* infection. The remaining 20% result from infection by *Klebsiella, Enterobacter, Proteus, Pseudomonas, Serratia, Streptococcus, Staphylococcus,* or diphtheroids, which are contaminants from normal flora of the urethra. These organisms probably spread to the prostate gland in one of four ways:

- from the bloodstream
- from ascending urethral infection
- from invasion by rectal bacteria through the lymphatic vessels
- from reflux of infected urine from the bladder into prostatic ducts.

Chronic prostatitis is usually caused by bacterial invasion from the urethra. Less common means of acute or chronic infection are urethral procedures performed with instruments, such as cystoscopy and catheterization, and infrequent or excessive sexual intercourse.

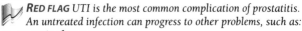 **RED FLAG** *UTI is the most common complication of prostatitis. An untreated infection can progress to other problems, such as:*

- *prostatic abscess*
- *acute urine retention from prostatic edema*
- *inflammation of the kidney (pyelonephritis)*
- *inflammation of the epididymis, where spermatozoa are stored (epididymitis).*

Signs and symptoms

Signs and symptoms vary with the type of prostatitis. In acute bacterial prostatitis, the patient has a sudden onset of fever, chills, lower back pain, muscle pain (myalgia), pelvic area (perineal) fullness, joint pain (arthralgia), urinary urgency and frequency, cloudy urine, painful urination (dysuria), nocturia, and transient erectile dysfunction. Some degree of urinary obstruction also may occur. The bladder may feel distended when palpated. Rectal palpation finds the prostate to be tender, abnormally hard, swollen, and warm.

Chronic bacterial prostatitis may develop from acute prostatitis that doesn't clear up with antibiotics. Some patients are symptom-free, but most have the same signs and symptoms as in the acute form, although to a lesser degree. Other signs and symptoms may include urethral discharge and painful ejaculation, leading to sexual dysfunction. The prostate may feel soft, and palpation may produce a dry, crackling sound or sensation (crepitation) if prostatic calculi are present.

A patient with nonbacterial prostatitis usually complains of dysuria, mild perineal or lower back pain, and nocturia. The patient also may have pain on ejaculation. The prostate gland usually feels normal during palpation.

Test results

A firm diagnosis of prostatitis depends on urine cultures, rectal examination, and cultures for bacterial growth. These tests confirm the diagnosis.

- X-ray of the pelvis may show prostatic calculi.
- Smears of prostatic secretions reveal inflammatory cells but usually no causative organism in nonbacterial prostatitis.
- Urodynamic evaluation may reveal detrusor muscle hyperreflexia and pelvic floor myalgia from chronic spasms.

Treatment

Treatment for prostatitis may include drug therapy, supportive measures, or surgery. Drugs used to treat prostatitis include:

- aminoglycosides, given with penicillins or cephalosporins in severe acute cases
- co-trimoxazole (Bactrim) to prevent chronic prostatitis
- co-trimoxazole, carbenicillin (Geocillin), nitrofurantoin (Macrobid), erythromycin (Erythrocin), or tetracycline (Sumycin) for *E. coli* infection
- anticholinergics, analgesics, and minocycline (Minocin), doxycycline (Vibramycin), or erythromycin for nonbacterial prostatitis.

Supportive therapy includes bed rest, plenty of fluids, sitz baths, and stool softeners. To promote drainage of prostatic secre-

TEACHING FOCUS

Prostatitis teaching topics

● Teach the patient about prescribed drugs. Tell him to take them exactly as ordered and to complete the prescribed drug regimen.

● Instruct the patient to drink at least eight 8-oz glasses of fluid daily.

● If the patient has chronic prostatitis, recommend that he stay sexually active and ejaculate regularly to promote drainage of prostatic secretions. Tell him to use a condom during sexual intercourse when he's having a bout of prostatitis.

tions, ejaculation or regular sexual intercourse using a condom is prescribed for chronic prostatitis. (See *Prostatitis teaching topics*.)

If drug therapy is unsuccessful, transurethral resection of the prostate may be done. This procedure may lead to retrograde ejaculation and sterility, so it usually isn't done on young men. Total prostatectomy is curative but may cause impotence and incontinence.

RENAL CALCULI

Renal calculi, or *kidney stones*, may form anywhere in the urinary tract, but they usually develop in the renal pelvis or calices. Calculi form when substances that normally dissolve in the urine precipitate. (See *A close look at renal calculi*.)

About 1 in 1,000 Americans need hospitalization at some time for renal calculi. They're more common in men than in women and rare in blacks and children.

Pathophysiology

Renal calculi are particularly prevalent in certain geographic areas such as the southeastern United States. Although their exact cause is unknown, there are several predisposing factors:

■ *dehydration*, because decreased water and urine excretion concentrates calculus-forming substances.

■ *infection*, because infected, scarred tissue provides a site for calculus development. Calculi may become infected if bacteria have formed the nucleus. Calculi that result from *Proteus* infection may destroy kidney tissue.

■ *changes in urine pH*, because consistently acidic or alkaline urine provides a favorable medium for calculus formation.

■ *obstruction*, because urine stasis allows calculus constituents to collect and adhere, forming calculi. Obstruction also encourages infection, which compounds the obstruction.

A close look at renal calculi

Renal calculi vary in size and type. Small calculi may stay in the renal pelvis or pass down the ureter, as shown on the left. A staghorn calculus, shown on the right, is a cast of the innermost part of the kidney—the calyx and renal pelvis. A staghorn calculus may develop from a calculus that stays in the kidney.

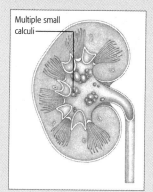

Multiple small calculi

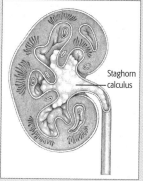

Staghorn calculus

- *immobilization,* because immobility from spinal cord injury or other disorders allows calcium to be released into the circulation and, eventually, to be filtered by the kidneys.
- *diet,* because increased intake of calcium or oxalate-rich foods encourages calculi formation.
- *metabolic factors,* because hyperparathyroidism, renal tubular acidosis, an elevated uric acid level (usually with gout), defective oxalate metabolism, a genetic defect in cystine metabolism, and excessive intake of vitamin D or calcium may predispose a person to renal calculi.

Renal calculi usually arise because the delicate excretory balance breaks down. Urine becomes concentrated with insoluble materials. Crystals form from these materials and then consolidate, forming calculi.

RED FLAG Calculi either remain in the renal pelvis and damage or destroy renal parenchyma, or they enter the ureter; large calculi in the kidneys cause pressure necrosis. Calculi in some sites cause obstruction, with resulting hydronephrosis, and tend to recur. Intractable pain and serious bleeding also can result from calculi and the damage they cause. If left untreated, irreversible damage may occur.

Signs and symptoms

The key symptom of renal calculi is severe pain, which may travel from the lower back to the sides and then to the pubic region and external genitalia. Pain intensity fluctuates and may be excruciating at its peak. It's typically accompanied by nausea, vomiting and, possibly, fever and chills.

Other signs and symptoms include hematuria (when stones abrade a ureter), abdominal distention, and oliguria (from an obstruction in urine flow).

Test results

Diagnosis is based on clinical features and these tests.
■ KUB radiography reveals most renal calculi.
■ Excretory urography shows the size and location of calculi.
■ Kidney ultrasonography detects obstructions not seen on KUB radiography.
■ Urinalysis may indicate pus in the urine (pyuria), a sign of UTI.
■ A 24-hour urine collection reveals calcium oxalate, phosphorus, and uric acid levels. Three separate collections, along with blood samples, are needed for accurate testing.
■ Calculus analysis shows mineral content.

Treatment

Ninety percent of renal calculi are smaller than 5 mm in diameter and may pass naturally with vigorous hydration (more than 3 L/day). Other treatments may include drug therapy for infection or other effects of illness and measures to prevent the recurrence of calculi. If calculi are too large for natural passage, they may be removed by surgery or other means. (See *Renal calculi teaching topics.*)

DRUG THERAPY

Drugs used to treat renal calculi include:
■ antimicrobial drugs for infection
■ analgesics for pain
■ diuretics to prevent urinary stasis and further calculi formation
■ thiazides to decrease calcium excretion into the urine
■ methenamine (Hiprex) to suppress calculi formation when infection is present.

PREVENTIVE MEASURES

Measures to prevent recurrence of renal calculi include:

TEACHING FOCUS

Renal calculi teaching topics

- Encourage increased fluid intake. Tell the patient to immediately report symptoms of acute obstruction, such as pain or an inability to void.
- Urge the patient to follow a prescribed diet and comply with drug therapy to prevent recurrence of calculi.
- If surgery is needed, supplement and reinforce the physician's teaching. If the patient will have an abdominal or flank incision, teach deep-breathing and coughing exercises.

■ a low-calcium oxalate diet
■ oxalate-binding cholestyramine (Questran) for absorptive hyper-calciuria
■ parathyroidectomy for hyperparathyroidism
■ allopurinol (Zyloprim) for uric acid calculi
■ daily oral doses of ascorbic acid to acidify urine.

REMOVING CALCULI
Calculi lodged in a ureter may be removed by inserting a cystoscope through the urethra and then manipulating the calculi with catheters or retrieval instruments. A flank or lower abdominal approach may be needed to extract calculi from other areas, such as the kidney calyx or renal pelvis. Percutaneous ultrasonic lithotripsy and extracorporeal shock wave lithotripsy shatter the calculi into fragments for removal by suction or natural passage.

RENAL FAILURE, ACUTE
Acute renal failure is a sudden interruption of renal function. It can be caused by obstruction, poor circulation, or kidney disease. It may be reversible; however, untreated, permanent damage can lead to chronic renal failure.

Pathophysiology
Acute renal failure may be classified as prerenal, intrarenal, or postrenal. Each type has distinct causes. (See *Causes of acute renal failure,* page 382.)

With treatment, each type of acute renal failure passes through three distinct phases: oliguric, diuretic, and recovery.

The oliguric phase is marked by decreased urine output (less than 400 ml/24 hours). Prerenal oliguria results from decreased blood flow to the kidney. Before damage occurs, the kidney re-

Causes of acute renal failure

Acute renal failure is classified as prerenal, intrarenal, or postrenal. Prerenal failure results from a condition that impairs blood flow to the kidneys (renal hypoperfusion) and causes a decreased glomerular filtration rate and increased tubular reabsorption of sodium and water. Intrarenal failure results from damage to the kidneys themselves. Postrenal failure results from obstructed urine flow. This table shows the causes of each type of acute renal failure.

PRERENAL FAILURE	INTRARENAL FAILURE	POSTRENAL FAILURE
CARDIOVASCULAR DISORDERS • Arrhythmias • Cardiac tamponade • Cardiogenic shock • Heart failure • Myocardial infarction **HYPOVOLEMIA** • Burns • Dehydration • Diuretic overuse • Hemorrhage • Hypovolemic shock • Trauma **PERIPHERAL VASODILATION** • Antihypertensive drugs • Sepsis **RENOVASCULAR OBSTRUCTION** • Arterial embolism • Arterial or venous thrombosis • Tumor **SEVERE VASOCONSTRICTION** • Disseminated intravascular coagulation • Eclampsia • Malignant hypertension • Vasculitis	**ACUTE TUBULAR NECROSIS** • Ischemic damage to renal parenchyma from unrecognized or poorly treated prerenal failure • Nephrotoxins, including anesthetics such as methoxyflurane, antibiotics such as gentamicin, heavy metals such as lead, radiographic contrast media, and organic solvents • Obstetric complications, such as eclampsia, postpartum renal failure, septic abortion, and uterine hemorrhage • Pigment release, such as crush injury, myopathy, sepsis, and transfusion reaction **OTHER PARENCHYMAL DISORDERS** • Acute glomerulonephritis • Acute interstitial nephritis • Acute pyelonephritis • Bilateral renal vein thrombosis • Malignant nephrosclerosis • Papillary necrosis • Periarteritis nodosa (inflammatory disease of the arteries) • Renal myeloma • Sickle cell disease • Systemic lupus erythematosus • Vasculitis	**BLADDER OBSTRUCTION** • Anticholinergic drugs • Autonomic nerve dysfunction • Infection • Tumor **URETERAL OBSTRUCTION** • Blood clots • Calculi • Edema or inflammation • Necrotic renal papillae • Retroperitoneal fibrosis or hemorrhage • Surgery (accidental ligation) • Tumor • Uric acid crystals **URETHRAL OBSTRUCTION** • Prostatic hyperplasia or tumor • Strictures

sponds to decreased blood flow by conserving sodium and water. After damage occurs, the kidney's ability to conserve sodium is impaired. Untreated prerenal oliguria may lead to acute tubular necrosis. During this phase, BUN and creatinine levels rise, and the ratio of BUN to creatinine falls from 20:1 (normal) to 10:1. Hypervolemia occurs, causing edema, weight gain, and elevated blood pressure.

The diuretic phase is marked by urine output that can range from normal (1 to 2 L/day) to as high as 4 to 5 L/day. High urine volume results from the kidney's inability to conserve sodium and water and osmotic diuresis produced by a high BUN level. During this phase, BUN and creatinine levels slowly rise, and hypovolemia and weight loss result. This phase lasts several days to 1 week. These conditions can lead to deficits of potassium, sodium, and water that can be deadly if left untreated.

The recovery phase is reached when BUN and creatinine levels have returned to normal and urine output is 1 to 2 L/day.

RED FLAG Primary damage to renal tubules or blood vessels results in kidney failure (intrarenal failure). The causes of intrarenal failure are classified as nephrotoxic, inflammatory, or ischemic. When the damage is from nephrotoxicity or inflammation, the delicate layer under the epithelium (basement membrane) is irreparably damaged, commonly leading to chronic renal failure. Severe or prolonged ischemia may lead to renal damage (ischemic parenchymal injury) and excess nitrogen in the blood (intrinsic renal azotemia).

Signs and symptoms

Signs and symptoms of prerenal failure depend on the cause. If the underlying problem is a change in blood pressure and volume, the patient may have oliguria, tachycardia, hypotension, dry mucous membranes, flat jugular veins, and lethargy progressing to coma. A patient with heart failure will have decreased cardiac output and cool, clammy skin.

As renal failure progresses, the patient may show signs and symptoms of uremia, including confusion, GI complaints, fluid in the lungs, and infection.

About 5% of all hospitalized patients develop acute renal failure. It's usually reversible with treatment; untreated, it may progress to end-stage renal disease, excess urea in the blood, and death.

Test results

These tests are used to diagnose acute renal failure.

TEACHING FOCUS

Acute renal failure teaching topics

- Clearly explain all diagnostic tests, treatments, and procedures.
- Tell the patient about his prescribed drugs, and stress the importance of complying with the regimen.
- Stress the importance of following the prescribed diet and fluid allowance.
- Instruct the patient to weigh himself daily and immediately report changes of 3 lb (1.4 kg) or more.
- Advise the patient against overexertion. Tell him to report shortness of breath during normal activity.
- Teach the patient to recognize and report edema.

- Blood studies reveal elevated BUN, serum creatinine, and potassium levels and decreased hematocrit (HCT) and blood pH, bicarbonate, and hemoglobin levels.
- Urine specimens show casts, cellular debris, decreased specific gravity and, in glomerular diseases, proteinuria and urine osmolality close to serum osmolality. Urine sodium level is less than 20 mEq/L if oliguria results from decreased perfusion and more than 40 mEq/L if it results from an intrarenal problem.
- Creatinine clearance test measures the GFR and is used to estimate the number of remaining functioning nephrons.
- ECG shows tall, peaked T waves, a widening QRS complex, and disappearing P waves if the serum potassium (hyperkalemia) level is increased.
- Other studies that help determine the cause of renal failure include kidney ultrasonography, plain films of the abdomen, KUB radiography, excretory urography, renal scan, retrograde pyelography, computed tomography scan, and nephrotomography.

Treatment
Supportive measures for acute renal failure include:
- a high-calorie diet low in protein, sodium, and potassium
- maintaining fluid and electrolyte balance
- monitoring for signs and symptoms of uremia
- fluid restriction
- diuretic therapy during the oliguric phase
- prevention of infection
- renal-dose dopamine (Intropin) to improve renal perfusion. (See *Acute renal failure teaching topics*.)

Close electrolyte monitoring is needed to detect excess potassium in the blood (hyperkalemia). If symptoms occur, hypertonic glucose, insulin, and sodium bicarbonate are given I.V., and sodium polystyrene sulfonate (Kayexalate) is given by mouth or enema. If these measures fail to control uremia, the patient may need hemodialysis, continuous renal replacement therapy, or peritoneal dialysis.

RENAL FAILURE, CHRONIC

Chronic renal failure, a usually progressive and irreversible deterioration, is the end result of gradual tissue destruction and loss of kidney function. Occasionally, however, chronic renal failure results from a rapidly progressing disease of sudden onset that destroys the nephrons and causes irreversible kidney damage. (See *Effects of aging on kidney function,* page 386.)

Pathophysiology

Chronic renal failure typically progresses through four stages. (See *Stages of chronic renal failure,* page 387.) It may result from:

■ chronic glomerular disease, such as glomerulonephritis, which affects the capillaries in the glomeruli
■ chronic infections, such as chronic pyelonephritis and tuberculosis
■ congenital anomalies, such as polycystic kidney disease
■ vascular diseases, such as hypertension and nephrosclerosis, that cause hardening of the kidneys
■ obstructions such as renal calculi
■ collagen diseases such as lupus erythematosus
■ nephrotoxic agents such as aminoglycosides given long-term
■ endocrine diseases such as diabetic neuropathy.

Nephron damage is progressive. Damaged nephrons can no longer function. Healthy nephrons compensate for destroyed nephrons by enlarging and increasing their clearance capacity. The kidneys can maintain relatively normal function until about 75% of nephrons are nonfunctional. Eventually, the healthy glomeruli are so overburdened they become sclerotic and stiff, leading to their destruction as well. If this condition continues unchecked, toxins accumulate and produce potentially fatal changes in all major organ systems.

RED FLAG *Even if the patient can tolerate life-sustaining maintenance dialysis or a kidney transplant, he may still have anemia, peripheral neuropathy, cardiopulmonary and GI complications, sexual dysfunction, and skeletal defects.*

LIFE STAGES

Effects of aging on kidney function

Although chronic renal failure can occur from infancy to older adulthood, end-stage renal disease is most common in those older than age 65.

After age 40, renal function begins to decline. Decreased glomerular filtration is caused by age-related changes to nephrons and renal vasculature that disturb glomerular hemodynamics as well as by reduced cardiac output and atherosclerotic changes that reduce renal blood flow.

The kidneys' functional units (nephrons) disappear or become nonfunctional with aging. A person age 80 or older may have only half of the number of functioning nephrons that he had as a young adult. These changes predispose elderly patients to chronic renal failure and warrant close monitoring of their fluid and electrolyte status during drug therapy and operative procedures.

Signs and symptoms

Few symptoms develop until more than 75% of glomerular filtration is lost. Then the remaining normal tissue deteriorates progressively. Symptoms worsen as kidney function decreases. Profound changes affect all body systems. Major findings include:

■ anemia
■ azotemia
■ hyperkalemia
■ hyperphosphatemia
■ hypervolemia (abnormal increase in plasma volume)
■ hypocalcemia
■ metabolic acidosis
■ peripheral edema
■ peripheral neuropathy.

Other signs and symptoms vary by body system. Renal signs and symptoms include dry mouth, fatigue, nausea, hypotension, loss of skin turgor, listlessness that may progress to somnolence and confusion, decreased or dilute urine, irregular pulses, and edema. Cardiovascular signs and symptoms include hypertension, irregular pulse, life-threatening arrhythmias, and heart failure.

Respiratory signs and symptoms include infection, crackles, and pleuritic pain. GI signs and symptoms include gum sores and bleeding, hiccups, a metallic taste, anorexia, nausea, vomiting, an ammonia smell to the breath, and abdominal pain on palpation. Neurologic signs and symptoms include an altered level of consciousness, muscle cramps and twitching, and pain, burning, and itching in the legs and feet (restless leg syndrome).

Stages of chronic renal failure

Chronic renal failure may progress through four stages:
- Reduced renal reserve – The glomerular filtration rate (GFR) is 35% to 50% of normal.
- Renal insufficiency – The GFR is 20% to 35% of normal.
- Renal failure – The GFR is 20% to 25% of normal.
- End-stage renal disease – The GFR is less than 20% of normal.

Endocrine signs and symptoms include growth retardation in children, infertility, decreased libido, amenorrhea, and impotence. Hematologic signs and symptoms include GI bleeding, hemorrhage from body orifices, and easy bruising. Musculoskeletal signs and symptoms include fractures, bone and muscle pain, abnormal gait, and impaired bone growth and bowed legs in children. Integumentary signs and symptoms include a pallid, yellowish-bronze skin color; dry, scaly skin; thin, brittle nails; dry, brittle hair that may change color and fall out easily; severe itching; and white, flaky urea deposits (uremic frost) in critically ill patients.

The progression of chronic renal failure can sometimes be slowed, but it's ultimately irreversible, culminating in end-stage renal disease. Although it's fatal without treatment, dialysis or a kidney transplant can sustain life.

Test results

These tests are used to diagnose chronic renal failure.
- Blood studies show decreased arterial pH and bicarbonate levels, low hemoglobin level and HCT, and elevated BUN, serum creatinine, sodium, and potassium levels.
- Arterial blood gas analysis reveals metabolic acidosis.
- Urine specific gravity becomes fixed at 1.010; urinalysis may show proteinuria, glycosuria, RBCs, leukocytes, casts, or crystals, depending on the cause.
- X-ray studies, including KUB radiography, excretory urography, nephrotomography, renal scan, and renal arteriography, show reduced kidney size.
- Renal biopsy is used to identify underlying disease.
- EEG shows changes that indicate brain disease (metabolic encephalopathy).

Chronic renal failure teaching topics

● Teach the patient about prescribed medications. Suggest taking diuretics in the morning to avoid nocturia.

● Instruct an anemic patient to conserve energy by resting often.

● Tell the patient to report leg cramps or excessive muscle twitching. Stress the importance of keeping follow-up appointments to have electrolyte levels monitored.

● Tell the patient to avoid high-sodium and high-potassium foods. Encourage adherence to fluid and protein restrictions. To prevent constipation, stress the need for exercise and sufficient dietary fiber.

● If the patient needs dialysis, make sure he receives complete teaching about the procedure, complications, and post-procedure monitoring.

● Demonstrate how to care for the shunt, fistula, or other vascular access device. Discourage activity that might cause the patient to bump or irritate the access site.

● Suggest that the patient wear or carry medical identification.

Treatment

Treatment for chronic renal failure may consist of one or more of these treatments, depending on the stage of failure. (See *Chronic renal failure teaching topics.*)

CONSERVATIVE MEASURES

Conservative treatment includes:

■ a low-protein diet to reduce end-products of protein metabolism that the kidneys can't excrete
■ a high-protein diet for patients on continuous peritoneal dialysis
■ a high-calorie diet to prevent ketoacidosis (the accumulation of ketones, such as acetone, in the blood) and tissue atrophy
■ sodium and potassium restrictions
■ phosphorus restriction
■ fluid restrictions to maintain fluid balance.

DRUG THERAPY

Drugs used to treat chronic renal failure include:

■ loop diuretics, such as furosemide (Lasix), if some renal function remains, to maintain fluid balance
■ antihypertensives to control blood pressure and edema
■ antiemetics to relieve nausea and vomiting

- histamine$_2$ receptor antagonists, such as famotidine (Pepcid), to decrease gastric irritation
- stool softeners to prevent constipation
- iron and folate supplements or RBC infusion for anemia
- synthetic erythropoietin (Epogen) to stimulate the bone marrow to produce RBCs
- antipruritics, such as promethazine (Phenergan) or diphenhydramine (Benadryl), to relieve itching
- aluminum hydroxide gel (AlternaGEL) to lower serum phosphate levels
- supplementary vitamins, particularly B and D, and essential amino acids.

DIALYSIS

When the kidneys fail, kidney transplantation or dialysis may be the patient's only chance for survival. Dialysis options include hemodialysis, which filters blood through a dialysis machine, and peritoneal dialysis, in which dialysate is instilled through a catheter placed in the peritoneal cavity.

EMERGENCY MEASURES

Potassium level in the blood must be monitored to detect hyperkalemia. Emergency treatment includes dialysis; oral or rectal administration of cation exchange resins, such as sodium polystyrene sulfonate; and I.V. administration of calcium gluconate, sodium bicarbonate, 50% hypertonic glucose, and regular insulin. Cardiac tamponade caused by pericardial effusion may require emergency pericardiocentesis or surgery. Intensive dialysis and thoracentesis can relieve pulmonary edema and pleural effusion.

12

MUSCULOSKELETAL SYSTEM

Understanding the musculoskeletal system

The structures of the musculoskeletal system include muscles, bones, cartilage, joints, bursae, tendons, and ligaments. These structures work together to support the body and produce movement.

MUSCLES

There are three major muscle types: skeletal (voluntary striated muscles), smooth (involuntary muscles), and cardiac (involuntary striated muscles). This chapter focuses on skeletal muscle, which is attached to bone. Skeletal muscle cells are arranged in long bands or strips called *striations*. Skeletal muscle is *voluntary*, meaning it can be contracted at will. (See *A close look at skeletal muscles*, pages 392 and 393.) Smooth muscle, found in the internal organs, such as the gallbladder, lacks striations and is called *involuntary* because it can't be consciously controlled.

Muscle develops when existing muscle fibers grow. Exercise, nutrition, gender, and genetic factors account for variations in muscle strength and size among individuals.

BONES

There are 206 bones in the human body. (See *A close look at the bones*, pages 394 and 395.) They're classified by shape and location and include:

- long, such as arm and leg bones (the humerus, radius, femur, tibia, ulna, and fibula)
- short, such as wrist and ankle bones (the carpals and tarsals)
- flat, such as the shoulder blade (scapula), ribs, and skull

■ irregular, such as bones of the vertebrae and jaw (mandible)
■ sesamoid such as the kneecap (patella).

    Bones of the head and trunk—called the *axial skeleton*—include the facial and cranial bones, the hyoid bone (a U-shaped bone at the base of the tongue, beneath the thyroid cartilage), vertebrae, ribs, and the breast bone (sternum).

    Bones of the extremities—called the *appendicular skeleton*—include the collarbone (clavicle), scapula, humerus, radius, ulna, hand bones (metacarpals), pelvis, femur, patella, fibula, tibia, and foot bones (metatarsals).

    Bones perform many mechanical and physiologic functions. For instance, they protect internal tissues and organs. (For example, 33 vertebrae surround and protect the spinal cord.) They stabilize and support the body. They provide a surface for muscle, ligament, and tendon attachment. They allow movement, through lever action, when muscles contract. They produce red blood cells in the bone marrow (a process called *hematopoiesis*). And they store mineral salts (about 99% of the body's calcium stores, for instance).

CARTILAGE AND BONE FORMATION

Bones begin as cartilage. This dense connective tissue is made up of fibers embedded in a strong, gel-like substance that supports, cushions, and shapes body structures. It's avascular (bloodless) and isn't innervated (supplied with nerves), and it may be fibrous, hyaline, or elastic.

    Fibrous cartilage forms the symphysis pubis and the intervertebral disks. This type of cartilage provides cushioning and strength. Hyaline cartilage covers the articular bone surfaces (where one or more bones meet at a joint). It also appears in the trachea, bronchi, and nasal septum and covers the entire skeleton of the fetus. This type of cartilage cushions against shock. Elastic cartilage is located in the auditory canal, external ear, and epiglottis. It provides support with flexibility.

    At 3 months' gestation, the full fetal skeleton is made of cartilage. At about 6 months' gestation, the cartilage hardens (ossifies) into bony skeleton. The process whereby cartilage hardens into bone is called *endochondral ossification*. In endochondral ossification, bone-forming cells produce a collagenous material called *osteoid* that hardens. Note that *endochondral* means "occurring within cartilage." Some bones—especially those of the wrists and ankles—don't ossify until after a baby's birth.

    Bone-forming cells called *osteoblasts* deposit new bone. In other words, osteoblastic activity results in bone formation. Large cells

(Text continues on page 396.)

A close look at skeletal muscles

The human body has about 600 skeletal muscles. Each is classified by the kind of movement it allows. For example, flexors permit the bending of joints, or flexion. Extensors permit straightening of joints, or extension. These illustrations show some of the major muscles along with their interior structures.

ANTERIOR VIEW

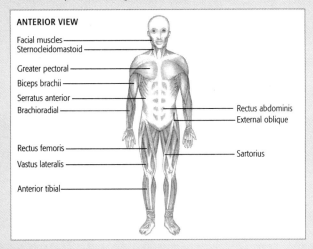

Facial muscles
Sternocleidomastoid

Greater pectoral

Biceps brachii

Serratus anterior

Brachioradial

Rectus abdominis
External oblique

Rectus femoris

Sartorius

Vastus lateralis

Anterior tibial

POSTERIOR VIEW

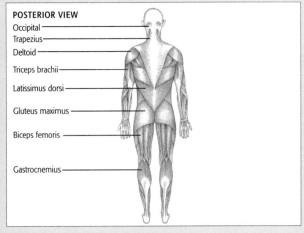

Occipital
Trapezius
Deltoid

Triceps brachii

Latissimus dorsi

Gluteus maximus

Biceps femoris

Gastrocnemius

MUSCLE STRUCTURE

Each muscle contains cells called *muscle fibers* that extend the length of the muscle. A sheath of connective tissues—called the *perimysium*—binds the fibers into a bundle, or fasciculus. A stronger sheath, the epimysium, binds fasciculi together to form the fleshy part of the muscle. Extending be- yond the muscle, the epimysium becomes a tendon. Each muscle fiber is surrounded by a plasma membrane, the sarcolemma. Inside the sacroplasm (or cytoplasm) of the muscle fiber lie tiny myofibrils. Arranged lengthwise, myofibrils contain still finer fibers, called thick fibers and thin fibers.

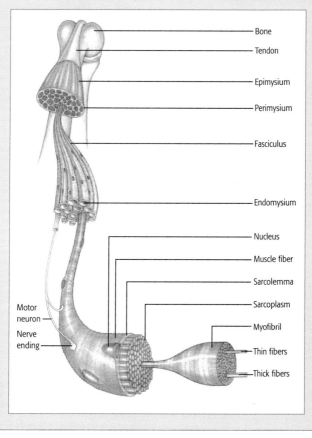

- Bone
- Tendon
- Epimysium
- Perimysium
- Fasciculus
- Endomysium
- Nucleus
- Muscle fiber
- Sarcolemma
- Sarcoplasm
- Myofibril
- Thin fibers
- Thick fibers

Motor neuron

Nerve ending

...ose look at the bones

The skeleton contains 206 bones; 80 form the axial skeleton and 126 form the appendicular skeleton. These illustrations show some major bones, bone groups, and the interior structure of a bone.

Bone consists of layers of calcified matrix containing spaces occupied by osteocytes (bone cells). Bone layers (lamellae) are arranged concentrically around central canals (haversian canals). Small cavities (lacunae) lying between the lamellae contain osteocytes. Tiny canals (canaliculi) connect the lacunae. These canals form the structural units and provide nutrients to bone tissue.

A TYPICAL LONG BONE

A typical long bone has a diaphysis (main shaft) and an epiphysis (end). The epiphyses are separated from the diaphysis with cartilage at the epiphyseal line. Beneath the epiphyseal articular surface lies the articular cartilage, which cushions the joint.

BENEATH THE BONE SURFACE

Each bone has an outer layer of dense compact bone containing haversian systems and an inner layer of spongy (cancellous) bone composed of thin plates, called *trabeculae* that interface to form a latticework. Red marrow fills the spaces between the trabeculae of some bones. Cancellous bone doesn't contain haversian systems.

Compact bone is located in the diaphyses of long bones and the outer layers of short, flat, and irregular bones. Cancellous bone

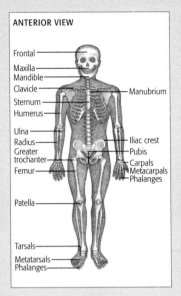

ANTERIOR VIEW

Frontal
Maxilla
Mandible
Clavicle
Sternum
Humerus
Ulna
Radius
Greater trochanter
Femur
Patella
Tarsals
Metatarsals
Phalanges

Manubrium
Iliac crest
Pubis
Carpals
Metacarpals
Phalanges

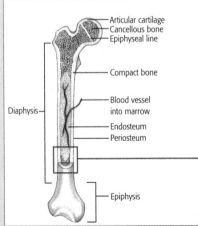

INTERNAL VIEW OF LONG BONE

Articular cartilage
Cancellous bone
Epiphyseal line

Compact bone

Blood vessel into marrow
Endosteum
Periosteum

Diaphysis

Epiphysis

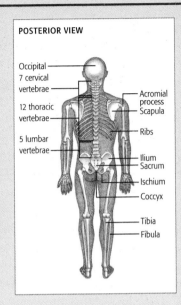

POSTERIOR VIEW

- Occipital
- 7 cervical vertebrae
- 12 thoracic vertebrae
- 5 lumbar vertebrae
- Acromial process
- Scapula
- Ribs
- Ilium
- Sacrum
- Ischium
- Coccyx
- Tibia
- Fibula

fills central regions of the epiphyses and the inner portions of short, flat, and irregular bones. Periosteum—specialized fibrous connective tissue—consists of an outer fibrous layer and an inner bone-forming layer. Endosteum (a membrane that contains osteoblast-producing cells) lines the medullary cavity (inner surface of bone, which contains the marrow).

Blood reaches bone by way of arterioles in haversian canals; vessels in Volkmann's canals, which enter bone matrix from the periosteum; and vessels in the bone ends and within the marrow. In children, the periosteum is thicker than in adults and has an increased blood supply to assist new bone formation around the shaft.

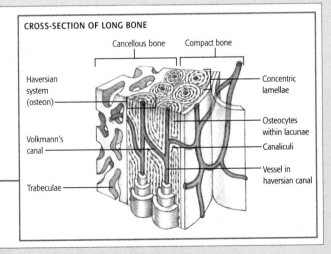

CROSS-SECTION OF LONG BONE

- Cancellous bone
- Compact bone
- Haversian system (osteon)
- Volkmann's canal
- Trabeculae
- Concentric lamellae
- Osteocytes within lacunae
- Canaliculi
- Vessel in haversian canal

called *osteoclasts* reabsorb material from previously formed bones, tearing down old or excess bone structure and allowing osteoblasts to rebuild new bone (a process called *resorption*). Osteoblastic and osteoclastic activity promotes longitudinal bone growth. This growth continues until adolescence, when bones stop lengthening. During adolescence, the epiphyseal growth plates located at bone ends close.

Osteoblasts and osteoclasts are responsible for remodeling — the continuous creation and destruction of bone in the body. When osteoblasts complete their bone-forming function and are located in the mineralized bone matrix, they transform into osteocytes (mature bone cells). Bone renewal continues throughout life, although it slows down with age.

Estrogen secretion plays a role in calcium uptake and release and helps regulate osteoblastic activity (bone formation). Decreased estrogen levels have been linked to decreased osteoblastic activity.

A person's sex, race, and age also influence bone mass, its ability to withstand stress, and bone loss. Men typically have denser bones than women; Blacks typically have denser bones than Whites. Bone density and structural integrity decrease after age 30 in women and after age 45 in men.

JOINTS

The union of two or more bones is called a *joint.* The body contains three major types of joints, classified by how much movement they allow. Synarthrosis joints allow no movement, such as the joints between skull bones. Amphidiarthrosis joints allow slight movement, such as the joints between vertebrae. Diarthrosis joints allow free movement, such as the ankle, wrist, knee, hip, and shoulder. Joints are further classified by shape and connective structure, such as fibrous, cartilaginous, and synovial.

In a free-moving joint, a fluid-filled space known as the *joint space* exists between the bones. The synovial membrane, which lines this cavity, secretes a viscous lubricating substance called *synovial fluid,* which allows two bones to move against one another without friction. Ligaments, tendons, and muscles help to stabilize the joint.

Bursae (small sacs of synovial fluid) are located at friction points around joints and between tendons, ligaments, and bones. In joints, such as the shoulder and knee, they act as cushions, easing stress on adjacent structures.

Ligaments are dense, strong, flexible bands of fibrous connective tissue that tie bones to other bones. Ligaments that connect the joint ends of bones either limit or facilitate movement. They also provide stability.

Tendons are bands of fibrous connective tissue that attach muscles to the fibrous membrane that covers the bones (the *periosteum*). Tendons enable bones to move when skeletal muscles contract.

MOVEMENT

Skeletal movement results mainly from muscle contractions, although other musculoskeletal structures also play a role. Here's a general description of how body movement takes place.

Skeletal muscle is loaded with blood vessels and nerves. To contract, it needs an impulse from the nervous system and oxygen and nutrients from the blood. When a skeletal muscle contracts, force is applied to the tendon that connects it to a bone. The force pulls one bone toward, away from, or around a second bone, depending on the type of muscle that contracted and the type of joint involved. Usually, one bone moves less than the other. The tendon's attachment to the more stationary bone is called the *origin;* the attachment to the more movable bone is the insertion site.

The 13 angular and circular musculoskeletal movements are:

■ circumduction — moving in a circular manner
■ flexion — bending, decreasing the joint angle
■ extension — straightening, increasing the joint angle
■ internal rotation — turning toward midline
■ external rotation — turning away from midline
■ abduction — moving away from midline
■ adduction — moving toward midline
■ supination — turning upward
■ pronation — turning downward
■ eversion — turning outward
■ inversion — turning inward
■ retraction — moving backward
■ protraction — moving forward.

Most movement involves groups of muscles rather than one muscle. Most skeletal movement is mechanical; the bones act as levers and the joints act as fulcrums (points of support for movement of the bones).

Musculoskeletal disorders

The musculoskeletal disorders discussed in this chapter include:

■ carpal tunnel syndrome
■ gout
■ osteoarthritis
■ osteomyelitis

- osteoporosis
- rhabdomyolysis.

CARPAL TUNNEL SYNDROME

The most common of the nerve entrapment syndromes, carpal tunnel syndrome results from compression of the median nerve at the carpal tunnel in the wrist. This nerve passes through the carpal tunnel, along with blood vessels and flexor tendons, to the fingers and thumb. The compression neuropathy causes sensory and motor changes in the hand, especially the palm and middle finger.

Carpal tunnel syndrome usually occurs between ages 30 and 60 and poses a serious occupational health problem. Those who use a computer often, assembly-line workers and packers, and people who repeatedly use poorly designed tools are most likely to develop this disorder. Any strenuous use of the hands — sustained grasping, twisting, or flexing — aggravates this condition.

Pathophysiology

The carpal tunnel is formed by the carpal bones and the transverse carpal ligament. Inflammation or fibrosis of the tendon sheaths that pass through the carpal tunnel typically causes edema and compression of the median nerve. (See *A close look at the carpal tunnel.*)

Many conditions can cause the contents or structure of the carpal tunnel to swell and press the median nerve against the transverse carpal ligament, including acromegaly, amyloidosis, benign tumors, diabetes mellitus, edema following Colles' fracture, hypothyroidism, menopause, myxedema, pregnancy, renal failure, rheumatoid arthritis, and tuberculosis.

Another source of damage to the median nerve is dislocation or an acute sprain of the wrist.

RED FLAG *Continued use of the affected wrist may increase tendon inflammation, compression, and neural ischemia, causing a decrease in wrist function. Untreated carpal tunnel syndrome can produce permanent nerve damage with loss of movement and sensation.*

Signs and symptoms

A patient with carpal tunnel syndrome usually complains of weakness, pain, burning, numbness, or tingling in one or both hands. This paresthesia affects the thumb, forefinger, middle finger, and half of the fourth finger. The patient can't clench his hand into a fist. The nails may be atrophic and the skin dry and shiny.

Symptoms are usually worse at night and in the morning. The pain may spread to the forearm and, in severe cases, as far as the

A close look at the carpal tunnel

The carpal tunnel is clearly visible in this cross-section of the right hand.

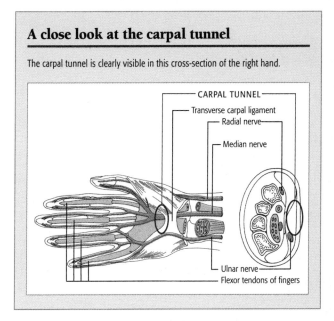

CARPAL TUNNEL
- Transverse carpal ligament
- Radial nerve
- Median nerve
- Ulnar nerve
- Flexor tendons of fingers

shoulder. The patient usually can relieve such pain by shaking his hands vigorously or dangling his arms at his side.

Test results
- Physical examination reveals decreased sensation to light touch or pinpricks in the affected fingers. Thenar (palm) muscle atrophy occurs in about half of those with carpal tunnel syndrome.
- The patient has a positive Tinel's sign (tingling over the median nerve on light percussion) and Phalen's wrist-flexion test (holding the wrists in complete flexion for 1 minute reproduces symptoms of carpal tunnel syndrome).
- A compression test supports the diagnosis. A blood pressure cuff inflated above systolic pressure on the forearm for 1 to 2 minutes provokes pain and paresthesia along the distribution of the median nerve.
- Electromyography detects a median nerve motor conduction delay of more than 5 milliseconds.
- Other laboratory tests may identify underlying disease.

TEACHING FOCUS
Carpal tunnel syndrome teaching topics

- Teach the patient how to apply a splint correctly. Tell her to remove it to perform gentle range-of-motion exercises daily.
- Advise the patient to occasionally exercise her hands in warm water. If she's using a sling, tell her to remove it several times a day to exercise her elbow and shoulder.
- If the patient needs surgery, explain preoperative and postoperative care.
- Suggest occupational counseling for a patient who has to change jobs because of carpal tunnel syndrome.

Treatment

Initial treatment should be conservative, such as resting the hands by splinting the wrists in neutral extension for 1 to 2 weeks. If a definite link has been established between the patient's occupation and the development of carpal tunnel syndrome, he should alter his work environment, if possible — or seek other work, if needed. Effective treatment also may require correction of an underlying disorder. (See *Carpal tunnel syndrome teaching topics.*)

DRUG THERAPY

Nonsteroidal anti-inflammatory drugs (NSAIDs) are commonly given to decrease inflammation around the nerve and relieve symptoms. Steroids may be injected directly into the carpal tunnel to decrease swelling and inflammation around the median nerve.

SURGICAL INTERVENTION

If conservative treatment fails, the only alternative is surgical decompression of the nerve by resecting the entire transverse carpal tunnel ligament or by using endoscopic surgical techniques. Neurolysis (freeing of the nerve fibers) also may be needed.

GOUT

This metabolic disease is marked by red, swollen, and acutely painful joints. Gout may affect any joint but is found mostly in joints of the feet, especially the great toe, ankle, and midfoot.

Pathophysiology

Primary gout usually occurs in men older than age 30 and in postmenopausal women who take diuretics. It follows an intermittent course. Between attacks, patients may be symptom-free for years.

The underlying cause of primary gout is unknown. In many patients it results from decreased excretion of uric acid by the kidneys. In a few patients, gout is linked to a genetic defect that causes overproduction of uric acid. This is called *hyperuricemia*.

Secondary gout may develop in the wake of another disease, such as obesity, diabetes mellitus, high blood pressure, leukemia and other blood disorders, bone cancer, and kidney disease. Secondary gout can also follow treatment with certain drugs, such as hydrochlorothiazide (Microzide) or pyrazinamide.

Untreated, gout progresses in four stages. During the first stage, the patient develops hyperuricemia; urate levels rise but don't produce symptoms. The second stage is marked by acute gouty arthritis, in which the patient experiences painful swelling and tenderness. Symptoms usually lead the patient to seek medical attention. The third stage, the interictal stage, may last for months to years. The patient may be asymptomatic or have flare-ups.

The fourth stage is the chronic stage. Without treatment, urate pooling may continue for years. Tophi may develop in cartilage, synovial membranes, tendons, and soft tissues. Tophi are clusters of urate crystals, typically surrounded by inflamed tissue. (See *A close look at gout tophi,* page 402.) They can deform and destroy hard and soft tissue. In joints, tophi lead to the destruction of cartilage and bone as well as other degeneration. This final unremitting stage of the disease is also known as *tophaceous gout.*

Tophi form in diverse areas, including the hands, knees, feet, the outer sides of the forearms, the pinna of the ear, and the Achilles tendon. Rarely, internal organs, such as the kidneys and heart, may be affected. Kidney involvement may cause kidney dysfunction.

Urates are uric acid salts. They predominate in the plasma, fluid around the cells, and synovial fluid. Hyperuricemia, the hallmark of gout, is a plasma urate concentration greater than 420 μmol/L (7 mg/dl). Hyperuricemia indicates increased total-body urate. Excess urates result from increased urate production, decreased excretion of uric acid, or a combination of the two. In hyperuricemia, plasma and extracellular fluids are supersaturated with urate. This leads to urate crystal formation. When crystals are deposited in other tissues, a gout attack occurs.

Many factors may provoke an acute attack of gout, including:

■ excessive intake of foods containing purine
■ hospitalization
■ infection
■ some drugs
■ starvation

A close look at gout tophi

In advanced gout, urate crystal deposits develop into hard, irregular, yellow-white nodules called *tophi*. These bumps commonly protrude from the great toe and the pinna, as shown.

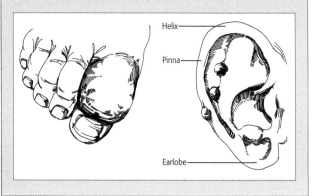

Helix

Pinna

Earlobe

■ stress
■ surgery
■ trauma
■ use of alcohol
■ weight reduction.

   A sudden increase in serum urate level may cause new crystals to form. A drop in serum and extracellular urate levels may cause previously formed crystals to partially dissolve and be excreted.

   Patients who receive treatment for gout have a good prognosis. ***RED FLAG*** *Potential complications include kidney disorders, such as renal calculi; infection that develops with tophi rupture and nerve damage; and circulatory problems, such as atherosclerotic disease, cardiovascular lesions, stroke, coronary thrombosis, and hypertension.*

Signs and symptoms

In some patients, serum urate levels increase but produce no symptoms. In symptom-producing gout, the first acute attack strikes suddenly and peaks quickly. Although it may involve only one or a few joints, the first acute attack causes extreme pain. Untreated gout attacks usually resolve in 10 to 14 days. Mild acute attacks usually subside quickly but tend to recur at irregular intervals. Severe attacks may last for days or weeks.

Patients with gout usually have no symptoms between attacks. Most have a second attack 6 months to 2 years after the first; in some patients, however, the second attack is delayed for 5 to 10 years. Delayed attacks, which may involve several joints, are more common in untreated patients. These attacks tend to last longer and produce more symptoms than initial episodes.

Chronic gout is marked by numerous, persistently painful joints. With tophi development, joints are typically swollen and dusky red or purple, with limited movement. Tophi — hard, irregular, yellow-white nodules — may be seen, especially on the ears, hands, and feet. Late in chronic gout, skin over the tophi may ulcerate and release a chalky white exudate or pus. Chronic inflammation and tophi lead to joint degeneration, deformity, and disability.

Warmth and extreme tenderness may be felt over the joint. The patient may have a sedentary lifestyle and a history of hypertension and renal calculi. The patient may wake during the night with pain in the great toe or other part of the foot. Initially moderate pain may grow so intense that eventually the patient can't bear the weight of bed linens or the vibrations of a person walking across the room. He may report chills and a mild fever.

Test results
These tests aid in the diagnosis of gout.
- Needle aspiration of synovial fluid (called *arthrocentesis*) or of tophi for microscopic examination reveals needlelike crystals of sodium urate in the cells and establishes the diagnosis. If test results identify calcium pyrophosphate crystals, the patient probably has pseudogout, a disease similar to gout.
- Blood and urine analysis reveal serum and urine uric acid levels.
- X-rays initially are normal. However, in chronic gout, X-rays show damage to cartilage and bone. Outward displacement of the overhanging margin from the bone contour characterizes gout.

Treatment
Treatment for gout varies, depending on whether gout is acute or chronic, and aims to terminate an acute attack, reduce uric acid levels, and prevent recurrent gout and renal calculi.

ACUTE ATTACKS
Treatment of an acute attack includes elevating the limb, when possible; immobilizing and protecting inflamed, painful joints; and lo-

cal application of cold. A bed cradle can be used to keep bed linens off sensitive, inflamed joints.

Analgesics, such as acetaminophen (Tylenol), relieve the pain of mild attacks. Acute inflammation requires NSAIDs or, if the patient is hospitalized, I.V. corticosteroids. Colchicine or oral corticosteroids are used occasionally to treat acute attacks, although they don't affect uric acid levels. Because acute gout can attack 24 to 96 hours after surgery — even minor surgery — colchicine may be given before and after surgery as prevention. The patient also should drink plenty of fluids (at least 2 qt [2 L]/day) to help prevent renal calculi.

CHRONIC GOUT
To treat chronic gout, serum uric acid levels are reduced to less than 6.5 mg/dl using various drugs, depending on whether the patient overproduces or underproduces uric acid. If he overproduces uric acid, he may be given allopurinol (Zyloprim). If he underproduces uric acid, he may be treated with probenecid (Benemid) or sulfinpyrazone (Anturane).

Serum uric acid levels should be monitored regularly and sodium bicarbonate or other agents given to alkalinize the urine.

ADJUNCTIVE THERAPY
Adjunctive therapy emphasizes avoiding alcohol (especially beer and wine) and purine-rich foods (which raise urate levels), such as anchovies, liver, sardines, kidneys, sweetbreads, and lentils. Dietary

restriction and weight loss also may be part of care. (See *Gout teaching topics.*) Obese patients should begin a weight-loss program to decreases uric acid levels and stress on painful joints. To diffuse anxiety and promote coping, the patient should be encouraged to express his concerns about his condition.

OSTEOARTHRITIS

Osteoarthritis, the most common form of arthritis, is widespread and equally common among men and women. It's most common after age 40; its earliest symptoms typically begin in middle age and may progress with advancing age.

Primary osteoarthritis, a normal part of aging, results from many things, including metabolic factors, genetics, and chemical and mechanical factors. Secondary osteoarthritis usually follows an identifiable predisposing event — most commonly trauma, congenital deformity, or obesity — and leads to degenerative changes.

Pathophysiology

Osteoarthritis is chronic, causing deterioration of the joint cartilage and formation of reactive new bone at the margins and subchondral (below the cartilage) areas of the joints. This degeneration results from a breakdown of chondrocytes (cartilage cells), most commonly in the hips and knees.

RED FLAG Osteoarthritis can cause flexion contractures, subluxation and deformity, ankylosis, bony cysts, gross bony overgrowth, central cord syndrome (with cervical spine osteoarthritis), nerve root compression, and cauda equina syndrome.

Signs and symptoms

The most common symptom of osteoarthritis is a deep, aching joint pain, particularly after exercise or weight bearing, that's usually relieved by rest. Other signs and symptoms of osteoarthritis include stiffness in the morning and after exercise (relieved by rest), aching during changes in weather, "grating" of the joint during motion, altered gait contractures, and limited movement. These changes increase with poor posture, obesity, and occupational stress.

Osteoarthritis in the fingers produces irreversible changes in the joints. (See *A close look at the effects of osteoarthritis,* page 406.)

Test results

A thorough physical examination confirms typical symptoms, and the absence of systemic symptoms rules out an inflammatory joint disorder. No laboratory test is specific for osteoarthritis.

A close look at the effects of osteoarthritis

Involvement of the interphalangeal (finger bone) joints produces irreversible changes in the distal joints (Heberden's nodes) and proximal joints (Bouchard's nodes), as shown. These nodes can be painless at first, with gradual progression to or sudden flare-ups of redness, swelling, tenderness, and impaired sensation and dexterity.

HEBERDEN'S NODE

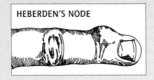

BOUCHARD'S NODE

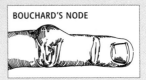

X-rays of the affected joint help confirm the diagnosis but may be normal in the early stages. Diagnosis may require many views, and X-rays typically show:
- bony growths at weight-bearing areas
- cystlike bony deposits in the joint space and margins
- fusion of joints
- joint deformity from degeneration or articular damage
- narrowing of the joint space or margins
- sclerosis of the subchondral space.

Treatment

The goal of osteoarthritis treatment is to relieve pain, maintain or improve mobility, and minimize disability. It may include drug therapy, other noninvasive interventions, and surgical interventions.

DRUG THERAPY

Drugs used to treat osteoarthritis include acetaminophen (Tylenol), aspirin (Genuine Bayer) or other nonopioid analgesics, celecoxib (Celebrex), ibuprofen (Motrin), and meloxicam (Mobic).

In some cases, intra-articular injections of corticosteroids given every 4 to 6 months may delay development of nodes in the hands.

NONINVASIVE INTERVENTIONS

Additional treatments may include weight loss to help decrease stress on joints. Also, strengthening exercises for muscles around the knee and hip help stabilize these joints and improve alignment of the articular surfaces, preventing further cartilage deterioration.

TEACHING FOCUS

Osteoarthritis teaching topics

- Caution the patient against overexertion. Explain that he should take care to stand and walk correctly, to minimize weight-bearing activities, and to be especially careful when bending over.
- Instruct him to take drugs exactly as prescribed. Tell him which adverse reactions to report immediately.
- Recommend that safety devices be installed in the home such as grab bars in the bathroom.

- Teach the patient to do gentle range-of-motion exercises.
- Advise maintaining proper body weight to minimize strain on joints.
- Teach the patient how to use crutches or other orthopedic devices properly. Stress the importance of proper fitting and regular professional adjustment of such devices. Warn that impaired sensation might allow tissue damage from these aids without discomfort.

Exercise may help with weight management as well. (See *Osteoarthritis teaching topics*.) Treatment also may include supporting or stabilizing the joint with crutches, braces, a cane, a walker, a cervical collar, or traction.

SURGICAL INTERVENTIONS
Surgical treatment, reserved for patients with severe disability or uncontrollable pain, may include the following:
- arthroplasty — replacing the deteriorated part of a joint with a prosthesis
- arthrodesis — surgically fusing bones, usually in the spine (laminectomy)
- osteoplasty — scraping and lavage of deteriorated bone from a joint
- osteotomy — changing bone alignment to relieve stress by excising a bone wedge or cutting a bone.

OSTEOMYELITIS
Osteomyelitis is a bone infection characterized by progressive inflammatory bone destruction after formation of new bone. It may be acute or chronic and commonly results from a combination of local trauma — usually trivial but causing a hematoma — and an acute infection originating elsewhere in the body. Although osteomyelitis typically remains localized, it can spread through the bone to the marrow, cortex, and periosteum.

Acute osteomyelitis is usually a blood-borne disease and most commonly affects rapidly growing children. Chronic osteomyelitis, which is rare, is characterized by draining sinus tracts and widespread lesions. (See *Age and osteomyelitis*.)

Pathophysiology

The most common causative organism in osteomyelitis is *Staphylococcus aureus*. Other organisms that can cause it include:

■ *Streptococcus pyogenes*
■ pneumococcus
■ *Pseudomonas aeruginosa*
■ *E. coli*
■ *Proteus vulgaris*
■ *Pasteurella multocida* (part of the normal mouth flora of cats and dogs).

Typically, these organisms begin multiplying in a hematoma (from recent trauma) or in a weakened area, such as the site of local infection, and travel through the bloodstream to the metaphysis, the section of a long bone that's continuous with the epiphysis plates, where blood flows into sinusoids.

RED FLAG Osteomyelitis may lead to chronic infection, skeletal deformities, joint deformities, disturbed bone growth (in children), differing leg lengths, and impaired mobility.

Signs and symptoms

Signs and symptoms of acute osteomyelitis may include:

■ rapid onset (acute osteomyelitis) of sudden pain in the affected bone along with tenderness, heat, swelling, erythema, guarding of the affected area of the limb, and restricted movement
■ chronic intermittent infection persisting for years, flaring after minor trauma or persisting as drainage of pus from an old pocket in a sinus tract (usually chronic osteomyelitis, although acute form may progress to this)

TEACHING FOCUS

Osteomyelitis teaching topics

- Explain all tests and treatment procedures.
- Review prescribed drugs. Discuss possible adverse reactions, and instruct the patient or parent to report them.
- Before surgery, explain preoperative and postoperative procedures to the patient and his family.
- Teach the patient techniques for promoting rest and relaxation.

- Before discharge, teach the patient or parent how to protect and clean the wound site and how to recognize signs of recurring infection.
- Urge the patient or parent to schedule follow-up examinations and to seek treatment for possible sources of recurrent infection, such as blisters, boils, sties, and impetigo.

- fever
- dehydration in children
- irritability and poor feeding in infants.

Test results
These test results help diagnose osteomyelitis.
- White blood cell count shows leukocytosis.
- Erythrocyte sedimentation rate is elevated.
- Blood cultures reveal the causative organism.
- Magnetic resonance imaging (MRI) delineates bone marrow from soft tissue to show the extent of the infection.
- X-rays show bone involvement after the disease has been active for 2 to 3 weeks.
- Bone scan detects early infection.

Treatment
Treatment should begin as soon as osteomyelitis is suspected. (See *Osteomyelitis teaching topics.*) For acute osteomyelitis, it includes drug therapy and other interventions. Drugs include I.V. antibiotics after blood cultures are obtained, analgesics to relieve pain, and intracavity instillation of antibiotics. Other interventions may include surgical drainage to relieve pressure and abscess formation, I.V. fluids to maintain hydration, and immobilization of the affected body part.

For chronic osteomyelitis, treatment may include surgery to remove dead bone and aid drainage, hyperbaric oxygen to stimulate healing, and skin, bone, and muscle grafts to increase blood supply.

OSTEOPOROSIS

Osteoporosis is a metabolic disorder in which the rate of bone resorption increases and the rate of bone formation decreases. The result is decreased bone mass. Bones affected by this disease lose calcium and phosphate and become porous, brittle, and abnormally prone to fracture. Osteoporosis is four times more common in women than in men. White and Asian women are more likely to develop the disease than Black or Hispanic women.

Pathophysiology

Osteoporosis may be a primary disorder or occur secondary to an underlying disease. The cause of primary osteoporosis is unknown. However, contributing factors include:

■ mild but prolonged lack of calcium from poor dietary intake or an age-related decrease in absorption by the intestine
■ hormonal imbalance caused by endocrine dysfunction
■ faulty metabolism of protein from estrogen deficiency
■ a sedentary lifestyle. (See *Primary osteoporosis classifications*.)

Secondary osteoporosis may result from:

■ alcoholism
■ bone immobilization or disuse, such as paralysis
■ hyperthyroidism
■ lactose intolerance
■ liver disease
■ malabsorption of calcium
■ malnutrition
■ osteogenesis imperfecta (an inherited condition that causes brittle bones)
■ prolonged therapy with steroids or heparin
■ rheumatoid arthritis
■ scurvy
■ smoking
■ trauma leading to atrophy in the hands and feet, with recurring attacks (Sudeck's disease).

Osteoporosis is characterized by a reduction in the bone matrix and in remineralization, resulting in soft bones that fracture easily. Bone mass is lost because of an imbalance between bone resorption and formation. Cancellous bone, the inner layer of spongy bone, is composed of trabeculae, which are sharp, needlelike structures forming a meshwork of interconnecting spaces. Trabeculae have a larger surface volume than compact bone (the outer layer of dense bone) and therefore are lost more rapidly as bone mass decreases. This loss leads to fractures.

Primary osteoporosis classifications

Primary osteoporosis is classified as one of three types:

● Postmenopausal osteoporosis (type I) usually affects women ages 51 to 75. It's related to the loss of estrogen and its protective effect on bone and is characterized by vertebral and wrist fractures.

● Senile osteoporosis (type II) occurs mostly between ages 70 and 85.

It's related to osteoblast or osteoclast shrinkage or decreased physical activity and characterized by fractures of the humerus, tibia, femur, and pelvis.

● Premenopausal osteoporosis (type III) involves higher estrogen levels that may inhibit bone resorption by affecting the sensitivity of osteoclasts to parathyroid hormone.

> **RED FLAG** *Bone fractures are the major complication of osteoporosis. They occur most commonly in the vertebrae, femoral neck, and distal radius.*

Signs and symptoms

Redness, warmth, and new sites of pain may indicate new fractures.

The patient is typically postmenopausal or has one of the conditions that cause secondary osteoporosis. She may report that she heard a snapping sound and felt a sudden pain in her lower back when she bent down to lift something. Or, she may say that the pain developed slowly over several years. If the patient has vertebral collapse, she may describe a backache and pain radiating around the trunk. Movement or jarring aggravates the pain.

The patient may have a humped back (dowager's hump); the curvature worsens with repeated vertebral fractures. The abdomen eventually protrudes to compensate for the changed center of gravity. The patient commonly reports a gradual loss of height, decreased exercise tolerance, and trouble breathing. Height may be reduced as much as 7″. Palpation may reveal muscle spasm. The patient also may have decreased spinal movement, with flexion more limited than extension.

Test results

A diagnosis excludes other causes of bone disease, especially those that affect the spine, such as cancer or tumors. These tests help confirm a diagnosis of osteoporosis.

- X-rays show characteristic degeneration in the lower vertebrae. Loss of bone mineral appears in later disease.
- Serum calcium, phosphorus, and alkaline phosphatase levels remain within normal limits; parathyroid hormone (PTH) levels may be elevated.
- Bone biopsy allows direct examination of changes in bone cells.
- Computed tomography (CT) scan allows accurate assessment of spinal bone loss.
- Radionuclide bone scans display injured or diseased areas as darker portions.
- Dual photon or dual energy X-ray absorptiometry can detect bone loss in a safe, noninvasive test.
- Bone density measurements confirm the diagnosis.

Treatment

Treatment focuses on a physical therapy program of gentle exercise and activity and drug therapy to slow the disease's progress. Care seeks to control bone loss, prevent fractures, and control pain.

Measures may include supportive devices, such as a back brace, and possible surgery to correct fractures. Estrogen (Premarin) may be prescribed within 3 years after menopause to decrease the rate of bone resorption. A balanced diet should be rich in nutrients, such as vitamin D, calcium, and protein, to support skeletal metabolism. Low-impact, weight-bearing exercises can help stimulate osteoblast formation. Heat may be applied to relieve pain.

Drugs used to treat osteoporosis include:
- analgesics to relieve pain
- alendronate (Fosamax), risedronate (Actonel), or raloxifene (Evista) to treat and prevent osteoporosis
- calcium and vitamin D supplements to support normal bone metabolism
- calcitonin (Calcimar) to reduce bone resorption and slow the decline in bone mass
- etidronate (Didronel), the first agent proved to increase bone density and restore lost bone by inhibiting osteoblast activity
- teriparatide (Forteo), an injectable form of human PTH, for postmenopausal women and men with osteoporosis who are at high risk for developing fractures; the drug stimulates bone formation in the spine and hips.

Preventing falls is the top priority. Safety precautions include keeping side rails up on the patient's bed and always moving the patient gently and carefully. (See *Osteoporosis teaching topics*.) Caution ancillary staff about how easily the patient's bones can fracture.

Osteoporosis teaching topics

- Thoroughly explain osteoporosis to the patient and her family.
- Explain all treatments, tests, and procedures. Make sure the patient and her family clearly understand the prescribed drug regimen. Teach them to recognize and immediately report significant adverse reactions.
- If the patient takes a calcium supplement, encourage liberal fluid intake to help maintain adequate urine output and thereby avoid renal calculi, hypercalcemia, and hypercalciuria.

- Tell the patient to report new pain sites immediately, especially after trauma.
- Demonstrate proper body mechanics. Show the patient how to stoop before lifting anything and how to avoid twisting movements and prolonged bending.
- Encourage adequate dietary calcium intake and regular exercise to help prevent some forms of osteoporosis.

RHABDOMYOLYSIS

Rhabdomyolysis, a disease involving the breakdown of muscle tissue, may cause myoglobinuria, in which varying amounts of muscle protein (myoglobin) appear in urine. It usually follows major muscle trauma, especially a crush injury. Long-distance running, certain severe infections, and exposure to electric shock also can cause extensive muscle damage and excessive release of myoglobin.

The prognosis is good if contributing causes are discovered and eliminated or if the disease is stopped before damage has become irreversible. Unchecked, rhabdomyolysis can cause renal failure.

Pathophysiology

Possible causes of rhabdomyolysis include:
- alcohol abuse and use of illicit drugs
- anesthetics, such as halothane, that cause intraoperative rigidity
- cardiac arrhythmias
- drugs, including HMG-CoA reductase inhibitors (especially with nicotinic acid), cyclosporine (Sandimmune), itraconazole (Sporanox), erythromycin (E-Mycin), colchicine, zidovudine (Retrovir), and corticosteroids
- electrolyte disturbances
- excessive muscle activity caused by status epilepticus, electroconvulsive therapy, or high-voltage electric shock
- familial tendency
- heatstroke
- infection and inflammatory processes
- strenuous exertion.

TEACHING FOCUS

Rhabdomyolysis teaching topics

- Explain rhabdomyolysis to the patient and his family. Also explain all needed tests, treatments, and procedures.
- Urge the patient to report pain or numbness in the extremities.

RED FLAG Trauma that compresses tissue causes ischemia and necrosis. Local edema further increases compartment pressure and tamponade; pressure from severe swelling causes blood vessels to collapse, leading to tissue hypoxia, muscle infarction, and neural damage in the area. Myoglobin, potassium, creatine kinase, and urate are released from the necrotic muscle fibers into the circulation.

Signs and symptoms

Local signs and symptoms include pain, tenderness, swelling, and muscle weakness caused by muscle trauma and pressure. Systemic signs and symptoms include urine that darkens and becomes reddish brown as myoglobin enters it, fever, malaise, nausea, vomiting, confusion, agitation, delirium, and anuria.

Test results

These diagnostic tests help confirm rhabdomyolysis.
- Urine myoglobin level is greater than 0.5 mg/dl.
- Creatine kinase level is severely elevated.
- Serum potassium, phosphate, and creatinine levels are elevated.
- Calcium level declines in early stages and rises in later stages.
- CT scan, MRI, and bone scintigraphy reveal muscle necrosis.
- Intracompartmental venous pressure measurements are elevated.

Treatment

Therapy for rhabdomyolysis typically includes treating the underlying disorder and measures to prevent renal failure. (See *Rhabdomyolysis teaching topics.*) These measures may be used for treatment:
- analgesics to relieve pain
- anti-inflammatory drugs
- bed rest
- corticosteroids in extreme cases
- if compartment venous pressure exceeds 25 mm Hg, immediate fasciotomy and debridement to reduce pressure and aid circulation
- I.V. hydration started as early as possible.

Less common disorders

Selected references

Index

Less common disorders

DISEASES AND CAUSES	PATHOPHYSIOLOGY	SIGNS AND SYMPTOMS
AMYLOIDOSIS • Pressure caused by accumulation and infiltration of amyloid that leads to atrophy of nearby cells; abnormal immunoglobulin synthesis and reticuloendothelial cell dysfunction possible • Familial inheritance in persons with Portuguese ancestry • May occur with tuberculosis, chronic infection, rheumatoid arthritis, multiple myeloma, Hodgkin's disease, paraplegia, brucellosis, and Alzheimer's disease	A rare, chronic disease of abnormal fibrillar scleroprotein (a waxy, starch-like glycoprotein) accumulation that infiltrates body organs and soft tissues. Perireticular type affects inner coats of blood vessels; pericollagen type affects outer coats. Amyloidosis can result in permanent, even life-threatening, organ damage.	• Proteinuria, leading to nephrotic syndrome, eventually to renal failure • Heart failure from cardiomegaly, arrhythmias, and amyloid deposits in subendocardium, endocardium, and myocardium • Stiffness and enlargement of tongue, decreased intestinal motility, malabsorption, bleeding, abdominal pain, constipation, and diarrhea • Peripheral neuropathy • Liver enlargement, commonly with azotemia, anemia, albuminuria and, rarely, jaundice
ANKYLOSING SPONDYLITIS • Cause unknown; strongly linked to presence of human leukocyte antigen B27 • Familial inheritance	Fibrous tissue of the joint capsule is infiltrated by inflammatory cells that erode bone and fibrocartilage. Repair of cartilaginous structures begins with the proliferation of fibroblasts, which synthesize and secrete collagen. The collagen forms fibrous scar tissue that eventually undergoes calcification and ossification, causing the joint to fuse or lose flexibility.	• Intermittent low-back pain that's most severe in the morning and after activity • Stiffness, limited lumbar spine motion • Chest pain and limited expansion • Peripheral arthritis in shoulders, hips, and knees • Kyphosis in advanced stages • Hip deformity and limited range of motion • Mild fatigue, fever, and anorexia or weight loss • Dyspnea if costovertebral joints are involved

DISEASES AND CAUSES	PATHOPHYSIOLOGY	SIGNS AND SYMPTOMS
ANTHRAX • Infection of the skin, lungs, or GI tract that results from contact with *Bacillus anthracis* spores	After infection, bacterium produces toxins that enter susceptible cells, leading to cell death; mechanism unknown.	• Incubation is 12 hours to 5 days • Red-brown bump on skin enlarges and swells around edges; a black scab forms after the bump blisters and hardens • Swollen lymph nodes • Muscle ache and headache • Nausea, vomiting, fever *In pulmonary anthrax:* • Respiratory problems that may progress to respiratory failure • Shock and coma *In GI anthrax (rare):* • Extensive bleeding; tissue death • Fatal if enters bloodstream
ASPERGILLOSIS • Fungal infection from *Aspergillus* species; transmitted by inhalation of fungal spores or invasion of spores through wounds or injured tissue • Usually occurs in immunocompromised people	*Aspergillus* species produce extracellular enzymes, such as proteases and peptidases, that contribute to tissue invasion, leading to hemorrhage and necrosis.	• Incubation is a few days to weeks • May produce no symptoms or mimic tuberculosis, causing a productive cough and purulent or blood-tinged sputum, dyspnea, empyema, and lung abscesses *Allergic aspergillosis:* • Wheezing, dyspnea, pleural pain, and fever *Aspergillosis endophthalmitis:* • Appears 2 to 3 weeks after eye surgery • Cloudy vision, eye pain, and reddened conjunctiva • Purulent exudate on exposure to anterior and posterior chambers of the eye

DISEASES AND CAUSES	PATHOPHYSIOLOGY	SIGNS AND SYMPTOMS
BELL'S PALSY ● Idiopathic facial paralysis that may have an infectious cause	Blockage of the seventh cranial nerve from inflammation around the nerve where it leaves bony tissue that leads to unilateral or bilateral facial weakness or paralysis. The blockage may result from hemorrhage, tumor, meningitis, or local trauma.	● Unilateral facial weakness or paralysis, with aching at the jaw angle ● Drooping mouth, causing salivation ● Distorted taste ● Impaired ability to close the eye on the affected side ● Loss of taste ● Tinnitus
BOTULISM ● Paralytic illness caused by an endotoxin produced by *Clostridium botulinum;* commonly caused by consumption of inadequately cooked, contaminated foods	The endotoxin acts at the neuromuscular junction of skeletal muscle, preventing acetylcholine release and blocking neural transmission, eventually resulting in paralysis.	● Appears 12 to 36 hours after digesting food; severity depends on amount consumed *Initial signs:* ● Dry mouth, sore throat, weakness, dizziness, vomiting, and diarrhea *Cardinal signs:* ● Acute symmetrical cranial nerve impairment, followed by weakness and muscle paralysis ● Mental or sensory processes not typically affected; if affected, usually with fever
BRONCHIECTASIS ● Conditions linked to continued damage to bronchial walls and abnormal mucociliary clearance causing tissue breakdown to adjacent airways; such conditions include cystic fibrosis, immunologic disorders, and recurrent bacterial respiratory tract infections	Inflammation and destruction of the structural components of the bronchial wall lead to chronic abnormal dilation.	*In early stages:* ● Asymptomatic with frequent pneumonia or hemoptysis ● Chronic cough producing copious, foul-smelling, mucopurulent secretions, hemoptysis ● Coarse crackles during inspiration ● Wheezing, dyspnea, sinusitis, fever, chills *In advanced stage:* ● Chronic malnutrition and right-sided heart failure from hypoxic pulmonary vasoconstriction

DISEASES AND CAUSES	**PATHOPHYSIOLOGY**	**SIGNS AND SYMPTOMS**
BRONCHIOLITIS ● Acute viral infection of the lower respiratory tract; infection with respiratory syncytial virus or parainfluenza virus most common cause; may be linked to specific diseases or conditions, such as bone marrow, heart, or lung transplants; rheumatoid arthritis; lupus erythematosus; and Crohn's disease	Infection or other unknown factors cause necrosis of the bronchial epithelium and destruction of ciliated epithelial cells. As the submucosa becomes edematous, cellular debris and fibrin form plugs in the bronchioles.	*Subacute symptoms:* ● Fever, persistent nonproductive cough, dyspnea, malaise, and anorexia ● Physical assessment reveals dry crackles *Less common:* ● Tachypnea, tachycardia, intercostal and subcostal retractions ● Productive cough, hemoptysis, chest pain, general aches, and night sweats ● Wheezing and respiratory distress in late stages
CELIAC DISEASE ● Results from a complex interaction of dietary, genetic, and immunologic factors	The body can't hydrolyze peptides contained in gluten. Ingestion of gluten injures the villi in the upper small intestine, leading to a decreased surface area and malabsorption of most nutrients. Inflammatory enteritis also results, leading to osmotic and secretory diarrhea.	● Recurrent diarrhea, abdominal distention, stomach cramps, weakness, muscle wasting, or increased appetite without weight gain ● Normochromic, hypochromic, or macrocytic anemia ● Osteomalacia, osteoporosis, tetany, and bone pain in lower back, rib cage, pelvis ● Peripheral neuropathy, paresthesia, or seizures ● Dry skin, eczema, psoriasis, dermatitis herpetiformis, and acne rosacea ● Amenorrhea, hypometabolism, and adrenocortical insufficiency ● Extreme lethargy, mood changes, and irritability

DISEASES AND CAUSES	PATHOPHYSIOLOGY	SIGNS AND SYMPTOMS
CHOLERA • Acute enterotoxin-mediated GI infection from gram-negative bacillus (*Vibrio cholerae*) that's transmitted through water and food contaminated with the fecal material of carriers or people with active infections	Following ingestion of a significant inoculum, colonization occurs in the small intestine. The secretion of a potent entero toxin results in a massive outpouring of isotonic fluid from the mucosal surface of the small intestine. Profuse diarrhea, vomiting, and fluid and electrolyte loss occur and may lead to hypovolemic shock, metabolic acidosis, and death.	• Incubation period is several hours to 5 days • Acute, painless, profuse watery diarrhea and vomiting • Intense thirst, weakness, loss of skin tone; dehydration; electrolyte imbalances; oliguria • Muscle cramps • Cyanosis • Tachycardia • Falling blood pressure, fever, and hypoactive bowel sounds
CREUTZFELDT-JAKOB DISEASE • Rare form of dementia • Prion infection	Organism infects the central nervous system (CNS), leading to myelin destruction and neuronal loss.	• Myoclonic jerking, ataxia, aphasia, vision disturbances, paralysis, and early abnormal EEG
ENDOCARDITIS • Infection of the endocardium of the heart caused by bacteria, viruses, fungi, rickettsiae, and parasites	Endothelial damage allows microorganisms to adhere to the surface, where they proliferate and promote endocardial vegetation.	• Weakness and fatigue • Weight loss, fever, night sweats, and anorexia • Arthralgia, splenomegaly, and new systolic murmur
ESOPHAGEAL VARICES • Portal hypertension	Shunting of blood to the vena cavae by portal hypertension leads to a complex of enlarged, swollen, and tortuous veins at the lower end of the esophagus.	• Hemorrhage and subsequent hypotension • Compromised oxygen supply • Altered level of consciousness • Hematemesis

DISEASES AND CAUSES	PATHOPHYSIOLOGY	SIGNS AND SYMPTOMS
FANCONI SYNDROME • Inherited renal tubular transport disorder • May result from exposure to certain environmental toxins such as heavy metals	Changes in the proximal renal tubules from atrophy of epithelial cells and loss of proximal tube volume results in a shortened connection to glomeruli by an unusually narrow segment. Malfunction of the proximal renal tubules leads to hyperkalemia, hypernatremia, glycosuria, phosphaturia, aminoaciduria, uricosuria, acidosis, retarded growth, and rickets.	• Mostly normal appearance at birth with slightly lower birth weights • After 6 months: Weakness, failure to thrive, dehydration, cystine crystals in the corners of the eye, and retinal pigment degeneration • Yellow skin with little pigmentation • Slow linear growth
HYPERSPLENISM • Increased activity of the spleen, where all types of blood cells are removed from circulation due to chronic myelogenous leukemia, lymphomas, Gaucher's disease, hairy cell leukemia, and sarcoidosis	Spleen growth may be stimulated by an increase in its workload such as the trapping and destroying of abnormal red blood cells (RBCs).	• Enlarged spleen • Cytopenia • Abdominal pain on left side • Fullness after eating very little amounts of food
IDIOPATHIC PULMONARY FIBROSIS • Chronic progressive lung disease with inflammation and fibrosis • No known cause	Interstitial inflammation consists of an alveolar septal infiltrate of lymphocytes, plasma cells, and histiocytes. Fibrotic areas are composed of dense acellular collagen. Areas of honeycombing are composed of cystic fibrotic air spaces, commonly lined with bronchiolar epithelium and filled with mucus. Smooth muscle hyperplasia may occur in areas of fibrosis and honeycombing.	• Dyspnea • Nonproductive cough • Chest heaviness • Wheezing • Anorexia • Weight loss

Diseases and causes	Pathophysiology	Signs and symptoms
KAPOSI'S SARCOMA • Malignant, acquired immunodeficiency syndrome–related cancer	A cancer arising from vascular endothelial cells, Kaposi's sarcoma affects endothelial tissue, which compromises all blood vessels.	• Red-purple or brown circular lesions, slightly raised on the face, arms, neck, and legs • Internal lesions, especially in GI tract, identified by biopsy
KERATITIS • Inflammation of cornea caused by microorganisms, trauma, or autoimmune disorders	Bacterial infection leads to ulceration of the cornea.	• Decreased visual acuity • Pain • Photophobia
KYPHOSIS • Excessive anteroposterior curving of the spine caused by a congenital anomaly, tuberculosis, syphilis, malignant or compression fracture, arthritis, or rickets	Pathophysiology is related to causative factor.	• Abnormally rounded thoracic curve
LATEX ALLERGY • Hypersensitivity to products containing natural latex	Latex protein allergens trigger release of histamine and other mediators of the systemic allergic cascade in sensitized persons.	• Local dermatitis to anaphylactic reaction
LEGIONNAIRES' DISEASE • Infection caused by gram-negative bacillus, *Legionella pneumophila*	Transmission follows inhalation of organism in aerosols produced by air-conditioning units, water faucets, shower heads, humidifiers, and contaminated respiratory equipment.	• Dry cough • Myalgia • GI distress, diarrhea • Pneumonia • Cardiovascular collapse
LEPROSY • Infection caused by *Mycobacterium leprae*	Chronic, systemic infection with progressive cutaneous lesions, attacks the peripheral nervous system.	• Skin lesions • Anesthesia • Muscle weakness • Paralysis

Diseases and causes	Pathophysiology	Signs and symptoms
MEDULLARY SPONGE KIDNEYS • Genetic disorder	Collecting ducts in the renal pyramids dilate, forming cavities, clefts, and cysts that produce complications of calcium oxalate stones and infections.	• Renal calculi • Hematuria • Infection (fever, chills, and malaise)
MYOCARDITIS • Inflammation of the myocardium caused by bacterial, fungal, viral, or protozoal infections; heatstroke; ionizing radiation; rheumatic fever; or diphtheria	Initial infection triggers an autoimmune, cellular and, possibly, humoral response resulting in myocardial inflammation and necrosis.	• Rapid, irregular, and weak pulse • Chest tenderness • S_1 resembles S_2 • Fatigue
NEUROFIBROMATOSIS • Inherited autosomal dominant disorder	Group of developmental disorders of the nervous system, muscles, bones, and skin that affects the cell growth of neural tissue.	• Café-au-lait spots • Multiple, pediculated, soft tumors (neurofibromas) • Hearing loss • Bone changes, skeletal deformities
OSGOOD-SCHLATTER DISEASE • Probably results from trauma before complete fusion of the epiphysis to the main bone (ages 10 to 15); such trauma may be a single violent action or repeated knee flexion against a tight quadriceps muscle	This disorder is a painful, incomplete separation of the epiphysis of the tibial tubercle from the tibial shaft and is most common in active adolescent boys. Severe disease may cause permanent tubercle enlargement.	• Constant aching and pain and tenderness below kneecap • Obvious soft-tissue swelling and localized heat and tenderness
PEDICULOSIS • Infestation by lice	Lice attach to hair shafts and feed on blood several times daily; they reside close to the scalp to maintain body temperature. Itching may be from an allergic reaction or irritation to louse saliva.	• Itching, inflammation • Eczematous dermatitis • Tiredness, irritability, weakness • Lice present in hair (head, axilla, and pubic)

DISEASES AND CAUSES	PATHOPHYSIOLOGY	SIGNS AND SYMPTOMS
PHEOCHROMOCYTOMA • Polyglandular multiple endocrine neoplasia	Tumor of the chromaffin cells of the adrenal medulla that increases catecholamine production.	• Hypertension, high blood sugar and lipid levels • Headache, palpitations, sweating, dizziness, syncope, anxiety, constipation
PLEURISY • Several causes, including lupus, rheumatoid arthritis, and tuberculosis	This disorder is an inflammation of the visceral and parietal pleurae that line the inside of the thoracic cage and envelop the lungs.	• Chills, fever • Sharp, stabbing chest pain • Suppressed cough • Dyspnea • Pallor
POLYCYTHEMIA VERA • Cause unknown; possibly a multipotential stem cell defect	Increased production of RBCs, neutrophils, and platelets inhibits blood flow to microcirculation, resulting in intravascular thrombosis.	• Signs and symptoms usually absent in early stages; in later stages, related to expanded blood volume and system affected • Weakness, headache, light-headedness, vision disturbances, fatigue • Hepatomegaly, splenomegaly • Maroon or plum-color skin and mucous membranes • Hypertension
PYLORIC STENOSIS • Congenital; cause unknown	Pyloric sphincter muscle fibers thicken and become inelastic, narrowing the opening. The extra peristaltic effort needed leads to hypertrophied muscle layers of the stomach.	• Progressive nonbilious vomiting, leading to projectile vomiting at ages 2 to 4 weeks
RETINAL DETACHMENT • Caused by trauma, after cataract surgery, severe uveitis, and primary or metastatic choroidal tumors; also may follow age-related changes in the vitreous chamber	The neural retina separates from the underlying retinal pigment epithelium.	• Floaters, flashing lights, scotoma in peripheral visual field (painless) and, eventually, a curtain or veil in the field of vision

DISEASES AND CAUSES	PATHOPHYSIOLOGY	SIGNS AND SYMPTOMS
RETINITIS PIGMENTOSA ● Autosomal recessive disorder in 80% of affected children ● Less commonly transmitted as an X-linked trait	Slow, degenerative changes in rods cause the retina and pigment epithelium to atrophy. Irregular black deposits of clumped pigment are in equatorial region of the retina and eventually in the macular and peripheral areas.	● Progressive night blindness, visual field constriction with ring scotoma, and loss of acuity progressing to blindness
REYE'S SYNDROME ● No known cause ● Viral agents and drugs (especially salicylates) have been implicated	Mitochondrial dysfunction and fatty vacuolization of the liver and renal tubules leads to hepatic injury and CNS damage.	● Vomiting ● Change in mental status progressing from lethargy to disorientation to coma
ROCKY MOUNTAIN SPOTTED FEVER ● Infection caused by *Rickettsia rickettsii* carried by several tick species	*R. rickettsii* multiplies in endothelial cells and spreads in the bloodstream. Focal areas of infiltration lead to thrombosis and leakage of RBCs into surrounding tissue.	● Fever, headache, mental confusion, and myalgia ● Rash developing as small macules that progress to maculopapules and petechiae; starting on wrists and ankles and spreading to trunk; diagnostic rash on palms and soles ● Constipation and abdominal distention
SARCOIDOSIS ● Cause unknown ● May result from exaggerated cellular immune response to limited class of antigens	Organ dysfunction results from an accumulation of T lymphocytes, mononuclear phagocytes, and nonsecreting epithelial granulomas, which distort normal tissue architecture.	● Mainly generalized, most commonly involving lung with resulting respiratory symptoms ● Fever, fatigue, and malaise

DISEASES AND CAUSES	PATHOPHYSIOLOGY	SIGNS AND SYMPTOMS
SCABIES • Human itch mite (*Sarcoptes scabiei* var. *hominis*)	Mite burrows superficially beneath stratum corneum and deposits eggs that hatch, mature, and reinvade the skin. Sensitization reaction against mite excreta results.	• Occurring from sensitization reaction against excreta that mites deposit • Intense itching, worsens at night • Threadlike lesions on wrists, between fingers, and on elbows, axillae, belt line, buttocks, and male genitalia • Possible secondary bacterial infection
SJÖGREN'S SYNDROME • Autoimmune rheumatic disorder of unknown cause; genetic and environmental factors may be involved	Lymphocytic infiltration of exocrine glands causes tissue damage that results in xerostomia and dry eyes.	*In xerostomia:* • Dry mouth; trouble swallowing and speaking; ulcers of tongue, buccal mucosa, and lips; severe dental caries *In ocular involvement:* • Dry eyes; gritty, sandy feeling; decreased tearing; burning, itching, redness, photosensitivity *Extraglandular:* • Arthralgia, Raynaud's phenomenon, lymphadenopathy, and lung involvement
STRABISMUS • Eye malalignment that's commonly inherited; controversy over whether amblyopia is caused by or results from strabismus	In paralytic (nonconcomitant) strabismus, paralysis of one or more ocular muscles may be from an oculomotor nerve lesion. In nonparalytic (concomitant) strabismus, unequal ocular muscle tone is caused by a supranuclear abnormality within the CNS.	• Noticeable eye malalignment by external eye examination, ophthalmoscopic observation of the corneal light reflex in center of pupils, diplopia, and other vision disturbances • Visual acuity declines with decreased use of an eye

DISEASES AND CAUSES	PATHOPHYSIOLOGY	SIGNS AND SYMPTOMS
THROMBOCYTHEMIA ● *Primary:* no known cause ● *Secondary:* caused by chronic inflammatory disorders, iron deficiency, acute infection, neoplasm, hemorrhage, and postsplenectomy	A clonal abnormality of a multipotent hematopoietic stem cell results in increased platelet production, although platelet survival is usually normal. If combined with degenerative vascular disease, may lead to serious bleeding or thrombosis.	● Weakness, hemorrhage, nonspecific headache, paresthesia, dizziness, and easy bruising
THROMBOPHLEBITIS ● Caused by endothelial damage, accelerated blood clotting, and reduced blood flow	Alteration in epithelial lining causes platelet aggregation and fibrin entrapment of RBCs, white blood cells, and additional platelets. The thrombus starts an inflammatory process in the vessel epithelium that leads to fibrosis, which may occlude the vessel lumen or embolize.	● Varies with site and length of affected vein ● Affected area usually extremely tender, swollen, red, and warm to touch
TRIGEMINAL NEURALGIA ● Cause unknown, possibly a compression neuropathy ● At surgery or autopsy, the intracranial arterial and venous loops are found to compress the trigeminal nerve root at the brain stem	Painful disorder along the distribution of one or more of the trigeminal nerve's sensory divisions, typically the maxillary.	● Searing or burning pain lasting seconds to 2 minutes at trigeminal nerve distribution ● Touching trigger point commonly elicits pain
VITILIGO ● Cause unknown; usually acquired but may be familial (autosomal dominant) ● Possible immunologic and neurochemical basis	Destruction of melanocytes (humoral or cellular) and circulating antibodies against melanocytes results in hypopigmented areas.	● Progressive, symmetrical areas of complete pigment loss with sharp borders, generally appearing in periorificial areas, flexor wrists, and extensor distal extremities

DISEASES AND CAUSES	PATHOPHYSIOLOGY	SIGNS AND SYMPTOMS
WILSON'S DISEASE ● Inherited copper toxicosis	Defective mobilization of copper from hepatocellular lysosomes for excretion by way of bile allows excessive copper retention in the liver, brain, kidneys, and corneas, leading to tissue necrosis and subsequent hepatic and neurologic disorders.	● Kayser-Fleischer ring: Rusty brown ring of pigment at periphery of corneas ● Signs of hepatitis leading to cirrhosis ● Tremors, unsteady gait, muscular rigidity, inappropriate behavior, and psychosis ● Hematuria, proteinuria, and uricosuria

Selected references

ACC Atlas of Pathophysiology, 2nd ed. Philadelphia: Lippincott Williams & Wilkins, 2005.

Anderson, S.C., and Poulsen, K.B. *Anderson's Atlas of Hematology.* Philadelphia: Lippincott Williams & Wilkins, 2003.

Bartlett, J.G. *2004 Pocket Book of Infectious Disease Therapy,* 12th ed. Philadelphia: Lippincott Williams & Wilkins, 2004.

Camacho, P.M., et al. *Evidence-Based Endocrinology.* Philadelphia: Lippincott Williams & Wilkins, 2003.

Cardiovascular Care Made Incredibly Easy. Philadelphia: Lippincott Williams & Wilkins, 2004.

DeSevo, M.R. "Would You Suspect This Genetic Disorder?" *RN* 68(3):47-50, March 2005.

Handbook of Pathophysiology, 2nd ed. Philadelphia: Lippincott Williams & Wilkins, 2004.

Itano, J.K., and Taoka, K.T. *Core Curriculum for Oncology Nursing,* 4th ed. Philadelphia: W.B. Saunders Co., 2005.

Kahn, C.R., et al. *Joslin's Diabetes Mellitus,* 14th ed. Philadelphia: Lippincott Williams & Wilkins, 2003.

Mayhall, C.G. *Hospital Epidemiology and Infection Control,* 3rd ed. Philadelphia: Lippincott Williams & Wilkins, 2004.

Ochs, H.D., et al., eds. *Primary Immunodeficiency Disease.* New York: Oxford University Press, 2004.

Pass, H.I. *Lung Cancer: Principles and Practice,* 3rd ed. Philadelphia: Lippincott Williams & Wilkins, 2004.

Porth, C.M. *Pathophysiology: Concepts of Altered Health States,* 7th ed. Philadelphia: Lippincott Williams & Wilkins, 2004.

Respiratory Care Made Incredibly Easy. Philadelphia: Lippincott Williams & Wilkins, 2005.

Rodgers, G.P., and Young, N.S. *Bethesda Handbook of Clinical Hematology.* Philadelphia: Lippincott Williams & Wilkins, 2004.

Skeel, R.T. *Handbook of Cancer Chemotherapy,* 6th ed. Philadelphia: Lippincott Williams & Wilkins, 2003.

Smith, G. *Gastrointestinal Nursing.* Cambridge, Mass.: Blackwell Scientific Pubs., 2003.

Weiner, H.L., et al. *Neurology,* 7th ed. Philadelphia: Lippincott Williams & Wilkins, 2004.

Woods, S.L., et al., eds. *Cardiac Nursing.* Philadelphia: Lippincott Williams & Wilkins, 2005.

Yamada, T., et al. *Atlas of Gastroenterology,* 4th ed. Philadelphia: Lippincott Williams & Wilkins, 2003.

Index

i refers to an illustration; t refers to a table.

i refers to an illustration; t refers to a table.

i refers to an illustration; t refers to a table.

i refers to an illustration; t refers to a table.

i refers to an illustration; t refers to a table.

i refers to an illustration; t refers to a table.

---

i refers to an illustration; t refers to a table.

i refers to an illustration; t refers to a table.

---

i refers to an illustration; t refers to a table.